CHURCHILL'S POCKETBOOK OF
Diabetes

To my family

Commissioning Editor: Michael Parkinson
Project Development Manager: Siân Jarman
Design Direction: Erik Bigland
Project Manager: Frances Affleck

CHURCHILL'S POCKETBOOK OF
Diabetes

Andrew J. Krentz

Consultant in Diabetes and Endocrinology and Honorary Senior Lecturer in Medicine, Southampton University, Southampton, UK

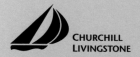

EDINBURGH LONDON NEW YORK PHILADELPHIA ST LOUIS SYDNEY TORONTO 2000

CHURCHILL LIVINGSTONE
An imprint of Harcourt Publishers Limited

© Harcourt Publishers Limited 2000

⟁ is a registered trademark of Harcourt Publishers
Limited

The right of Andrew J. Krentz to be identified as
author of this work has been asserted by him in
accordance with the Copyright, Designs and Patents
Act 1988

First published 2000
  Reprinted 2002

ISBN 0 443 06118 1

British Library Cataloguing in Publication Data
A catalogue record for this book is available from the
British Library

Library of Congress Cataloging in Publication Data
A catalog record for this book is available from the
Library of Congress

Note
Medical knowledge is constantly changing. As new
information becomes available, changes in treatment,
procedures, equipment and the use of drugs become
necessary. The author and the publishers have, as far
as it is possible, taken care to ensure that the
information given in this text is accurate and up to
date. However, readers are strongly advised to
confirm that the information, especially with regard
to drug usage, complies with the latest legislation
and standards of practice.

The
publisher's
policy is to use
**paper manufactured
from sustainable forests**

Printed in China

Preface

This book was conceived as an accessible guide for health care professionals confronted with questions relating to the care of patients with diabetes.

The structure of the book is as follows: an outline of the key biochemical defects of diabetes is followed by a discussion of recent changes in classification and diagnosis. Aspects of the management of diabetes and its acute and chronic complications are then addressed; the emerging roles of novel pharmacological agents such as the thiazolidinediones and insulin analogues are considered. Summaries of major clinical trials which have influenced clinical practice, e.g. the Diabetes Control and Complications Trial and the United Kingdom Prospective Diabetes Study, are presented; relevant trials of antihypertensive and lipid-modifying therapy are also discussed. These summaries are highlighted in Evidence-Based Medicine boxes.

The emphasis throughout is on clinical management, anchored in an appreciation of the underlying pathophysiology. The aim has been to provide a balanced view reflecting current clinical practice coupled with an awareness of the relevant scientific evidence on which this is based.

Southampton
2000   A.J.K.

Acknowledgements

The results of discussions with the multidisciplinary Southampton Local Diabetes Advisory Group have been incorporated into many parts of this book. Particular thanks also go to the staff of the Department of Teaching Media, Southampton General Hospital and to colleagues who provided some of the colour plates. Jim Killgore and Siân Jarman of Harcourt Health Sciences supervised the project with skill and patience.

A.J.K.

Contents

Abbreviations

ACE	angiotensin-converting enzyme		**GI**	gastrointestinal
ADA	American Diabetes Association		**GP**	general practitioner
AGE	advanced glycation endproduct		**HDL**	high density lipoprotein
ATP	adenosine triphosphate		**HIV**	human immuno-deficiency virus
			HLA	human-lymphocyte-associated
BDA	British Diabetic Association (Diabetes UK from 2000)		**HMG-CoA**	hydroxymethyl glutaryl-coenzyme A
BMI	body mass index		**IDDM**	insulin-dependent diabetes mellitus
BP	blood pressure		**IPPV**	intermittent positive pressure ventilation
BUN	blood urea nitrogen			
CAPD	continuous ambulatory peritoneal dialysis		**IUGR**	intrauterine growth retardation
CHD	coronary heart disease			
CoA	coenzyme A		**LADA**	latent autoimmune diabetes in adults
CT	computerized tomography		**LDL**	low density lipoprotein
DCCT	US Diabetes Control and Complications Trial		**MHC**	major histocompatibility complex
DIGAMI	Diabetes Mellitus Insulin Glucose Infusion in Acute Myocardial Infarction study		**MI**	myocardial infarction
			MODY	maturity-onset diabetes of the young
DKA	diabetic ketoacidosis		**MRI**	magnetic resonance imaging
ECG	electrocardiogram		**NAD**	nicotinamide adenine dinucleotide
GAD	glutamic acid decarboxylase		**NDDG**	US National Diabetes Data Group

NIDDM	non-insulin-dependent diabetes mellitus	**UKPDS**	UK Prospective Diabetes Study
NSAID	non-steroidal anti-inflammatory drug	**VLDL**	very low density lipoprotein
RCT	randomized controlled trial	**WHO**	World Health Organization

BIOCHEMISTRY AND CLASSIFICATION

THE SYNDROME OF DIABETES MELLITUS

Logical treatment of diabetes mellitus is grounded in an appreciation of the principal biochemical disturbances which characterize this complex and heterogeneous syndrome. Diabetes is a collection of disorders characterized by defective regulation of carbohydrate, lipid and protein metabolism. The biochemical hallmark of diabetes mellitus is chronic hyperglycaemia which results from an absolute or relative deficiency of insulin. Impairment of insulin action in target tissues (see insulin resistance, p. 28) is an important component of type 2 diabetes.

 Chronic hyperglycaemia is the sine qua non of diabetes mellitus.

The clinical manifestations of diabetes mellitus range from asymptomatic type 2 diabetes (see p. 18) to the dramatic life-threatening conditions of diabetic ketoacidosis (DKA) (see p. 168) and hyperosmolar non-ketosis (see p. 185). The principal determinant of the presentation is the degree of insulin deficiency although additional factors may also be important. In addition pathological hyperglycaemia sustained over several years may produce functional and structural changes within certain tissues (see pp. 7–9); these microvascular complications, which ultimately become irreversible, are a major cause of morbidity and premature mortality:

- Retinopathy.
- Nephropathy.
- Neuropathy.

In addition, patients with diabetes are at increased risk of atherosclerotic complications (see p. 9).

 Diabetes mellitus is characterized by the risk of long-term micro- and macrovascular complications.

The degree of hyperglycaemia and disposition to ketosis (see p. 168) may fluctuate over time; at diagnosis it can sometimes be difficult to predict precisely how a patient will respond in the future. For example, insulin may be required temporarily during pregnancy in some women hitherto well controlled with oral antidiabetic agents (see insulin resistance, p. 28; and p. 270); conversely, some patients may present with major metabolic decompensation yet can subsequently be successfully treated with oral agents. Such difficulties notwithstanding, the majority of patients can be classified as belonging to one or other major subgroups according to the aetiology of their diabetes (see p. 9). However, such classification is based mainly on clinical and biochemical features; only in a small minority of patients is it presently possible to make a precise diagnosis using molecular genetic techniques (see maturity-onset diabetes of the young (MODY), p. 26).

BIOCHEMISTRY OF DIABETES

GLUCOSE METABOLISM

Insulin (Fig. 1.1) is the principal anabolic hormone of the body exerting myriad actions on intermediary metabolism, ion transport and gene expression (Table 1.1). Insulin is synthesized and secreted by the B-cells of the pancreatic islets in response to glucose and other secretagogues such as aminoacids. The secretion of insulin is inhibited by some other hormones, notably adrenaline and somatostatin. By contrast, insulin secretion is enhanced by other hormones (e.g. glucagon). Insulin may also exert autocrine effects, inhibiting its own secretion. Furthermore, the metabolic actions of insulin at tissue level may be antagonized by the so-called counter-regulatory hormones:

- Glucagon.
- Catecholamines.
- Growth hormone.

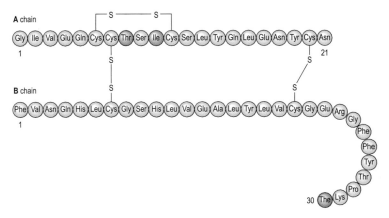

Fig. 1.1 Primary structure (amino acid sequence) of human insulin.

TABLE 1.1 Main physiological actions of insulin

Metabolic actions (mainly acute effects)
— Suppression of hepatic glucose production
— Stimulation of glucose uptake by muscle and adipose tissue
— Promotion of glucose storage as glycogen
— Suppression of adipocyte lipolysis and hepatic ketogenesis
— Regulation of protein turnover
— Effects on electrolyte balance

Other actions (longer-term effects)
— Regulation of growth and development (e.g. in utero)
— Regulation of expression of certain genes

These hormones enter their anti-insulin actions through direct tissue effects and, in the case of the catecholamines, by inhibition of insulin secretion.

THE INSULIN RECEPTOR

The actions of insulin are mediated via binding of the hormone to specific receptors located in the membrane of almost all mammalian cells. Certain tissues are regarded as classical targets for insulin:

- Hepatocytes.
- Skeletal myocytes.
- Adipocytes.

Key post-binding events include autophosphorylation at tyrosine sites within the β-subunit of the receptor induced by conformational alterations (Fig. 1.2). This, in turn, leads to a cascade of post-receptor signalling events which remain only partially elucidated. The best-characterized substrate for the insulin receptor is insulin-receptor substrate-1. Further phosphorylation/dephosphorylation events lead ultimately to the activation of enzymes such as glycogen synthase. Impaired actions of insulin (see insulin resistance, p. 28) may result from two main mechanisms:

- *Receptor defects.* A reduced number of insulin receptors or a reduction in their affinity for insulin. This may occur in response to chronic hyperinsulinaemia (so-called down-regulation). Lesser degrees of obesity and glucose intolerance (see p. 10) are associated with receptor defects which may be largely reversible with treatment. Inherited severe receptor defects are rare (see p. 33).

- *Post-receptor defects.* Defects in intracellular events distal to the binding of insulin account for insulin resistance in most patients with type 2

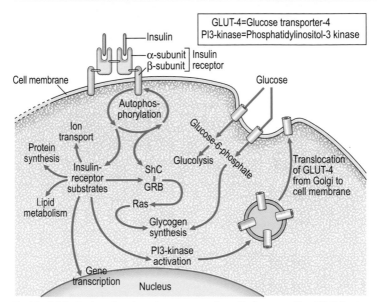

Fig. 1.2 Cellular binding of insulin to its receptor and post-binding events. Key: GLUT-4, glucose transporter-4; PI3-kinase, phosphatidyl inositol-3 kinase.

diabetes; the maximal response to insulin is impaired and is usually only partially reversible, even with insulin-sensitizing thiazolidinedione drugs (see p. 127). The precise nature of these defects has not yet been identified.

Secretion of insulin is very tightly matched to circulating glucose concentrations. Insulin is secreted at a low background (or basal) level throughout the day; this accounts for approximately 50% of insulin secretion. The remainder is secreted in close temporal association to the rise in portal plasma glucose following meals. In health, venous plasma glucose concentrations are strictly maintained in the range of approximately 5–7 mmol/L. At any time point, the plasma glucose concentration reflects the net balance between:

- Rate of appearance of glucose in the circulation.
- Rate of disappearance from the circulation.

The glucose-lowering effects of insulin (Fig. 1.3) result primarily from:

- Suppression of hepatic glucose production (reducing the rate of glucose released into the blood).
- Stimulation of glucose disposal (principally by skeletal muscle and, to a lesser degree, adipose tissue, i.e. clearance from the circulation).

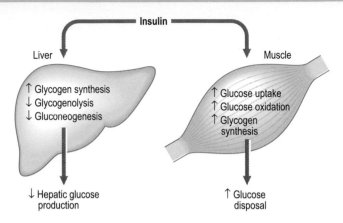

Fig. 1.3 Regulation of glucose metabolism by insulin.

• *Hepatic glucose production.* In the post-absorptive state (i.e. after an overnight fast), the rate at which glucose enters the circulation glucose from the liver is the main determinant of plasma glucose concentrations. This glucose is derived from breakdown of stored glycogen and synthesis of de novo glucose molecules from 3-carbon precursors (gluconeogenesis). As glycogen stores become depleted, gluconeogenesis assumes a quantitatively greater role. Suppression of hepatic glucose production is a major regulatory action of insulin.

 Hepatic glucose production is the principal determinant of fasting blood glucose concentration.

• *Glucose disposal.* Stimulation of glucose uptake (and subsequently metabolism or storage as glycogen) requires higher plasma insulin concentrations than are necessary for suppression of hepatic glucose production. A major action of insulin is to stimulate translocation of facilitative glucose transporters (GLUT-4 transporters) to the cell membrane for this purpose (see Fig. 1.2). Other isoforms of glucose transporters (e.g. GLUT-1 at the blood–brain and blood–retinal barriers, GLUT-2 in islet B-cells) do not require insulin to transfer glucose into cells. Lactate metabolism (including the Cori cycle) is considered on pages 188–189.

LIPOLYSIS AND KETONE BODY METABOLISM

The crucial role of insulin in inhibiting the breakdown of adipose tissue stores of triglyceride to non-esterified fatty acids (and the gluconeogenic precursor, glycerol) is considered in more detail on pages 28–35. Fatty acids are the principal substrate for ketogenesis within the liver. Thus, via control of plasma fatty acid levels and other effects, insulin is a major regulator of ketogenesis (Fig. 1.4). Both fatty acids and ketones can be used as alternative fuels, e.g. during starvation and prolonged exercise. The pathophysiological roles of ketone bodies are described in the section on DKA (p. 171).

BIOCHEMISTRY OF DIABETIC TISSUE COMPLICATIONS

MICROVASCULAR DISEASE

While the acute symptoms of diabetes can usually be controlled with appropriate therapy, diabetes is also associated with the insidious development of specific organ damage primarily affecting the retina, renal glomerulus and peripheral nervous system (see Section 5). These tissues are freely permeable to glucose and the small vessel (microvascular) complications of diabetes are closely linked to glycaemic control. The ultimate clinical sequelae of diabetic microvascular disease include:

- Visual impairment.
- Chronic renal failure.
- Neuropathic foot ulceration.

Studies in animal models have provided insights into the biochemical mechanisms responsible for the chronic complications of diabetes which are discussed in detail in Section 5. The principal hypotheses which link long-term exposure to high glucose concentrations and tissue damage are:

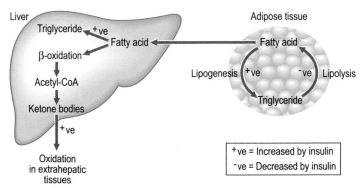

Fig. 1.4 Regulation of lipolysis and ketone body metabolism by insulin (+ve = increased by insulin; –ve = decreased by insulin).

● *Polyol pathway*. Increased activity of this ubiquitous biochemical pathway leads to intracellular accumulation of osmotically-active sorbitol (and fructose) through the action of the enzyme aldose reductase; depletion of *myo*-inositol and impairment of Na^+-K^+-ATPase activity are associated disturbances which have been implicated particularly in the pathogenesis of diabetic neuropathy (see p. 205). Alterations in cellular redox state resulting from the following reactions may also be relevant:

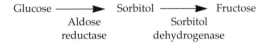

$$\text{Glucose} \xrightarrow[\substack{\text{Aldose} \\ \text{reductase}}]{} \text{Sorbitol} \xrightarrow[\substack{\text{Sorbitol} \\ \text{dehydrogenase}}]{} \text{Fructose}$$

● *Protein kinase C activity*. Accumulation of diacylglycerol resulting from high intracellular glucose concentrations causes activation of protein kinase C-β in endothelial cells. This results in pathological changes via alterations in vascular permeability and increased basement membrane synthesis, the latter being an important, early, histological feature of the microvascular complications of diabetes.

↑ Glucose ⟶ ↑ Diacylglycerol ⟶ ↑ Protein kinase C-β

Secondary increases in the expression of growth factors with effects on vascular permeability may contribute to neovascularization in the retina (see p. 201).

● *Non-enzymatic glycation*. The long-term modification of proteins such as collagen and nucleic acids by non-enzymatic glycation (i.e. attachment of glucose to the amino groups of proteins at a rate proportional to the mean glucose concentration) may also contribute to tissue damage. Physical cross-linking of biochemically-altered proteins alters structure and function, e.g. in the vascular wall. The earliest biochemical changes are reversible with restoration of good glycaemic control. However, with continuing hyperglycaemia, the alterations ultimately become irreversible culminating in the formation of so-called advanced glycation endproducts (or AGEs).

Glucose + Protein ⟶ Schiff base ⟶ Amadori product ⟶ AGEs

This process is the basis of glycated haemoglobin assays for the determination of medium-term glycaemic control (see p. 71).

Drugs (respectively: aldose reductase inhibitors, protein kinase C inhibitors and aminoguanidine) that block these metabolic pathways can prevent the development of complications in animal models of diabetes. However, the most studied of these – aldose reductase inhibitors – have proved disappointing in studies of human diabetes.

At present, therefore, good metabolic control remains fundamental to the prevention and retardation of the microvascular complications of diabetes (see Sections 2 and 5).

MACROVASCULAR DISEASE

Diabetes is also associated with an increased mortality from atherosclerotic complications, particularly coronary heart disease (CHD). These metabolic and vascular complications are major (and growing) causes of morbidity and mortality on a global scale. Atherosclerotic disease is the principal cause of death in patients with diabetes with age-adjusted rates 2—4-fold higher than for non-diabetics (see p. 228). Conventional risk factors for atherosclerosis (p. 228) appear to have an even greater impact in the presence of diabetes. The glycaemic threshold for atheroma is lower than that for microvascular complications such as retinopathy; thus, patients with impaired glucose tolerance (see p. 10) share some of the increased risk of macrovascular disease.

 NB Macrovascular disease is the principal cause of death in patients with diabetes.

CLASSIFICATION OF DIABETES MELLITUS

In 1980, the World Health Organization (WHO) proposed a classification of diabetes mellitus based on recommendations of the US National Diabetes Data Group (NDDG). This classification (revised in 1985) reflected advances in knowledge concerning the aetiology and pathogenesis of diabetes. The descriptive terms 'juvenile-onset' and 'maturity-onset' diabetes were rendered obsolete, being replaced with insulin-dependent and non-insulin dependent diabetes, respectively.

In 1997, the American Diabetes Association (ADA) reclassified diabetes and revised their diagnostic criteria introducing the new category of impaired fasting glucose (see p. 43). This new classification attempted to classify patients according to the aetiology of the diabetes rather than whether insulin is required at some stage. For example, a sizeable proportion of patients with type 2 diabetes ultimately require insulin to maintain adequate glycaemic control (see p. 148).

 NB The 1997 American Diabetes Association classification is based on aetiology rather than therapy.

At the same time, WHO initiated a consultative period arriving at similar diagnostic criteria. However, WHO continues to support the use of the oral glucose tolerance test (see p. 48).

AMERICAN DIABETES ASSOCIATION CLASSIFICATION

The ADA (1997) classification is outlined in Table 1.2.

TABLE 1.2 Aetiological classification of diabetes mellitus (American Diabetes Association, 1997)

I *Type I diabetes*
(previously 'insulin-dependent diabetes')
- Islet B-cell destruction usually leading to absolute insulin deficiency
  A. Immune-mediated
  B. Idiopathic

II *Type 2 diabetes*
(previously 'non-insulin-dependent diabetes')
- Accounts for >85% of cases worldwide
- Heterogeneous – Ranging from predominantly insulin resistance to predominantly insulin deficiency

III *Other specific forms*
  A. Genetic defects of B-cell function, e.g MODY syndromes
  B. Genetic defects in insulin action, e.g. leprechaunism
  C. Diseases of the exocrine pancreas, e.g. pancreatitis
  D. Secondary to endocrinopathies, e.g. acromegaly
  E. Drug- or chemical-induced, e.g. glucocorticoids
  F. Infections, e.g. congenital rubella
  G. Uncommon forms of immune-mediated diabetes, e.g. 'stiff man' syndrome
  H. Other genetic syndromes associated with diabetes, e.g. Down's syndrome

IV *Gestational diabetes*
- Diabetes diagnosed in pregnancy – includes pre-existing diabetes and diabetes which develops during pregnancy (see p. 278)

NB All patients with type I diabetes require lifelong insulin treatment. Patients in categories II, III and IV may also require insulin treatment. Thus, use of insulin per se does not classify the patient's diabetes.

IMPAIRED GLUCOSE TOLERANCE

The 1979/1980 reclassification introduced the intermediate diagnostic category of impaired glucose tolerance in recognition of an area of diagnostic uncertainty between normality and diabetes. Patients with stable, impaired glucose tolerance are not at risk of developing microvascular complications of diabetes. However, they are at increased risk of developing:

- Type 2 diabetes.
- Macrovascular disease.

Impaired glucose tolerance and impaired fasting glucose, both of which are asymptomatic, are discussed in more detail in Section 2 (pp. 43 and 47).

 NB Impaired glucose tolerance represents an intermediate category between normality and diabetes.

TYPE 1 DIABETES

EPIDEMIOLOGY

The incidence of type 1 diabetes shows considerable geographic variation. The highest rates are in Finland, Norway, Sweden and Denmark with Japan having the lowest incidence amongst developed countries. In England, Scotland, Finland and Poland, the incidence has been rising in recent years; other countries have also reported increasing rates.

 NB The incidence of type 1 diabetes under the age of 16 years has doubled during recent years in the UK.

Variable incidence rates between and within populations are cited as evidence of pathogenetic environmental factors (e.g. viruses, toxins). The peak age of presentation is 11–13 years; however, type 1 diabetes can affect any age group, even the very elderly. In some populations, up to 20% of patients diagnosed initially with type 2 diabetes prove to have evidence of autoimmune activity more typical of type 1 diabetes (see p. 109); such patients respond poorly to oral antidiabetic agents having an early requirement for insulin therapy. Reports of circulating antibodies directed to glutamic acid decarboxylase (GAD) in such patients point to progressive B-cell destruction. This form has been called 'latent autoimmune diabetes in adults' (LADA).

PATHOPHYSIOLOGY

Type 1 diabetes is characterized by autoimmune, cell-mediated, selective destruction of the insulin-producing B-cells of the pancreatic islets in genetically predisposed individuals. Histological examination of islets shows infiltration by lymphocytes ('insulitis'). As a consequence, patients are completely reliant upon exogenous insulin to prevent ketosis and thereby preserve life. This accounts for the main clinical and biochemical features presented in Table 1.3.

TABLE 1.3 Cardinal clinical and biochemical features of type 1 diabetes

- Autoimmune aetiology
- Islet B-cell destruction
- Absolute insulin deficiency
- Abrupt onset of symptoms
- Weight loss
- Ketosis
- Dependence on exogenous insulin to sustain life
- Tissue complications absent at diagnosis

Plasma levels of C-peptide (a marker of endogenous insulin secretion) cannot be pharmacologically stimulated above 0.6 nmol/L in established type 1 diabetes. However, C-peptide responses are not measured routinely (being predominantly used in research, e.g. in prevention studies of type 1 diabetes (see below)). Stimulated C-peptide levels can also provide evidence of endogenous insulin secretion which may be of use in deciding whether discontinuation of insulin therapy might be feasible in the occasional patient in whom the diagnosis of type 1 diabetes is in doubt (see p. 151). For example, some younger patients with other syndromes (e.g. MODY, p. 26) may be treated with insulin from the outset because the young age at diagnosis was taken as evidence supporting a diagnosis of type 1 diabetes; insulin may be successfully withdrawn in carefully selected cases.

AETIOLOGY

Class II major histocompatibility complex (MHC) factors' genes on the short arm of chromosome 6 (*IDDM 1* locus) are responsible for most of the genetic susceptibility to the disease with 95% of patients being positive for human-lymphocyte-associated (HLA) antigens DR3 or DR4 (compared with 40% of controls). The highest risk is in DR3/DR4 heterozygotes, whereas DR2 is protective. Certain DQ alleles are more common amongst patients with type 1 diabetes. In addition, non-MHC genes (e.g. the insulin gene on the short arm of chromosome 11 – *IDDM 2*) modify risk.

Environmental factors

The concordance rate of less than 100% for monozygotic twins (reported rates ranging from 35–70%) points to factors other than those inherited from parents. Nonetheless, the greater risk for monozygotic than for dizygotic twins underlines the importance of the genetic influence which appears to be the principal determinant of autoimmunity. Putative environmental factors implicated in the aetiology of type 1 diabetes include viruses (rubella, coxsackie B4, cytomegalovirus; see p. 260) and certain foods (early exposure to cow's milk in infancy, ingestion of smoked food products containing nitrosamines). To date, however, no common, precipitating, environmental factor has been identified with certainty. Reports of a rising incidence in several countries (see p. 11) also argue in favour of an environmental modifier of risk.

Non-autoimmune type 1 diabetes

Serological markers of autoimmunity, e.g. islet cell antibodies, GAD antibodies and insulin antibodies may be detected in approximately 90% of patients with classical type 1 diabetes at presentation; these tests are usually reserved for research studies. Of interest, and clinical relevance, are a small subgroup of patients who appear to have features of insulin-dependence (e.g. ketosis) yet whose requirements for insulin fluctuate markedly with time. Following an episode of ketoacidosis such patients may subsequently be well controlled with oral agents. These patients, usually of Black or East Asian origin, do not have serological evidence of autoimmunity. However, a cautious approach is indicated erring on the use of insulin if there is any doubt.

PREDICTION AND PREVENTION

Combinations of genetic, immunological and metabolic markers have been used to identify high-risk individuals for intervention trials of using agents such as nicotinamide or even low-dose, prophylactic insulin to limit B-cell loss. These trials utilize the knowledge that type 1 diabetes has a long, asymptomatic prodrome during which B-cells are gradually being destroyed. It held that only when the majority of B-cells (approximately 90%) have been destroyed does the patient present with typical clinical symptoms. Thus, the aim has been to identify siblings at particularly high risk in order to test interventional strategies in the setting of randomized controlled trials (RCTs).

> **NB** Type 1 diabetes has a long, asymptomatic, prodromal period during which B-cells are selectively destroyed.

However, since only around 10% of patients have a first-degree relative with the disorder, general population screening is not feasible with present strategies. Moreover, prediction, even in higher-risk groups, is imperfect and the complex methodology is not available other than for clinical trials. For relatives of a patient with type 1 diabetes, approximate risks for developing the syndrome are as follows:

- Sibling affected – 10% risk overall.
- Mother affected – 2–3% (risk to offspring varies with age that mother developed diabetes – higher with younger-onset).

- Father affected – 5–10%.
- Both parents affected – 30%.

Approximately 30–50% of identical (monozygotic) twins and up to 20% of non-identical (dizygotic) twins will ultimately develop type 1 diabetes if the other twin is affected. Experimental interventions to limit B-cell damage using potentially toxic immunosuppressive agents, e.g. cyclosporin, at diagnosis have proved to be, at best, only partially effective; this reflects the extensive and irreversible loss of B-cells by the time of presentation.

CLINICAL PRESENTATION

In established type 1 diabetes, endogenous insulin secretion is negligible; there is certainly marked insulin deficiency at presentation, any residual insulin secretion declining with time. Plasma glucagon and catecholamine levels are elevated but return towards normal with insulin therapy. Insulin deficiency has major implications for fat and protein metabolism. Adipocyte lipolysis (the breakdown of triglyceride to non-esterified fatty acids and glycerol) is disinhibited and fatty acids taken up by the liver are converted into ketone bodies. Ketonuria (along with hyperglycaemia) indicates marked insulin deficiency since lipolysis is inhibited at relatively low plasma insulin levels. Protein synthesis is decreased while breakdown of structural proteins contributes to loss of body weight at presentation.

Clinic presentation is nearly always with marked classical symptoms (see pp. 38–40). Importantly, children (see Section 6, p. 262) and young adults, in particular, may present with ketoacidosis.

TREATMENT

This is considered in more detail in Sections 2, 3 and 4.

- *Insulin therapy*. Patients with type 1 diabetes are dependent on exogenous insulin treatment to avoid ketosis and thereby preserve life.

 Insulin treatment is life-sustaining in type 1 diabetes.

The risks of major metabolic decompensation, DKA (see p. 168) and iatrogenic hypoglycaemia (see p. 156) are ever-present for the patient with type 1 diabetes. Following initiation of insulin, and particularly in children, a variable period of very good control may be attainable with small or minimal doses of insulin. This is known as the 'honeymoon' period and may last from days to, less commonly, several years. Partial recovery of endogenous insulin secretion is responsible although this usually fades again with time; insulin requirements then increase and remain at a higher level thereafter. Alleviation of putative deleterious effects of hyperglycaemia may be relevant to the temporary improvement of endogenous insulin secretion with treatment (see glucose toxicity, p. 29). True remission occurring after many years of type 1 diabetes is essentially unknown; factitious remission with surreptitious insulin administration is rare (see p. 165).

• *Pancreatic transplantation.* This is generally reserved for patients with end-stage renal failure who also require a kidney transplant (see Sections 3 and 5); the availability of the procedure varies considerably in different parts of the world, with the USA leading.

• *Experimental therapies.* Islet cell transplantation remains largely experimental (see p. 153). Gene therapy and other strategies such as implantable, glucose, sensor-insulin delivery systems are possible future options.

• *Intervention trials.* See page 13.

PROGNOSIS

The overall mortality associated with type 1 diabetes is still increased several-fold compared with the non-diabetic population; the excess risk is particularly high for patients presenting in childhood (see p. 262). The main causes of this excess mortality are:

• Renal failure.
• CHD.

In fact, these complications are closely linked through complex mechanisms. DKA (see p. 168) remains a significant cause of premature death. The syndrome of sudden death in patients with type 1 diabetes is considered on pages 156–165.

TYPE 2 DIABETES

EPIDEMIOLOGY

The cardinal clinical and biochemical features of type 2 diabetes are presented in Table 1.4. Type 2 diabetes accounts for >85% of diabetes on a global basis although rates vary between populations. In the UK (and elsewhere), the prevalence increases with age; up to 20% of the over-80s are diabetic (see p. 268). Rates of diabetes have reached epidemic proportions in some parts of the world; the increase appears to be closely associated with the development of obesity.

TABLE 1.4 Clinical and metabolic features of type 2 diabetes

- Presentation usually in middle age or later life
- Obesity common (present in >75%)
- Symptoms often mild, absent or unrecognized
- Relative rather than absolute insulin deficiency
- Insulin resistance common
- Ketosis-resistant
- Progressive disorder – even with antidiabetic therapy
- Insulin treatment often required to maintain long-term glycaemic control
- Other features of the 'insulin resistance syndrome' often present, e.g. hypertension, dyslipidaemia
- High risk of macrovascular complications – main cause of premature mortality
- Tissue damage often present at diagnosis

NB The global prevalence of type 2 diabetes is projected to double within the next 15 years to 200 million cases.

The lowest prevalences (<3%) have been reported in the least-developed countries; by contrast, the highest prevalence rates (30–50% of adults) are observed in populations (e.g. North American Indians, Pacific Islanders, Australian Aborigines) who have undergone radical changes from traditional to Westernized lifestyles (see below). The Pima Indians of Arizona have the highest prevalence with over 50% of adults aged 35 years or older having diabetes. The prevalence of diabetes is also high in migrant populations, e.g. South Asians in the UK have a 4-fold higher rate than that of the indigenous white population. Thus, type 2 diabetes represents an enormous – and rapidly expanding – global public health problem. In the USA, the increasing incidence of type 2 diabetes in the young, predominantly in ethnic minorities, has been described as an emerging epidemic.

PATHOPHYSIOLOGY

A relative deficiency of endogenous insulin in the presence of impaired insulin action leads to increased hepatic glucose production and decreased insulin-mediated glucose uptake due to post-receptor defect (see below) in muscle. Type 2 diabetes is regarded as a heterogeneous syndrome with the relative contributions of these defects varying between individuals and possibly between different populations.

- *Defective insulin secretion*. Patients with type 2 diabetes secrete enough insulin to prevent ketosis but insufficient to maintain normal glucose metabolism. A 30–40% reduction in insulin-mediated glucose disposal leads to progressive compensatory fasting hyperinsulinaemia until fasting plasma glucose exceeds approximately 7 mmol/L; thereafter, endogenous insulin secretion progressively fails. Islet mass is reduced with deposition of islet amyloid polypeptide; the latter produces striking histological changes within the islets, yet its role in the initiation and progression of type 2 diabetes is disputed. Increased plasma levels of proinsulin-like molecules indicate B-cell dysfunction; this is an early feature, being demonstrable prior to the development of diabetes in high-risk groups. Transient gestational diabetes (see p. 278) is a potent risk factor for the subsequent development of permanent type 2 diabetes. This may reflect the effect of increasing insulin resistance during pregnancy acting to unmask a predisposition to diabetes.

● *Insulin resistance*. Obesity is common (>75%) and is a prominent feature of some animal models of type 2 diabetes such as the *ob/ob* mouse which is deficient in an adipocyte-derived satiety-promoting protein – leptin (see p. 92). The metabolic effects of leptin are the subject of intense research activity. Abdominal or visceral fat deposits are associated with features of the insulin resistance syndrome (see p. 28) including type 2 diabetes; waist girth has been proposed as a simple marker of risk to health (see p. 89). However, there is controversy about the magnitude of the contribution made by visceral adipose tissue to whole body insulin resistance. The importance of insulin resistance in relation to cardiovascular risk – which is greatly increased in patients with type 2 diabetes (see p. 29) – is considered in Section 5.

AETIOLOGY

The high concordance rate for identical twins (~90%) is cited as evidence of either a strong genetic component (generally non-HLA linked, c.f. type 1 diabetes) or, more controversially, of a shared predisposing intrauterine environment – the fetal origins hypothesis.

Environmental factors

● *The fetal origins hypothesis*. Briefly, this challenges the more established (but unproven) thrifty genotype hypothesis of Neel (see below). David Barker and colleagues propose that relative intrauterine malnutrition leads to metabolic 'programming' with a reduced complement of islet B-cells together with insulin resistance in skeletal muscle. Studies in populations in whom birthweight has been carefully recorded have demonstrated an inverse correlation between birthweight and risk of type 2 diabetes in middle age. The risk appears to be particularly high if obesity (a major environmental factor) develops in adulthood. Other cardiovascular risk factors, including hypertension, have also been linked to low birthweight.

Genetic factors

● *Genetics of type 2 diabetes.* A family history of type 2 diabetes is common; the lifetime risk associated with having a single parent with type 2 diabetes is approximately 40% and 50% or more if both parents are affected. In contrast to type 1 diabetes, however, unravelling the genetics of type 2 diabetes has proved to be much more problematic. While studies of an uncommon form of non-insulin-dependent diabetes – MODY – have yielded important evidence for single gene defects (discussed below), the genetics of the common form of type 2 diabetes remain obscure; a polygenic inheritance is proposed for the majority of cases. Many plausible (candidate) genes, e.g. the insulin receptor, have been excluded; increasingly attention is being directed to the regulation of the insulin gene. Difficulties in differentiating the insulin resistance attributable to type 2 diabetes per se from that associated with obesity may be relevant to these difficulties.

● *The thrifty genotype hypothesis.* In 1962, J.V. Neel proposed that some populations have genetic traits which once conferred survival advantages but which have been rendered detrimental by abundant food supplies and reduced habitual levels of physical activity.

CLINICAL PRESENTATION

Patients are usually over 40 years at diagnosis; younger onset may be observed in high prevalence populations or with two affected parents. Presentation of type 2 diabetes is usually with typical symptoms although weight loss is infrequent. Many asymptomatic cases are diagnosed at screening (particularly targeted screening as indicated by other risk factors, see p. 42) or after presentation with associated disorders (e.g. myocardial infarction, MI); on close enquiry, a history of unrecognized symptoms may be obtained.

 NB Many asymptomatic patients with type 2 diabetes are diagnosed by opportunistic testing or screening.

Since the disease is often subclinical for many years before it becomes clinically apparent, careful evaluation may reveal established complications (see Section 5); in the UK Prospective Diabetes Study (UKPDS) (see p. 65) approximately 50% of patients had evidence of diabetes-related tissue damage at diagnosis.

PREDICTION AND PREVENTION

It is impossible to accurately predict who will develop type 2 diabetes. Major gaps in understanding of the aetiology of this heterogeneous disorder need to be filled before this might become feasible. However, it is possible to define groups at higher-than-average risk of developing type 2 diabetes. Factors which have been identified include:

- Affected first degree relative – parent or sibling.
- Ethnicity – high-risk populations.
- Middle age to elderly (earlier in high-risk, ethnic groups).
- Glucose intolerance.
- Obesity (especially visceral adiposity).
- Certain endocrinopathies.
- Treatment with diabetogenic drugs.
- Sedentary lifestyle.
- Cigarette smoking.
- History of gestational diabetes.
- Other features of the insulin resistance syndrome.
- Small birthweight (fetal origins hypothesis).

Clinical studies have suggested that the risk of progression from a high-risk group such as impaired glucose tolerance (see p. 43) to type 2 diabetes may be averted (or at least postponed) by measures such as supervised physical training and dietary advice (e.g. the Malmö Study in Sweden and encouraging preliminary results from the Diabetes Prevention Study in Finland). Large trials evaluating the impact of pharmacological adjuncts (e.g. the US Diabetes Prevention Program) may clarify the efficacy and safety of this more interventional approach which is not currently recommended (the troglitazone-treatment arm of the latter study because of reports of serious hepatotoxicity, see p. 129). For the present, sensible 'lifestyle' advice for higher-risk individuals includes:

- Avoidance of obesity.
- Regular aerobic exercise.
- Avoiding cigarettes.
- Avoidance of diabetogenic drugs (e.g. high dose corticosteroids).

TREATMENT

This is considered in greater detail in Sections 2 and 3.

• *Non-pharmacological measures.* Weight reduction and increased levels of physical exercise are the cornerstones of treatment. These act primarily to partially counter insulin resistance.

• *Pharmacological agents.* Initially as monotherapy and subsequently in combination, are required by most patients. The main modes of action (see also pp. 106–131) are enhanced insulin secretion (sulphonylureas and other secretagogues), amelioration of insulin resistance (metformin, thiazolidinediones) or a reduction in hepatic glucose production (metformin). Alpha-glucosidase inhibitors (see p. 125) mainly reduce post-prandial glucose elevations; they may also reduce the putative adverse metabolic effects of hyperglycaemia (see glucose toxicity, p. 29).

● *Exogenous insulin*. A significant proportion of patients will ultimately progress to insulin in order to maintain long-term metabolic control. This reflects the progressive nature of type 2 diabetes, even when treated with currently available therapy (see UKPDS, p. 65)

● *Reducing cardiovascular risk*. Prevention of atherosclerotic cardiovascular disease requires a therapeutic assault on other modifiable risk factors, including hypertension and dyslipidaemia (see pp. 240 and 250).

PROGNOSIS

Life expectancy is reduced by an average of 5–10 years in patients when type 2 diabetes is diagnosed in middle age. The majority of deaths (approximately 70%) are attributable to macrovascular disease, principally CHD (see p. 228).

 Type 2 diabetes diagnosed in middle age is associated with a reduced life expectancy.

SECONDARY FORMS OF DIABETES

Diabetes mellitus may arise as a consequence of a number of hereditary and acquired diseases and secondary to treatment with certain drugs. It should be noted that patients with secondary diabetes are at risk of chronic complications as is the case for the major primary forms of diabetes.

 Patients with secondary diabetes are also at risk of long-term complications.

PANCREATIC DISEASE

● *Acute pancreatitis*. Transient hyperglycaemia may require insulin therapy but diabetes is rarely permanent following a single episode.

● *Chronic pancreatitis*. This may be complicated by glucose intolerance or diabetes and, at least in Western countries, is often attributable to chronic alcoholism. Pancreatic calcification may be evident on plain radiographs or computerized tomography (CT). Associated malabsorption and glucagon deficiency (the latter arising from destruction of islet A-cells) may contribute to a tendency to hypoglycaemia in patients requiring insulin treatment.

● *Carcinoma of the pancreas.* This may be more common in patients with pre-existing diabetes and should be suspected in elderly patients presenting with a short history of diabetes which includes the following features:

● Marked rapid weight loss.
● Upper abdominal pain (especially radiating to the back).
● Jaundice with features of biliary obstruction.

Diabetes developing de novo with pancreatic carcinoma is not a consequence of insulinopenia arising from destruction of islets; insulin resistance is implicated and glucose tolerance may improve with resection of the tumour.

● *Pancreatectomy.* This is sometimes required for chronic pain resulting from pancreatitis and if greater than 80–90% necessitates lifelong insulin therapy. Large doses (>30–40 U daily) are rarely necessary, reflecting the associated loss of glucagon secretion. Sulphonylureas are ineffective. Lesser distal resection (including those performed on living-related donors of segmental pancreatic graft recipients, see p. 153) cause variable degrees of glucose intolerance, including diabetes.

● *Cystic fibrosis.* Diabetes mellitus may complicate cystic fibrosis, especially in disease of long duration; with increased survival of affected individuals, this is emerging as an important complication of this chronic and disabling disorder. Diabetes usually appears in the late teens or early 20s. Recurrent chest infections and intestinal malabsorption may complicate management. Insulin is ultimately required in most patients although sulphonylureas may be useful as an interim measure.

● *Haemochromatosis.* This autosomal dominant inborn error of metabolism is characterized by excessive iron deposition in a number of organs; diabetes develops in approximately 50% of cases. Insulin therapy is usually required. It is a rare cause of diabetes. The alternative name 'bronzed diabetes' derives from cutaneous pigmentation, partly caused by melanin. The diagnosis should be suspected in patients with hepatomegaly or other features such as suspicious pigmentation, pituitary or testicular failure, cardiomyopathy or chondrocalcinosis. Investigations include measurement of serum iron and ferritin, hepatic imaging and liver biopsy. A search for the most common mutations causing the disorder is now possible. Hepatocellular carcinoma (which, incidentally, may be associated with hypoglycaemia secondary to production of insulin-like growth factor-II) develops in approximately 15% of cases. Treatment is by regular venesection and the prognosis is good if adequate and started prior to the development of cirrhosis; family members of the proband should be screened.

• *Malnutrition-related diabetes*. This encompasses rare ketosis-resistant subtypes of 'fibrocalculous diabetes' or 'protein-deficient pancreatic diabetes' encountered in the tropics. The syndrome has a number of other synonyms. Cyanide toxicity (derived from cassava) has been hypothesized; however, this has been challenged. Some patients may require high doses of insulin (>200 units daily).

DRUG-INDUCED DIABETES

Many drugs are associated with the development of glucose intolerance or with a deterioration in glycaemic control in patients with pre-existing diabetes. Some show dose-dependent effects. For example, anti-inflammatory doses of corticosteroids may necessitate use of insulin in patients hitherto controlled with oral agents; major metabolic decompensation, e.g. hyperosmolar pre-coma or coma, may ensue (see p. 186). Indeed, such therapy not infrequently precipitates diabetes in middle-aged or elderly individuals with no history of glucose intolerance. A subclinical, partial defect in insulin secretory capacity is postulated in such individuals, the diabetes being unmasked by drug-induced insulin resistance. This is difficult to predict although a family history of type 2 diabetes may alert the clinician to the possibility of a predisposition to diabetes. Patients with a prior history of glucose intolerance, e.g. gestational diabetes, are at particularly high risk. Thus, when high-dose corticosteroids are used, routine monitoring of plasma glucose concentrations is a sensible precaution.

 High-dose corticosteroids may precipitate diabetes mellitus in predisposed individuals.

The diabetogenic effects of drugs may also involve impairment of endogenous insulin secretion in some cases. The most commonly implicated drugs include:

• *Corticosteroids*. Especially high doses of synthetic corticosteroids, e.g. dexamethasone, via post-receptor insulin resistance; activation of the glucose–fatty acid cycle (see p. 30) may contribute.

• *Diuretics*. Particularly thiazides at high doses; insulin resistance and hypokalaemia-induced impairment of insulin secretion. Loop diuretics are less diabetogenic.

• *Beta-blockers*. Especially non-selective drugs (see p. 245). Patients with hypertension often have other features of the insulin resistance syndrome (p. 31). Both beta-blockers and thiazide diuretics have been implicated in the development of diabetes mellitus in patients with essential hypertension, particularly when used in combination. Nonetheless, the clinical benefits of lowering elevated blood pressure (BP) levels in non-diabetics and in patients with established diabetes outweigh putative metabolic disadvantages (see p. 247). Modern prescribing utilizes lower doses of thiazides (≤2.5mg bendrofluazide, or equivalent) with the objective of minimizing adverse metabolic effects.

● *Beta–adrenergic agonists.* Especially parenteral (used in premature labour, e.g. ritodrine, see p. 278).

● *Oral contraceptives.* Minor metabolic effects with modern low-dose oestrogen preparations (see pp. 281–282) and minimal with progesterone-only preparations.

● *Cyclophilin immunosuppressants.* Immunosuppression is required for organ transplantation (e.g. renal transplantation for diabetic nephropathy, see p. 227). Cyclosporin is associated with insulin resistance and B-cell toxicity; similar but greater metabolic derangements have been observed with the newer agent, tacrolimus. Concomitant corticosteroid therapy exacerbates these effects.

● *Diazoxide.* The inhibitory effect on insulin secretion of the infrequently used, antihypertensive vasodilator, diazoxide, has been exploited in the medical management of insulinoma and severe sulphonylurea-induced hypoglycaemia (see p. 167); the drug has potent diabetogenic effects in non-diabetics.

NB Beta-blockers and thiazide diuretics are implicated in the development of diabetes in patients with essential hypertension.

ENDOCRINOPATHIES

Pathological chronic hypersecretion of hormones which antagonize the actions of insulin (i.e. the counter-regulatory hormones, p. 5) are frequently associated with glucose intolerance and/or diabetes mellitus. Deteriorating glycaemic control may be the presenting feature of such an endocrinopathy developing in a diabetic patient. The most common of these is Graves' disease, an autoimmune form of thyrotoxicosis which, incidentally, is more prevalent in patients with type 1 diabetes. Cutaneous markers of autoimmunity such as vitiligo or alopecia may be present in affected patients.

NB Patients with type 1 diabetes are at increased risk of developing other autoimmune endocrinopathies.

Other less common examples include:

● *Acromegaly*. Approximately 30% of patients have impaired glucose tolerance with another 30% having diabetes mellitus; insulin resistance may make control of pre-existing diabetes problematic.

● *Cushing's syndrome*. Especially with high cortisol levels secondary to ectopic corticotrophin (ACTH) secretion; post-receptor insulin resistance (pp. 4–5).

● *Conn's syndrome*. Primary hyperaldosteronism; glucose intolerance in ~50%; effects of hypokalaemia on insulin secretion is implicated.

● *Phaeochromocytoma*. Rare; insulin resistance and α-adrenergic inhibition of insulin secretion by adrenaline.

● *Glucagonoma*. Very rare; characteristic clinical and metabolic syndrome, including rash – necrolytic migratory erythema; insulin resistance.

● *Somatostatinoma*. Very rare; inhibition of endogenous insulin secretion; characteristic syndrome includes cholelithiasis.

Prolactinomas, the most common functioning pituitary tumours, may be associated with hyperinsulinaemia although glucose intolerance is usually unimpaired; insulin resistance is rarely, if ever, clinically evident. Insulin resistance has also been reported in association with hyperparathyroidism.

Endocrine deficiency states
By contrast, the following autoimmune disorders, which are also more frequently encountered in patients with type 1 diabetes mellitus as part of a pluriglandular syndrome (type II), are associated with enhanced insulin sensitivity. Clinically, this may be associated with a decrease in insulin requirements; in non-diabetic patients a tendency to fasting hypoglycaemia is well recognized in patients with untreated hypoadrenalism:

● *Primary hypothyroidism*. Common. Reduced metabolic rate and impaired insulin clearance.

● *Addison's disease*. Rare. Lifelong corticosteroid replacement therapy is required.

In addition, the development of hypopituitarism (low levels of growth hormone and cortisol) in an insulin-treated patient will lead to increased insulin sensitivity, thereby increasing the risk of hypoglycaemia.

● *'Stiff man' syndrome*. This rare condition presents as a progressive spastic paraparesis with acute exacerbations precipitated by sudden noises. Polyglandular endocrine involvement is a prominent feature. Anti-GAD65 antibodies, a marker for type 1 diabetes, are diagnostic; approximately 30% of patients develop type 1 diabetes.

Finally, another autoimmune disorder which is more common in patients with type 1 diabetes – gluten enteropathy or coeliac disease – may also lead to hypoglycaemia through intestinal malabsorption. The presentation may include diarrhoea which may be mistakenly attributed to autonomic neuropathy (see p. 209). Anti-gliaden antibodies are specific; the diagnosis is confirmed by duodenal biopsy. Institution of a gluten-free diet may lead to an increase in insulin requirements. Both children and adults may be affected.

GENETIC SYNDROMES ASSOCIATED WITH DIABETES MELLITUS

The incidence of diabetes (mainly with ketosis-resistant, non-insulin-dependent phenotypes) is increased in a number of inherited syndromes:

CHROMOSOMAL DEFECTS

- *Down's syndrome*. Trisomy or translocation of chromosome 21.

- *Turner's syndrome*. Karyotype 45 XO; mosaics.

- *Klinefelter's syndrome*. Karyotype 47 XXY; mosaics.

- *Prader–Willi syndrome*. Deletion or translocation of chromosome 15.

    Other unusual inherited syndromes include:

- *Bardet–Biedl syndrome*. Autosomal recessive; main features are retinitis pigmentosa, polydactyly, central obesity, mental retardation, diabetes and hypogonadism. Genetic loci on chromosome 11 have been described.

- *Alstrom syndrome*. Pigmentary retinal degeneration, sensorineural deafness, obesity, diabetes, hyperlipidaemia and nephropathy. Disease-causing defect mapped to chromosome 2p.

- *Neonatal diabetes*. This is defined as hyperglycaemia occurring during the first 6 weeks of life in term infants and has an incidence in the UK of 1 in 400 000 live births. Inheritance of both copies of genetic material on chromosome 6 from a single parent (paternal isodisomy) is implicated. There are no unusual phenotypical features of this form of neonatal diabetes although intrauterine growth retardation (IUGR) is usual.

- *Wallcott–Rallison syndrome*. Multiple epiphyseal dysplasia with neonatal diabetes. Autosomal recessive; rare.

NEURODEGENERATIVE DISORDERS

- *Myotonic dystrophy*. This is an autosomal dominant multisystem disorder which arises from expansion of a trinucleotide repeat on chromosome 19. It is associated with insulin resistance; however, overt diabetes is relatively uncommon.

● *Friedreich's ataxia.* Autosomal recessive. This is also associated with diabetes. Both insulin resistance and impaired insulin secretion have been reported.

MITOCHONDRIAL SYNDROMES

Mitochondria are intracellular organelles responsible for the generation of energy by oxidative phosphorylation. Defects in the mitochondrial genome associated with diabetes were first recognized in the 1990s. Mitochondrial DNA is exclusively maternally inherited.

● *Wolfram syndrome.* This is a rare autosomal recessive neurodegenerative syndrome comprising **D**iabetes **I**nsipidus, **D**iabetes **M**ellitus (with a tendency to ketosis), **O**ptic **A**trophy and sensorineural **D**eafness (hence, alternative name: **DIDMOAD**). The deafness may not be clinically evident; many patients also develop hydronephrosis, ataxia and psychiatric disturbances. Abnormalities in mitochondrial DNA have been described. Death occurs in the third to fifth decade.

● *Maternally inherited diabetes.* Syndromes associated with mitochondrial DNA mutations account for only a small proportion (<1%) of diabetes in the UK. Families have been described with maternal transmission of non-insulin-dependent diabetes associated with sensorineural deafness. A point mutation in mitochondrial DNA at position 3243 in the tRNA$^{LEU(UUR)}$ gene has been identified. This is the same mutation responsible for another rare syndrome of '**M**yopathy, **E**ncephalopathy, **L**actic **A**cidosis and **S**troke-like episodes' (**MELAS**); however, diabetes is not usually a feature of the latter syndrome, indicating heterogeneity of the phenotype.

MATURITY-ONSET DIABETES OF THE YOUNG (MODY)

This uncommon form of diabetes is a heterogeneous autosomal dominant disorder characterized by hyperglycaemia and relative insulinopenia which presents before the age of 25 years. Offspring with both parents affected by type 2 diabetes have generally been excluded from molecular genetic studies. Such studies have elucidated the aetiology of this syndrome in recent years.

> **NB** There is a 50% risk of diabetes in the offspring of a patient with MODY.

The main features which distinguish MODY from the common form of type 2 diabetes are presented in Table 1.5. The two syndromes differ in several important aspects.

TABLE 1.5 Comparison of type 2 diabetes with MODY syndromes

	Type 2 diabetes	MODY
Age of onset	Middle to old age	Childhood to young adult
Pathophysiology	B-cell dysfunction/ insulin resistance	B-cell dysfunction
Role of environment	Considerable	Minimal
Obesity	Frequent	Rare
Inheritance	Polygenic/ heterogeneous	Monogenic/ autosomal dominant

Several distinct genetic subtypes have been identified to date, the first in 1992:

- *MODY 1.* Mutations in the gene encoding hepatic nuclear factor 4-α (5% of cases).
- *MODY 2.* Mutations in the gene encoding the putative 'glucose-sensing' B-cell enzyme glucokinase (10% of cases).
- *MODY 3.* Mutations in the gene encoding hepatic nuclear factor 1-α (65% of cases).
- *MODY 4.* Insulin promoter gene mutation.
- *MODY 5.* Other mutations.

Mutations in the gene encoding for B-cell (and liver) glucokinase lead to a reduction of insulin secretion by a mechanism which can be interpreted as a shift in the dose–response curve for the secretion of insulin. Thus, for any specified plasma glucose concentration less insulin is secreted. Fasting plasma glucose concentrations are typically around 7 mmol/L, with post-prandial levels <10 mmol/L; this is a stable defect which is probably present from birth and which shows little or no progression with time.

Patients who are started on insulin at diagnosis appear to be in a chronic 'honeymoon' state (see p. 14) requiring less than 0.5 U/kg/day insulin. Glycaemic control is good in many patients without pharmacological therapy. The major exception to this rule is pregnancy; here, insulin may be required temporarily in order to ensure optimal control (see p. 271). Many cases are diagnosed during pregnancy (see p. 279). The minor biochemical disturbance is not usually associated with a significant risk of chronic microvascular complications.

MODY 2 accounts for approximately 10% of mutations in UK families tested to date. This benign subtype contrasts with the hepatic nuclear factor mutations which cause progressive hyperglycaemia. Accordingly, oral agents and even insulin may prove necessary and there is a significant risk of long-term complications. The precise molecular mechanism responsible for diabetes in MODY 1 and MODY 3 remains uncertain. Other mutations appear to await discovery since approximately 20% of families do not have any of the mutations identified to date.

Molecular genetic testing

Knowledge of the genotype in the unaffected child of a patient with this syndrome offers the possibility of a firm diagnosis, or, importantly, exclusion of the possibility of diabetes in later life. If the genetic testing is negative, no screening will be necessary and individuals and their families can be reassured. If an unaffected offspring is found to have a MODY-2 mutation, then annual testing of fasting plasma glucose and, for females, awareness of the importance of excellent glycaemic control before conception are required. Identification of a MODY-1 or MODY-3 genotype necessitates more rigorous, regular screening through childhood, adolescence and early adult life to detect the development of diabetes since pharmacological treatment, including insulin, is likely to prove necessary. Such testing raises ethical issues and it has been suggested that it should be offered only after appropriate genetic counselling. Whether such knowledge will ultimately allow intervention to prevent or retard the appearance of diabetes is presently uncertain.

INSULIN RESISTANCE

Insulin resistance may be defined in generic terms as:

A reduced biological response to a physiological amount of insulin.

The presence of insulin resistance is implied by normo- or hyperglycaemia in concert with hyperinsulinaemia. For research purposes, insulin action can be quantified using laborious techniques such as the hyperinsulinaemic glucose clamp. This involves simultaneous infusions of insulin and hypertonic dextrose and is widely regarded as the gold standard for quantifying insulin action. Briefly, the more dextrose that is required to maintain euglycaemia during the sustained hyperinsulinaemia produced by the insulin infusion, the more insulin-sensitive the individual.

NB Fasting hyperinsulinaemia in the presence of a normal or elevated plasma glucose level implies insulin resistance.

Clamp studies have suggested a defect in insulin action distal to the interaction of the hormone with its membrane receptor (see p. 5); the nature of this defect remains obscure. In clinical practice, the presence of insulin resistance is usually inferred from the presence of obesity (although there is evidence of heterogeneity within the obese population). It is asymptomatic unless metabolic decompensation occurs leading to diabetes.

 NB Insulin resistance per se is asymptomatic.

There is a broad range of insulin sensitivity in apparently healthy populations. Up to 25% have unrecognized insulin resistance to degrees similar to patients with glucose intolerance or type 2 diabetes; the clinical significance of this insulin resistance is presently uncertain. However, the prevalence of cardiovascular risk factors (see p. 228) increases along with increasing plasma insulin concentrations.

NB Insulin resistance is a prominent metabolic feature of type 2 diabetes.

Various drugs may induce insulin resistance. Reduced insulin sensitivity is also observed in certain physiological situations, notably:

- Puberty.
- Pregnancy (second and third trimesters, p. 272).

Compensatory insulin secretion usually ensures that the insulin resistance associated with puberty or pregnancy remains subclinical. However, in patients with diabetes, increased insulin requirements (or need for insulin in patients hitherto controlled by diet ± oral agents) may be necessary (see p. 277). Other factors which may influence insulin sensitivity include:

- *Sex.* Men and women normally have approximately equal insulin sensitivity if factors such as differences in body composition (women have more adipose tissue) and aerobic capacity (lower in women) are taken into account.

- *Ageing.* The effect of ageing, per se, on insulin sensitivity is disputed (see p. 268). However, glucose tolerance generally deteriorates with age.

GLUCOSE TOXICITY

Importantly, from a therapeutic standpoint, there is evidence that hyperglycaemia per se may adversely affect both insulin action and endogenous insulin secretion. These effects have been termed 'glucose toxicity'. The clinical implication is that reducing the level of hyperglycaemia (whether by non-pharmacological measures, oral agents or insulin) may produce secondary improvements in intermediary metabolism.

LIPOTOXICITY

Disturbed fatty acid metabolism has been documented in patients with type 2 diabetes and lesser degrees of glucose intolerance. Experimental data indicate that elevated fatty acid concentrations may:

- Impair insulin-mediated glucose disposal and oxidation (via the glucose-fatty acid or Randle cycle).
- Accelerate hepatic glucose production.
- Inhibit endogenous insulin secretion.
- Contribute to hypertriglyceridaemia (see p. 251).

   These effects may be regarded conceptually as evidence for a toxic effect of fatty acids. Indeed, recent data suggest that under experimental conditions at least, fatty acids may induce apoptosis (programmed cell death) in islet B-cells. Tumour-necrosis factor-α produced by adipocytes has also been implicated in the production of insulin resistance in glucose metabolism via inhibitory effects on insulin signalling. In addition, elevated circulating fatty acid concentrations have also been implicated in the pathogenesis of hypertension.

REGIONAL ADIPOCITY

While insulin action is often reduced in the presence of obesity, inverse correlations have been observed in some glucose clamp studies between insulin sensitivity and visceral or abdominal fat deposits, independently of body mass index. This form of obesity is commonly observed in men although some women also have upper body obesity rather than the more common, lower body obesity. The insulin resistance, which is associated with an increased risk of type 2 diabetes, has been linked to increased metabolic activity of the adipocytes in this area. Visceral adipocytes, whose principal function is storage of triglycerides, have been shown to have altered responses to certain hormones when compared to adipocytes from subcutaneous depots:

- *Insulin*. Visceral adipocytes are relatively resistant to the actions of insulin (which inhibits triglyceride hydrolysis).

- *Catecholamines*. Visceral adipocytes exhibit greater sensitivity to the lipolytic effect of these hormones.

   This combination serves to increase the rate of lipolysis resulting in increased portal delivery of non-esterified fatty acids to the liver (see p. 7). However, visceral adipocytes account for only 5–10% of total adipose tissue mass and some investigators have not confirmed a unique contribution of visceral adipocity to whole body insulin sensitivity.

HYPERTENSION AND INSULIN RESISTANCE

Hypertension is common among patients with type 2 diabetes (see p. 240). Moreover, many patients with essential hypertension have features of the insulin resistance syndrome (see below). Hypotheses linking insulin resistance with hypertension in patients with type 2 diabetes include:

- Insulin-induced sympathetic activation leading to vasoconstriction and increased peripheral vascular resistance.
- Insulin-stimulated renal sodium retention.

However, these are speculative and the cause of hypertension in patients with type 2 diabetes, the prevalence of which is also influenced by factors such as age and obesity, remains uncertain. Reported BP-lowering effects of insulin-sensitizing dugs such as metformin and troglitazone (see pp. 123 and 129) merit further investigation.

THE INSULIN RESISTANCE SYNDROME

This has a number of synonyms: 'Syndrome X'; 'Reaven's syndrome'; and the 'metabolic syndrome'. Insulin resistance has been implicated in a number of pathological states which frequently co-segregate in affected individuals and which are associated with an increased risk of atherosclerotic disease, principally CHD. The key features of the syndrome, as originally described by Reaven in 1988 include:

- Decreased insulin-mediated glucose disposal.
- Glucose intolerance or diabetes mellitus.
- Hyperinsulinaemia.
- Hypertriglyceridaemia.
- Low plasma HDL-cholesterol levels.
- Essential hypertension.

However, there is currently no consensus on the definition of the syndrome and the following features have been added:

- Visceral obesity.
- Hyperuricaemia.
- Impaired fibrinolysis.
- Microalbuminuria.

Environmental factors such as physical inactivity and possibly cigarette smoking may exacerbate insulin resistance. The following criteria have been proposed for non-diabetic individuals by the European Group for the Study of Insulin Resistance (1999):

- Fasting plasma insulin levels in the highest 25% for the population, together with two of the following:

— Fasting glucose >6.1 mmol/L.
— Hypertension (BP $\geq$ 140/90 mmHg (or treated)).
— Dyslipidaemia: plasma triglycerides >2.0 mmol/L or HDL-cholesterol <1.0 mmol/L.
— Central obesity: waist circumference >94 cm in men and >80 cm in women.

Note that obesity per se is not a component, nor is microalbuminuria included. There are practical difficulties with such definitions, however, particularly in relation to paucity of population-derived reference ranges for plasma insulin concentrations.

Clinical implications

Components of the insulin resistance syndrome are frequently present in combination in patients with impaired glucose tolerance and type 2 diabetes. Whether insulin resistance is the fundamental metabolic defect which links these abnormalities together is uncertain. There is considerable epidemiological and experimental evidence that insulin resistance syndrome confers an increased risk of cardiovascular disease. Importantly, the magnitude of the risk associated with a combination of factors is greater than would be expected by simple addition, i.e. the effects are synergistic. Finally, there is evidence from longitudinal studies that these metabolic risk factors:

a. Worsen continuously across the spectrum of glucose intolerance and
b. Are present many years before diagnosis of type 2 diabetes.

> **NB** Modifiable risk factors greatly magnify the risk of atherosclerosis when present in combination.

Taking a different perspective, a substantial proportion of patients with essential hypertension have one or more additional components of the syndrome which contribute to their risk of cardiovascular events. It has been recommended that management of high-risk patients, such as those with hypertension in conjunction with other features of the syndrome, with non-pharmacological and pharmacological measures should take account of these factors which can be identified by routine clinical and biochemical tests. There is an emerging consensus that reduction of cardiovascular risk demands attention to all modifiable factors (see Section 5).

> **NB** Other components of the insulin resistance syndrome should be sought in patients presenting with either diabetes, hypertension or dyslipidaemia.

SYNDROMES OF SEVERE INSULIN RESISTANCE

A number of rare syndromes are associated with defective cellular insulin receptor structure and function or post-receptor defects in insulin signalling (see p. 4). The molecular biology of some of these syndromes has been elucidated. The scientific importance of these syndromes derives principally from the insights they have provided about insulin action:

- *Leprechaunism.* Intrauterine growth retardation; homozygous or compound heterozygous mutations affecting the insulin receptor gene resulting in profound impairment of insulin action.

- *Rabson–Mendenhall syndrome.* Characteristic phenotypic features; insulin receptor defects.

Clinical features

Severe insulin resistance may be accompanied by physical stigmata such as the dermatological condition acanthosis nigricans (Plate 1). This is found in the axillae, around the nape of the neck and at other sites. Other features, present to variable degrees, include growth retardation, hyperandrogenism (with hirsutism), syndrome-specific features (e.g. pineal hyperplasia in Rabson–Mendenhall syndrome) and an appearance reminiscent of acromegaly in the absence of elevated growth hormone concentrations.

HYPERANDROGENISM AND INSULIN RESISTANCE

In women, polycystic ovary syndrome is a relatively common cause of insulin resistance which is associated with features of hyperandrogenism (hirsutism, oligomenorrhoea). Other biochemical features of the insulin resistance syndrome are reportedly more common, the implication being that the risk of cardiovascular disease may be increased. Retrospective studies also suggest that the risk of type 2 diabetes may be increased. Recent data suggest that there may be some overlap between gestational diabetes (see p. 278) and the polycystic ovary syndrome, women with previous gestational diabetes having a higher incidence of polycystic ovaries and hyperandrogenism.

> **NB** Women with polycystic ovary syndrome are at increased risk of developing type 2 diabetes.

Polycystic ovary syndrome appears to overlap with a much less common syndrome – type A severe insulin resistance. Of interest is the observation that hirsutism and cystic ovarian changes appear to be consistent associations of severe insulin resistance. It is hypothesized that hyperinsulinaemia stimulates ovarian androgen production.

Insulin acts as a gonadotrophin in polycystic ovary syndrome.

Plasma levels of sex-hormone binding globulin are reduced in the presence of insulin resistance; hyperinsulinaemia inhibits the hepatic production of this carrier protein. In turn, this results in lower binding of androgens, mainly testosterone, thereby increasing target tissue exposure to the unbound or free hormone; weight reduction increases the concentrations of the binding protein, thereby reducing the free testosterone levels.

 Reducing hyperinsulinaemia leads to a decrease in androgen levels in polycystic ovary syndrome.

Reduced levels of sex-hormone binding globulin are regarded as a biochemical marker for subclinical insulin resistance. Recent studies have suggested a potential role for metformin and thiazolidinediones in the management of polycystic ovary disease; however, the efficacy and safety of this approach require further evaluation. Weight loss may lead to improved insulin action and an improvement in hirsutism.

LIPODYSTROPHIC DIABETES

These are enigmatic disorders which may be classified as either:

- Congenital.
- Acquired (onset in early childhood).

The principal, phenotypic characteristic is partial or total absence of subcutaneous fat (Plate 2), variable degrees of insulin resistance and hyperlipidaemia (sometimes severe with risk of pancreatitis and atherosclerosis). The paucity of adipose tissue leads to striking clinical appearances and ketosis-resistant diabetes. The molecular defects responsible await elucidation. Cirrhosis and mesangioproliferative glomerulonephritis are recognized features of some forms.

PROTEASE-INHIBITOR-ASSOCIATED LIPODYSTROPHY

Recently, a syndrome has been described in patients with human immunodeficiency virus-1 (HIV-1) receiving treatment with protease-inhibitors or nucleoside-analogue reverse transcriptase inhibitors, the cardinal features of which are:

- Peripheral-acquired lipoatrophy (face, limbs).
- Central adiposity (abdomen and dorsocervical spine).
- Hyperlipidaemia.

- Glucose intolerance.
- Insulin resistance.

It is hypothesized that this syndrome may be a consequence of programmed cell death (apoptosis) of adipocytes induced by the drugs; mitochondrial toxicity has also been postulated. Type 2 diabetes has been reported in a minority of cases (<10%).

NON-ALCOHOLIC STEATOHEPATITIS

Recently, it has been suggested that fatty infiltration of the liver is associated with other features of the insulin resistance syndrome in some patients.

DIAGNOSIS, INITIAL MANAGEMENT AND EDUCATION

CLINICAL PRESENTATION OF DIABETES

Diabetes mellitus is a syndrome, i.e. a collection of disorders rather than a single pathological entity (see p. 2), its clinical presentation varies considerably between patients.

NB The clinical presentation of diabetes is heterogeneous.

Presentations may range from occasional, life-threatening, metabolic decompensation, i.e. ketoacidosis or the hyperosmolar syndrome (see pp. 168 and 185), to asymptomatic cases detected by opportunistic screening. Patients with type 2 diabetes are often identified by urinalysis in general practice, at health insurance checks or during attendance at hospital for an unrelated problem. This heterogeneity reflects not only the relevant diagnostic category into which the patient falls, i.e. type 1 vs type 2 (see p. 9), but also the point in the natural history of the disorder at which the diagnosis is made.

NB The presentation depends on the type of diabetes and the point reached in the natural history.

The clinical presentation may also be modified, precipitated or caused by intercurrent illness.

TYPE 1 DIABETES

The clinical presentation of type 1 diabetes in younger patients is usually acute with classical osmotic symptoms (Table 2.1).

TABLE 2.1 Presenting features of type 1 diabetes

Osmotic symptoms
- Thirst
- Polyuria
- Nocturia
- Weight loss
- Fatigue and lassitude

Associated symptoms
- Muscular cramps
- Blurred vision
- Fungal or bacterial infection – usually oro–genital and cutaneous, respectively

---

In general, symptoms will have been present only for a few weeks with osmotic symptoms; weight loss predominates and gradually increases in intensity. Weight loss in these circumstances reflects catabolism of protein and fat resulting from profound insulin deficiency (see p. 14) as well as dehydration if hyperglycaemia is marked. Associated symptoms, particularly blurred vision, are not uncommon although these are generally less prominent. While the islet B-cell destruction of type 1 diabetes is a process which occurs gradually over many years (see p. 12), it is very uncommon to detect type 1 diabetes during the early asymptomatic stages of the condition. Once symptoms appear, diagnosis may sometimes be usefully expedited by awareness of symptoms in other family members with diabetes. However, patients sometimes do not seek medical advice despite the presence of significant osmotic symptoms. A significant proportion (approximately 5–10%) of patients with type 1 diabetes continue to present in DKA (Table 2.2).

NB Approximately 5–10% of patients with type 1 diabetes present in DKA.

TABLE 2.2 Cardinal clinical features of diabetic ketoacidosis

- Marked polyuria and polydipsia
- Nausea and vomiting
- Dehydration
- Reduced level of consciousness
- Acidotic (Kussmaul) respiration

Diabetic ketoacidosis

The relatively high rate of presentation in DKA may reflect the rapidity with which metabolic decompensation may ensue when islet B-cell mass or function falls below a critical level. In these circumstances, intercurrent illnesses such as infections, to which diabetic patients may be predisposed, are likely to expose the patient's limited, endogenous insulin reserve; an abrupt ascent in plasma glucose concentration may ensue in concert with dehydration, ketosis, acidosis and electrolyte depletion.

NB Intercurrent illness, e.g. sepsis, may cause rapid metabolic decompensation in patients with type 1 diabetes.

DKA is a life-threatening, medical emergency requiring hospitalization for treatment with intravenous fluids and insulin. Patients with the features listed in Table 2.2 along with the following features should be admitted promptly to hospital for further assessment and treatment:

- Heavy glycosuria.
- Ketonuria (++ or greater).

The diagnosis and management of DKA are considered in more detail in Section 4 (pp. 168–185).

 Patients with clinical features suggestive of DKA must be admitted to hospital without delay.

TYPE 2 DIABETES

The majority of patients with type 2 diabetes are diagnosed at a relatively late stage of a long, pathological process which has its origins in the patient's genotype (or perhaps intrauterine experience) and develops and progresses over many years.

 Type 2 diabetes represents a late stage of a complex and progressive, pathological process.

The presenting clinical features of type 2 diabetes (Table 2.3) range from none at all to those associated with the dramatic and life-threatening, hyperglycaemic emergency of the hyperosmolar non-ketotic syndrome (see p. 185). In many patients with lesser degrees of hyperglycaemia, symptoms may go unnoticed or unrecognized for many years; however, such undiagnosed diabetes carries the risk of insidious tissue damage. It has been estimated that patients with type 2 diabetes have often had pathological degrees of hyperglycaemia for several years before the diagnosis is made; over 5 million people in the USA alone may have undiagnosed diabetes. In the USA, African–American, Hispanic and native populations have the highest rates of diabetes.

 Approximately 50% of patients in the UK with type 2 diabetes are undiagnosed.

Thus, although classical osmotic symptoms, albeit not necessarily pronounced, are the rule in type 2 diabetes – with the notable exception of significant weight loss – a high index of clinical suspicion must be maintained so that asymptomatic cases may be identified. The absence of

---

TABLE 2.3 Presenting features of type 2 diabetes

None – asymptomatic patients identified by screening

Osmotic symptoms
- Thirst
- Polyuria
- Nocturia
- Blurred vision
- Fatigue/lassitude

Infection
- Recurrent fungal infection (e.g. genital candidiasis)
- Recurrent bacterial infections (e.g. urinary tract)

Macrovascular complications
- Coronary artery disease (angina pectoris, acute MI)
- Cerebrovascular disease (transient ischaemic episodes, stroke)
- Peripheral vascular disease (intermittent claudication, rest pain, ischaemic ulceration)

Microvascular complications
- Retinopathy (acute or progressive visual impairment)
- Nephropathy (proteinuria, hypertension, nephrotic syndrome)
- Neuropathy (symptomatic sensory polyneuropathy, foot ulceration, amyotrophy, cranial nerve palsies, peripheral mononeuropathies, entrapment neuropathies)

Associated conditions
- Glaucoma
- Cataracts

---

weight loss reflects the presence of sufficient secretion of endogenous insulin to prevent catabolism of protein and fat. In fact, most patients with type 2 diabetes are overweight or obese, adding to their insulin resistance and hyperinsulinaemia (see p. 28).

Population screening for type 2 diabetes

In the UKPDS (see p. 65), the severity of diabetes-related tissue damage correlated with the glycated haemoglobin concentration at diagnosis. Thus, there is the prospect that earlier intervention in patients identified by screening of asymptomatic at-risk individuals may prevent or retard chronic diabetic complications. Although this has not been confirmed in clinical trials, type 2 diabetes satisfies the major criteria for a disorder for which screening would be appropriate.

> **NB** Tissue damage at diagnosis of type 2 diabetes reflects the degree and duration of preceding hyperglycaemia.

In 1997, the ADA recommended that testing be performed using fasting plasma glucose measurements every 3 years (Table 2.4). However, the cost-

---

TABLE 2.4 Criteria for testing for diabetes in asymptomatic, undiagnosed individuals aged <45 years (American Diabetes Association, 1997)

Testing every 3 years should be considered in subjects who have:
- First-degree relatives with diabetes
- Excess weight or obesity (especially abdominal obesity)
- Impaired glucose tolerance (on previous testing)
- Impaired fasting glucose
- Previous gestational diabetes or large baby (>4.5 kg)
- Polycystic ovary syndrome
- Essential hypertension
- Hypertriglyceridaemia
- Low HDL-cholesterol levels
- High-risk ethnic origin
- Premature cardiovascular disease
- Corticosteroid, beta-blocker, high-dose thiazide therapy
- Primary hyperuricaemia or gout
- Specific endocrinopathies (e.g. Cushing's disease and sydrome, acromegaly, phaeochromocytoma)
- Certain inherited disorders (e.g. Turner's syndrome, Down's syndrome or myotonic dystrophy)

---

effectiveness of universal testing is uncertain and would be expected to vary according to the demographics of the particular population.

The main determinant of the mode of presentation of type 2 diabetes, which in turn generally reflects the severity of osmotic symptoms (Table 2.3), is the degree to which insulin is deficient in either secretion or action in target tissues (see p. 4).

Effect of renal threshold for glucose

A high renal threshold for glucose, which is particularly common in elderly subjects, may attenuate the osmotic symptoms of hyperglycaemia. Thus, glycosuria may be minimal or absent despite diabetic plasma glucose concentrations (see below).

NB A high renal threshold for glucose may protect against osmotic symptoms, particularly in elderly subjects.

In addition to the intrinsic insulin resistance of type 2 diabetes, the metabolic actions of insulin (see pp. 3–7) may be further impaired by the secretion of antagonistic hormones. These are the counter-regulatory hormones – glucagon, adrenaline, noradrenaline, cortisol and growth hormone. They are secreted in response to physical and psychological stresses, and impair insulin action at cellular level. In addition, catecholamines can inhibit endogenous insulin secretion. The combination of effects may cause metabolic decompensation in patients with type 2 diabetes who have limited insulin secretory capacity. Thus, acute conditions such as MI, left ventricular failure or severe sepsis may unveil hitherto unrecognized diabetes. Patients with type 2 diabetes are predisposed to these complications by the diabetic state.

IMPAIRED GLUCOSE TOLERANCE

Impaired glucose tolerance denotes an intermediate stage between normality and diabetes. Since, by definition, plasma glucose levels are not raised to diabetic levels, osmotic symptoms are usually absent.

> **NB** Impaired glucose tolerance is usually asymptomatic.

Although some patients with impaired glucose tolerance may have a reduced renal threshold, osmotic symptoms are not a feature of this syndrome. Sometimes, therefore, the presence of asymptomatic glycosuria will result from impaired glucose tolerance rather than type 2 diabetes (Table 2.5). The diagnosis of impaired glucose tolerance relies on glucose tolerance testing (see below). Patients with impaired glucose tolerance, although not at direct risk of developing chronic microvascular disease, may be detected following the development of macrovascular complications:

- Ischaemic heart disease.
- Cerebrovascular disease.
- Peripheral vascular disease.

The presence of one of these conditions should therefore alert the clinician to the possibility of undiagnosed, impaired glucose tolerance or type 2 diabetes even in the absence of osmotic symptoms. Comparative, cross-sectional studies to date suggest that impaired glucose tolerance and the more recently introduced category of impaired fasting glucose (see p. 47) may not be synonymous in terms of pathophysiology and long-term implications; longitudinal studies will be necessary to test the hypothesis that these categories are clinically equivalent.

> **NB** The equivalence of impaired fasting glucose and impaired glucose tolerance has not been established in prospective studies.

A proportion of individuals who have impaired glucose tolerance diagnosed by an oral glucose tolerance test may revert to normal glucose tolerance on retesting.

ESTABLISHING THE DIAGNOSIS

WHO MAKES THE DIAGNOSIS?

In the UK, the diagnosis of diabetes is most commonly made in the general practitioner's (GP) surgery. Routine checks, insurance medicals and consultations with opticians or urologists also bring cases of type 2 diabetes to light. Diagnosis on the coronary care unit following an acute MI is not uncommon. Less commonly, the diagnosis is made when the patient presents with an established complication such as an infected neuropathic foot lesion or symptomatic diabetic retinopathy. Although the discovery of glycosuria may be an important clue, the diagnosis hinges on accurate determination of the blood glucose concentration.

GLYCOSURIA

Urine testing is a valuable pointer to diabetes but is insufficient to make the diagnosis.

> **NB** Diabetes cannot be diagnosed from the presence of glycosuria alone; accurate measurement of blood glucose is necessary.

Although glucose oxidase test strips are specific for glucose, glycosuria does not invariably indicate the presence of diabetes (Table 2.1); the converse is also true.

> **NB** Glycosuria may occur in the absence of diabetes; conversely, diabetes may be present without glycosuria.

TABLE 2.5 Causes of glycosuria

- Diabetes mellitus
- Impaired glucose tolerance
- Lowered renal threshold for glucose (e.g. during pregnancy, in children)

> **NB** Fluid intake, urine concentration and certain drugs may influence tests for glycosuria.

The diagnosis of diabetes relies on the demonstration of unequivocally elevated blood glucose levels which can be:

- Random – the first-line investigation.
- In the fasting state.
- In response to oral glucose challenge – if necessary.

 NB Measurement of random plasma glucose concentration is the first-line investigation for diagnosing diabetes mellitus.

Neither the confirmation nor exclusion of diabetes should rest on measurement of either:

- Glycated haemoglobin (see p. 71).
- Fructosamine (see p. 73).

Although of high specificity, these blood tests are not sufficiently standardized nor do they have sufficient sensitivity to be routinely used for this purpose; they are not available in all countries, being relatively expensive. False negative results are particularly likely with less marked degrees of hyperglycaemia, especially in patients with impaired glucose tolerance or impaired fasting glucose.

BLOOD GLUCOSE

A blood glucose measurement is the essential investigation in the diagnosis of diabetes; this should be performed by a clinical chemistry laboratory using a specific glucose assay to ensure accuracy. An appropriate sample must be collected, usually venous plasma in fluoride oxalate (as an inhibitor of glycolysis). If other samples, e.g. capillary or venous whole blood are taken, this will influence the glucose result.

 NB The type of glucose sample must be known; diagnostic levels vary according to the specimen.

While convenient and readily available, reagent test strips for monitoring of capillary glucose, even when used in conjunction with a reflectance meter, are unsuitable for securing the diagnosis of diabetes. Although the co-efficient of variation of such tests may be less than 5% under optimal conditions, there is potential for error (see below); a confirmatory laboratory measurement must therefore always be performed when test strips suggest the diagnosis. Usually, a random or fasting plasma glucose will be measured. In the presence of diabetic symptoms, this will usually be sufficient to establish the diagnosis.

CONFIRMATION OF THE DIAGNOSIS

In the absence of unequivocal hyperglycaemia with acute metabolic decompensation, the diagnosis should ideally be confirmed by a repeat measurement on a separate day which may be either a random or fasting glucose. This is especially important in individuals with minimal or absent symptoms of diabetes – the diagnosis **must** be confirmed with a second laboratory measurement of blood glucose. The diagnostic difficulties that may be posed by acute severe intercurrent illness are discussed below.

> **NB** The diagnosis of diabetes should always be confirmed by a repeat blood glucose measurement in asymptomatic individuals.

Note that an oral glucose tolerance test is rarely required to confirm the diagnosis and should not be regarded as a first-line investigation. Glucose tolerance tests are time-consuming, relatively labour intensive and less reproducible than measurements of fasting plasma glucose.

> **NB** The diagnosis of diabetes can usually be established using random or fasting glucose measurements; glucose tolerance testing is rarely required.

MAJOR METABOLIC DECOMPENSATION

Arrangements should be made to ensure that the blood glucose result is relayed by telephone or fax to the responsible medical practitioner as a matter of urgency in the presence of either:

- Marked osmotic symptoms.
- Ketonuria.

An unexpectedly high blood glucose level (>20 mmol/L) should prompt the laboratory to contact the clinician with the minimum of delay. Even if the patient is not in immediate danger of major decompensation this may ensue if appropriate therapeutic intervention is unduly delayed. In any case, the patient will almost certainly have osmotic symptoms which will be relieved by treatment.

 Plasma glucose concentrations >20 mmol/L should be communicated urgently to the responsible clinician.

DIAGNOSTIC CRITERIA

The revised ADA (1997) diagnostic criteria for diabetes are:

- Random plasma glucose ≥11.1 mmol/L.
- Fasting plasma glucose ≥7.0 mmol/L.

Note. The diagnostic fasting plasma glucose is lower than the previous NDDG (1979) and WHO (1980, 1985) criteria which specified a diagnostic fasting plasma glucose ≥7.8 mmol/L. The new figure reflects the results of cross-sectional and prospective studies which have identified this cut-off as being closely associated with the risk of microvascular complications of diabetes. Furthermore, ADA has placed emphasis on the equivalence of fasting glucose concentrations and the value 120 min following a 75 g oral glucose challenge; WHO in their reclassification have argued for the retention of the oral glucose tolerance test. Limited studies to date suggest that the ADA criteria are more likely to identify middle-aged, obese individuals with diabetes; the overall prevalence of diagnosed diabetes may also increase. Finally, US and European studies suggest that post-prandial hyperglycaemia, as identified using glucose tolerance tests, may more accurately predict mortality through identification of patients with impaired glucose tolerance (see p. 48).

IMPAIRED FASTING GLUCOSE

The 1997 ADA criteria introduced the new, intermediate category of impaired fasting glucose defined as:

- Fasting venous plasma 6.1–6.9 mmol/L.

This category denotes an abnormally high fasting glucose concentration which falls short of the diagnosis of diabetes. False positive diagnoses of diabetes or impaired fasting glucose may arise if the subject has prepared inadequately. This possibility is more likely following the reduction in the diagnostic threshold for diabetes based on fasting glucose in the 1997 criteria. Therefore the clinician must ensure that the subject understands the preparation required; this should be carefully explained verbally and with written instructions (Table 2.6).

TABLE 2.6 Preparation for a fasting blood test

- The subject should refrain from consuming any food or drink from midnight before the morning of the test
- Water alone is permitted for thirst
- Regular medication can generally be deferred until the sample has been taken
- The appropriate sample is taken between 0800–0900 h the following morning

This preparation is also required for a 75 g oral glucose tolerance test or for measurement of fasting blood lipids.

IMPAIRED GLUCOSE TOLERANCE

The diagnosis of impaired glucose tolerance can only be made using a 75 g oral glucose tolerance test; a random glucose measurement will often point to the diagnosis of impaired glucose tolerance when the result of casual measurement is found to be non-diagnostic, i.e. less than 11.1 mmol/L.

 The diagnosis of impaired glucose tolerance requires a 75 g oral glucose tolerance test; it cannot be made on a casual blood test.

Oral glucose tolerance test

The oral glucose tolerance test is the most robust means for establishing the diagnosis of diabetes. Cross-sectional studies in the USA and Europe indicate that there is disagreement in a substantial proportion of cases when fasting glucose levels and 120 min measurements (after a 75 g oral glucose load) are compared. For individuals – as opposed to epidemiological surveys – the WHO (1998) consultation paper (subsequently ratified) placed emphasis on the oral glucose tolerance test as the gold standard with both fasting and 120 min values being taken into consideration. Only when an oral glucose tolerance cannot be performed should the diagnosis rely on fasting levels.

 The WHO (1998) consultation document on the revised diagnostic criteria reaffirms the importance of the oral glucose tolerance test.

The ADA (1997), by contrast, proposes measurement of fasting glucose as the principal means of diagnosis. Glucose tolerance tests should be carried out under controlled conditions after an overnight fast. The patient is prepared as detailed in Table 2.6.

- Anhydrous glucose is dissolved in 250 mL water; flavouring with sugar-free lemon and chilling increase palatability and may reduce nausea. The patient sits quietly throughout the test.
- Blood glucose is sampled before (time 0) and at 120 min after ingestion of the drink, which should be completed within 5 min.
- Urinalysis may also be performed every 30 min although this is really only of interest if a significant alteration in renal threshold for glucose is suspected.

Interpretation of the results of a 75 g glucose tolerance test are presented in Table 2.7. Note that results apply to venous plasma – whole blood values are 15% lower than corresponding plasma values if haematocrit is normal. For capillary whole blood, the diagnostic cut-offs for diabetes are ≥6.1 mmol/L (fasting) and 11.1 mmol/L (i.e. the same as for venous plasma; Table 2.7). The range for impaired fasting glucose based on capillary whole blood is ≥5.6 and <6.1 mmol/L. Note that marked carbohydrate deprivation can impair glucose tolerance; the subject should have received adequate nutrition in the days preceding the test.

> **NB** To avoid false positive results, patients should receive an unrestricted diet containing adequate carbohydrate (>150 g daily) for 3 days prior to an oral glucose tolerance test.

TABLE 2.7 Interpretation of 75 g oral glucose tolerance test

	Venous plasma glucose (mmol/L)		
	Fasting		120 min-post glucose load
Normal	≤6.0		<7.8
Impaired fasting glucose	6.1–6.9		<7.8
Impaired glucose tolerance	6.1–6.9	and/or	7.8–11.0
Diabetes mellitus	≥7.0		>11.1

> **NB** In the absence of symptoms, diabetes must be confirmed by a second diagnostic test, i.e. fasting, random or repeat glucose tolerance test, on a separate day.

Intercurrent illness

Patients under the physical stress associated with surgical trauma, acute MI, acute pulmonary oedema or stroke may have transient elevations of plasma glucose which often settle rapidly without specific antidiabetic therapy. However, such clinical situations are also liable to unmask asymptomatic pre-existing diabetes or to precipitate diabetes in predisposed individuals. Such elevations, which may have short- and longer-term prognostic importance, should not be dismissed; as a minimum, appropriate follow-up and retesting is indicated following resolution of the acute illness. If there is doubt about the significance of hyperglycaemia:

● *Blood glucose*. This should be re-checked 30–60 min later and urine tested for ketones.

If hyperglycaemia is sustained, treatment with insulin may be indicated (see p. 283). More marked degrees of hyperglycaemia, particularly with ketonuria, demand vigorous treatment in an acutely ill patient.

HISTORY AND INITIAL PHYSICAL EXAMINATION

A thorough history and physical examination should be performed. The consultation should take place in appropriate and comfortable circumstances wherever possible.

- The mode of diagnosis and presence of symptoms, if any, are recorded.
- Family history of diabetes is carefully reviewed. For women, enquiry into obstetric (stillbirths, large babies, gestational diabetes) and menstrual history (oligomenorrhoea, especially with features of hyperandrogenism) may be relevant.
- A detailed drug history is required. Smoking habits and alcohol consumption are explored as well as enquiry into habitual physical activity and sporting interests.
- Height and weight are recorded and body mass index calculated. Waist–hip ratio may also be measured in patients with glucose intolerance or type 2 diabetes; values greater than 0.90 for men and 0.85 for women are considered undesirable.
- Associated conditions (see Section 1), predisposing and aggravating factors should be identified.
- Features of other endocrinopathies (see p. 23) may rarely be evident; signs of marked insulin resistance (Plate 1) are relatively uncommon; specific syndromes of diabetes such as the lipodystrophies are rare (Plate 2).
- BP is carefully measured; lying and standing pressures should be recorded if there is any suggestion of postural hypotension arising from autonomic neuropathy.
- Evidence of established diabetic complications should be diligently sought at diagnosis in patients with type 2 diabetes (see Section 5).
- Symptoms and signs of neuropathy (including autonomic dysfunction where appropriate) and foot disease are sought (see p. 213).
- Unless contraindications exist, notably angle-closure glaucoma, the fundi are examined through pharmacologically-dilated pupils in all patients with type 2 diabetes, as well as in patients with features which are not classical of autoimmune type 1 diabetes.

Physical examination of the patient with newly presenting type 1 diabetes is usually unremarkable although there may be evidence of recent weight loss and occasionally signs compatible with dehydration. Features of oro–genital candidiasis or cutaneous sepsis are not uncommon but are non-specific. Vitiligo should be sought (see pp. 56 and 258). The presence of chronic microvascular complications in the newly diagnosed patient with classical type 1 diabetes is virtually unknown, being much more likely in type 2 diabetes.

OCULAR COMPLICATIONS

Retinopathy
In patients with type 1 diabetes, the appearance of symptoms provides a fairly reliable indicator of the time of onset of pathological hyperglycaemia. Complications such as retinopathy are therefore absent at diagnosis. Visual symptoms such as blurred vision, which results from osmotic changes within the ocular lens, usually resolve within weeks; patients should be advised to defer obtaining prescription eyewear until the diabetes is stabilized.

Cataract
Cataracts may be present at diagnosis of type 2 diabetes and may rarely develop acutely in type 1 diabetes (see p. 203).

NEPHROPATHY

Proteinuria is the hallmark of diabetic nephropathy. As with the other microvascular complications of diabetes, the development of nephropathy is closely related to the duration of diabetes.

Type 1 diabetes
Tests for microalbuminuria (see p. 222) may be positive at diagnosis. This may simply reflect renal effects of uncontrolled hyperglycaemia and should not automatically be interpreted as evidence of nephropathy requiring specific therapy. The test should be deferred until the diabetes has been stabilized.

Type 2 diabetes
In addition to early nephropathy, the presence of microalbuminuria may reflect a further increase in risk of macrovascular disease (see p. 228). However, because nephropathy can develop during the asymptomatic phase preceding diagnosis, plasma creatinine should be checked, especially if Albustix-positive (indicative of urinary protein losses of 500 mg/day or more; see p. 223).

NEUROPATHY AND FOOT DISEASE

Evidence of these complications should be carefully evaluated at diagnosis in patients with type 2 diabetes as detailed on pages 204–219.

MACROVASCULAR DISEASE

The close relationship between the components of the insulin resistance syndrome (see p. 31) should prompt the identification and treatment, if clinically indicated, of associated risk factors for atherosclerosis such as:

- Hypertension.
- Dyslipidaemia.
- Microalbuminuria.
- Renal impairment.

As a minimum, clinical stigmata of hyperlipidaemia should be sought, pedal pulses palpated and signs of vascular insufficiency noted. Further investigations may be warranted.

INITIAL MANAGEMENT

Having confirmed the diagnosis of diabetes, the crucial clinical question is whether insulin treatment is required immediately. In the younger patient, i.e. aged <35 years, with acute symptoms, weight loss and ketonuria, the decision to start insulin is straightforward. Similarly, the overweight or obese, middle-aged or elderly patient with minor symptoms will usually be a candidate for a trial of dietary manipulation initially. Sulphonylureas might, however, be used from diagnosis, in addition to appropriate dietary measures, for symptomatic normal weight patients.

 In newly diagnosed diabetic patients, the first consideration is whether insulin treatment is required immediately.

An attempt should be made to place the diabetes within the classification system. Sometimes assignment to a particular category is not possible with certainty and only becomes clear later. Initial therapy does not, therefore, necessarily confirm the aetiology. This difficulty centres mainly around the degree of endogenous insulin deficiency at diagnosis and the rate at which this progresses. Thus, patients with what proves ultimately to be type 1 diabetes will sometimes be treated with a trial of oral antidiabetic drugs, usually because the clinical and biochemical features were not classical; conversely, patients with type 2 diabetes may need insulin temporarily at diagnosis, especially if there is significant intercurrent illness.

NB Initial treatment with insulin does not necessarily confirm a diagnosis of type 1 diabetes.

It can sometimes be difficult to decide whether a newly presenting, middle-aged, non-obese patient with moderately severe hyperglycaemia has type 2 diabetes which will respond adequately to oral, antidiabetic agents or whether the patient would be better treated with insulin from the outset. In this context, it should be remembered that, although relatively uncommon in the elderly, type 1 diabetes may present at any age.

 Type 1 diabetes may present at any age – even in nonagenarians.

The situation is complicated by increasing awareness of subtypes of diabetes in which insulin deficiency appears to be the predominant feature but which present less dramatically than classical type 1 diabetes. Moreover, even the presence of morbid obesity does not guarantee a diagnosis of type 2 diabetes; occasionally, obese patients present with marked osmotic symptoms and/or ketonuria indicative of insulin dependence.

 Features of type 1 diabetes sometimes develop in patients with morbid obesity; insulin is required.

A trial of insulin is probably the most sensible option under these circumstances. The continuing need for insulin is then reviewed after 2–3 months (see p. 148). Any intercurrent illness, e.g. sepsis, severe candidiasis, should be treated. Identification of patients with apparently autoimmune diabetes with a relatively slow onset can be problematic; the prevalence of this syndrome is not known but is perhaps underdiagnosed. The diagnosis is usually made retrospectively (often with a degree of continuing uncertainty) following the primary failure of treatment with oral antidiabetic agents (see Section 3, p. 106). Useful clinical pointers at diagnosis which suggest that insulin may be required include:

- Unintentional weight loss preceding diagnosis.
- Normal body weight or underweight for height at diagnosis.
- Presentation with osmotic symptoms of short duration.
- Marked fasting hyperglycaemia.

Of these pointers, weight loss is the most important. The degree of fasting hyperglycaemia is perhaps the least reliable; dietary manipulation ± oral agents may sometimes produce dramatic improvements. The issue of insulin dependence is particularly vexed in Black patients who may present with ketosis, even DKA, yet who ultimately prove to have diabetes which is controllable with oral agents or even diet alone. Caution is required in deciding whether to attempt withdrawal of insulin (see p. 151). If urinalysis reveals ketonuria, in concert with glycosuria, liaison with the local hospital diabetes team is advisable. Personal telephone contact is best to ensure that insulin treatment is initiated with the minimum of delay.

Can insulin treatment be deferred?

In the great majority of adult patients with type 1 diabetes, insulin treatment will be started in the community; the days of admitting all newly diagnosed patients in order to start insulin treatment have passed. The practicalities of initiating insulin treatment are considered on pages 131–152. With less pronounced degrees of ketonuria it is always difficult to predict whether metabolic decompensation will occur if insulin is deferred. If it is not possible to start insulin promptly in the community, it is probably best to admit the patient to hospital for a day or two. Clearly, avoidance of DKA should be paramount; patients will appreciate prompt alleviation of their osmotic symptoms.

> **NB** Insulin treatment should be initiated with the minimum delay in patients with newly diagnosed type 1 diabetes.

Ketonuria

Note that ketonuria (in concert with hyperglycaemia) usually suggests the presence of a marked degree of insulin deficiency. False positives due to certain drugs (containing free sulphydryl groups) should never be confidently assumed. In these circumstances, ketonuria results from:

- Accelerated breakdown of adipocyte triglycerides.
- Preferential hepatic β-oxidation of the liberated fatty acids to ketone bodies (3-hydroxybutyrate and acetoacetate).

Insulinopenia (absolute or, more commonly, relative) is primarily responsible for the acceleration of ketogenesis. Reduced ketone body clearance by peripheral tissues may also contribute as ketosis develops and this too is influenced by insulin. There is a common misconception that ketonuria is usually benign; ketonuria in diabetics is often erroneously attributed to fasting or decreased carbohydrate intake. Although ketonuria is a physiological response to fasting in non-diabetics, the crucial distinction in the diabetic patient is the combination of ketonuria in concert with hyperglycaemia (see Section 4).

> **NB** Ketonuria in concert with hyperglycaemia suggests marked insulinopenia.

In non-diabetic individuals, the plasma glucose concentration will be normal, or even marginally reduced, during fasting. In healthy subjects, the mobilization of fatty acids from adipocyte stores is a physiological response mediated by a reduction in endogenous insulin secretion (see pp. 5–7). However, there is some evidence that fasting may promote the development of ketosis in type 1 diabetes patients under circumstances of insulin deficiency. The combination of significant ketonuria together with glycosuria should be interpreted as evidence of a need for prompt insulin treatment.

 Significant ketosis is a contraindication to oral antidiabetic therapy – insulin is required.

Conversely, in patients with otherwise typical features of type 1 diabetes, especially weight loss, the absence of ketonuria at diagnosis should not be taken as unequivocal evidence that insulin therapy will not be required.

Autoimmune and non-autoimmune type 1 diabetes
A few young patients with hyperglycaemia but no ketonuria will prove to have relatively uncommon inherited forms of diabetes, e.g. MODY (see p. 26); such patients often receive insulin therapy from diagnosis, the assumption being that they have type 1 diabetes. A family history with an autosomal dominant inheritance and diagnosis under the age of 25 years are prerequisites for the diagnosis which may be confirmed in an affected family by genetic testing.

In the absence of significant obesity, i.e. in those with a body mass index <30 kg/m² or osmotic symptoms, it is prudent to treat all young patients with small doses of insulin initially; the dose of insulin can always be reduced, if glycaemic control allows or even withdrawn for a day or two, and substituted with a sulphonylurea, if there are continuing doubts about whether the patient is truly insulin-dependent.

In difficult cases, the presence of serum islet cell antibodies will confirm the diagnosis of type 1 diabetes (see p. 13). However, since a proportion of patients with type 1 diabetes test negative for islet cell antibodies the diagnosis may remain in doubt. Furthermore, although relatively uncommon, non-autoimmune forms of type 1 diabetes are recognized, albeit mainly in ethnic minorities.

Pluriglandular syndrome
The pluriglandular syndrome type II should be borne in mind in patients presenting with features suggesting autoimmune type 1 diabetes, particularly in those who are known to be positive for islet cell antibodies

(see p. 13). Consideration should be given to checking for other endocrine autoantibodies in the serum, particularly:

- Thyroid microsomal and thyroglobulin antibodies.
- Adrenal antibodies.

Antibody positivity does not predict future autoimmune disease with certainty. However, the prevalence of autoimmune thyroid disease, Addison's disease and other non-endocrine autoimmune disorders such as pernicious anaemia, coeliac disease and premature menopause is increased in patients with type 1 diabetes. Vitiligo is a useful cutaneous marker of autoimmune disease. Periodic checks of target organ function, e.g. thyroid function tests, serum B_{12} level, are indicated even in the absence of clinical features. Co-existing endocrinopathies may adversely affect metabolic stability (see p. 23).

INFLUENCE OF COMORBIDITY

The presence of significant physical or psychological disease may be important modifiers of the presentation and management of diabetes. For example, if malignancy severely limits life expectancy in a patient with diabetes (perhaps precipitated by high-dose dexamethasone), the primary goals of management will be (a) avoidance of osmotic symptoms and (b) major metabolic decompensation; concern about long-term microvascular complications would be misplaced. None the less, insulin may be the most appropriate therapy; considerations such as the likely inadequacy of oral agents or concomitant renal or hepatic impairment may preclude alternatives. The general point may be made that patients with diabetes are no less likely to encounter significant comorbidity and indeed are predisposed to the development of important complications which influence treatment.

> **NB** Diabetic patients are frequently affected by significant comorbidity.

PSYCHOLOGICAL IMPACT OF DIABETES

The diagnosis of diabetes carries a major emotional impact for many patients (and often for their immediate family). The precise nature of this for an individual will depend on many factors:

- The age of the patient (especially children).
- The type of diabetes (and hence the treatment required).

- The degree and type of self-monitoring required.
- The presence of significant long-term complications at diagnosis.
- The presence of comorbidity unrelated to diabetes.
- The implications of the diagnosis for employment prospects (see p. 288).

Important psychological factors will have a bearing not only on the initial reaction to the diagnosis but also to the patient's success in managing the disease in the longer term. These include:

- Personality.
- Temperament.
- Health beliefs.
- Cultural or religious conditioning.
- Acute and chronic psychological states.
- Intelligence.
- Educational achievement.
- Occupation.
- Philosophical attitudes.

Such factors may influence the response to diabetes education which aims to equip the patient with the knowledge and means to self-manage the disorder wherever possible (see p. 77). Family cohesion and marital satisfaction are also of relevance to immediate and long-term success in dealing with diabetes.

A sympathetic approach, tailored to the individual as appropriate, is therefore required from the diabetes health care team. For example, an overtly emotional response from a young girl facing a lifetime balancing food intake with insulin, avoiding extremes of hypo- and hyperglycaemia and aiming to minimize the risk of complications, is entirely understandable. In the months that follow diagnosis the patient will usually come to terms with the diagnosis and its implications. The process, common to the diagnosis of any chronic disease, has been compared with mourning.

DEPRESSION

The majority of patients cope well, some remaining remarkably stoical in the face of considerable problems. However, higher rates of depression have been recorded in adults with diabetes and may occur particularly in those with serious chronic tissue complications, notably sight-threatening retinopathy and macrovascular disease. Overall, however, the prevalence of depression is similar to that observed in other chronic diseases. Psychosocial pressures are often cited by patients as a reason for their failure (as they may see it) to attain or sustain glycaemic targets. The identification of serious psychiatric disturbance such as depression with suicidal intent demands an expert psychiatric opinion. Self-administered insulin overdose can have catastrophic consequences either by causing death or inflicting permanent intellectual or cognitive impairment. Chronic psychoses, habitual drug abuse or alcoholism may place considerable obstacles in the path to successful self-management. The issue of eating disorders in diabetic patients is considered on pages 266–267.

> **NB** Depression is more common in patients with diabetes mellitus.

AIMS OF TREATMENT

The main aims of treatment of diabetes may be summarized as:

- Relief of symptoms attributable to diabetes.
- Prevention (or at least amelioration) of micro- and macrovascular complications.
- Attainment of as near-normal life expectancy as possible.

Other considerations pertaining to special situations (e.g. children and pregnancy) are discussed in Section 6. These objectives are ideally attained with the minimum of disruption to normal daily living. In addition, avoidance of iatrogenic complications, especially hypoglycaemia, is an important aim wherever possible. Despite progress in recent years, areas of controversy still exist about optimal management. This difficulty reflects the limitations of current non-pharmacological and drug treatments, in particular the narrow therapeutic index of insulin therapy.

RELATIONSHIP BETWEEN GLYCAEMIC CONTROL AND COMPLICATIONS

MICROVASCULAR COMPLICATIONS

All forms of diabetes, be they primary or secondary (see Section 1), are characterized by a risk of the development of long-term complications (see Section 5). While there are differences in susceptibility between individual patients, perhaps reflecting genetic or other influences, the most important factors determining the risk of development and progression of chronic complications are:

- The magnitude of hyperglycaemia.
- The duration of diabetes.

Subclinical (or functional) abnormalities, e.g. increased retinal blood flow, delayed peripheral nerve conduction velocity, may be present at diagnosis. These usually remain asymptomatic (being detectable only with specialized techniques) and tend to improve as hyperglycaemia is controlled. In the longer term, sustained hyperglycaemia causes tissue damage via a number of postulated mechanisms (see Section 1).

 The risk of chronic microvascular complications is closely related to the degree and duration of hyperglycaemia.

GLUCOSE HYPOTHESIS

According to the glucose hypothesis of diabetic complications (see p. 2), permanent – and effectively irreversible – tissue damage is attributable to chronic exposure to pathological degrees of hyperglycaemia. This process usually takes years to become clinically apparent and may be influenced by additional genetic or environmental (e.g. smoking) factors.

 Factors such as hypertension and smoking have an adverse influence on the development and progression of diabetic complications.

The justification for aiming for the best possible, long-term metabolic control starts with clinical observations and builds logically to the results of definitive RCTs.

Type 1 diabetes

Anecdotal evidence abounds that better, long-term glycaemic control is associated with less severe microvascular and neurological complications; the converse is also sometimes only too apparent. Data from early retrospective and prospective observational studies suggested that there was a relationship between glycaemic control and chronic complications (although the latter really only came to prominence after the advent of insulin treatment in the 1920s). However, much of the early data were inadequate for meaningful analysis while other diligently performed observational studies were open to criticism on grounds of potential (if unintentioned) bias.

The lack of reliable methods for measuring long-term glycaemic control was also a major limitation of the early studies. Dissection of different (and not necessarily mutually exclusive) mechanisms required interventional trials wherein patients were randomly assigned to differing levels of glycaemic control. Building on the results of animal studies, clinical trials published in the 1980s provided tantalizing if somewhat inconsistent evidence that the progression of complications such as retinopathy could be lessened by efforts directed at improved control.

Doubt was finally laid to rest by the results of major RCTs initiated during the 1980s which utilized new insulin delivery systems to attain improved control by random allocation allied to measurements of glycated haemoglobin (see below). These culminated in publication, first, of the Stockholm Diabetes Intervention Study, and subsequently the larger and more definitive US multicentre Diabetes Control and Complications Trial (DCCT). Both studies confirmed a relationship between glycaemic control and the development and progression of microvascular complications in patients with type 1 diabetes.

> **NB** The DCCT confirmed that improved glycaemic control reduces the development and progression of microvascular complications in type 1 diabetes.

EVIDENCE-BASED MEDICINE 2.1

THE DIABETES CONTROL AND COMPLICATIONS TRIAL

(N Engl J Med 1993; 329: 977–986.)

In this multicentre RCT, 1441 relatively young (mean age 26 years) and otherwise healthy (normotensive, normal cholesterol), highly motivated patients with type 1 diabetes and either no retinopathy ('primary prevention' cohort) or minor retinopathy ('secondary intervention' cohort) were randomly allocated to continuing 'conventional' control or 'intensive' control. No children under the age of 13 years were included.

STUDY DESIGN

- *Conventional treatment.* This comprised once- or twice-daily insulin with daily blood or urine tests and a 3-monthly clinic review.

- *Intensive treatment.* This involved hospitalization for initiation of treatment, three- to four-times daily insulin by subcutaneous injection or continuous subcutaneous infusion with four-times daily, home glucose monitoring; education and support at monthly clinic visits were supplemented by expert telephone advice. Strict targets aiming for near-normoglycaemia, with the minimum of major hypoglycaemic episodes, were set.

→

RESULTS

Intensive therapy produced a decline of approximately 2% in HbA_{1c} whereas the conventional treatment group continued with a mean HbA_{1c} of approximately 9% (Fig. 2.1); only 5% of patients attained HbA_{1c} levels consistently within the non-diabetic range of <6.5%. At an average of 6.5 years follow-up, the reduction in HbA_{1c} was sufficient to produce the following mean reductions in risk in the intensively treated group:

- A 76% reduction in the development of any retinopathy ($P<0.001$; Fig. 2.2).
- A 54% reduction in progression of retinopathy ($P<0.001$).
- The need for laser photocoagulation was reduced by 56%.
- The appearance of microalbuminuria (34%; $P=0.04$) and clinical neuropathy at 5 years (69%; $P<0.006$) in the primary prevention cohort with intensified treatment.
- In the secondary intervention cohort, the risk of clinical nephropathy was reduced by 56% ($P=0.01$).

No threshold of HbA_{1c} could be identified at which the risk of progression of retinopathy increased; the inverse curvilinear relationship was continuous (Fig. 2.2).

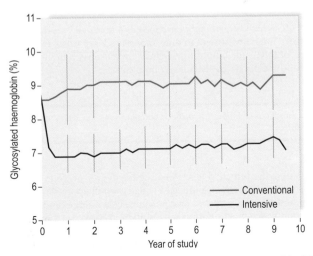

Fig. 2.1 Glycaemic control in the conventional and intensive treatment arms of the DCCT. (Reproduced with permission from The Diabetic Control and Complications Trial Research Group. N Engl J Med 1993; 329: 977–986.)

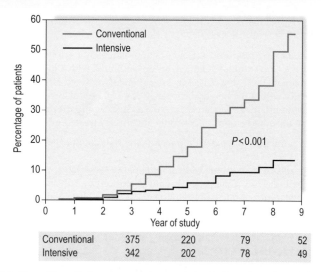

Conventional	375	220	79	52
Intensive	342	202	78	49

Fig. 2.2 Effect of intensified treatment on the appearance of retinopathy in the DCCT. (Reproduced with permission from The Diabetic Control and Complications Trial Research Group. N Engl J Med 1993; 329: 977-986.)

The DCCT, which is justifiably described as a landmark study, represented a huge investment in time, money and expertise. However, translation of the results into routine clinical practice with more limited expertise and resources presents many problems.

> **NB** No threshold of HbA_{1c} for diabetic complications has been reliably identified.

In particular, the principal factor limiting the degree of control attainable – a frequency of severe insulin-induced hypoglycaemia approximately 3-fold higher in the intensively treated group – represents a huge obstacle (Fig. 2.3). Severe hypoglycaemia was defined as resulting in coma, seizure or hospitalization or requiring treatment from a third party with parenteral glucose or glucagon. The risk increased as mean HbA_{1c} declined (Fig. 2.3), i.e. the better the control (and lower the risk of complications), the greater the risk of severe hypoglycaemia. Weight gain was the other major adverse effect of intensified insulin therapy.

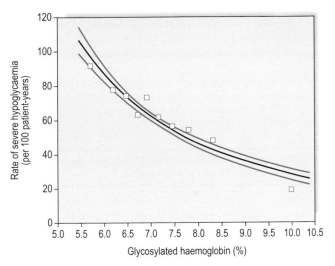

Fig. 2.3 Relationship between mean HbA_{1c} and risk of severe hypoglycaemia in the DCCT. (Reproduced with permission from The Diabetes Control and Complications Trial Research Group. N Engl J Med 1993; 329: 977–986.)

NB The risk of severe hypoglycaemia was increased 3-fold among the intensively treated patients in the DCCT.

Clearly the results of the DCCT (which selected participants very carefully) can be extrapolated only with caution to the generality of patients with type 1 diabetes. Moreover, intensive insulin therapy is contraindicated in certain groups in whom the risk of severe hypoglycaemia may exceed potential benefits (Table 2.8; see also Sections 3 and 4).

TABLE 2.8 Contraindications to intensive insulin therapy in patients with type 1 diabetes

- Young children (<13 years)
- Patients unable or unwilling to comply with intensive self-monitoring
- Patients with major tissue complications, e.g. diabetic nephropathy
- Patients with recurrent severe hypoglycaemia
- Patients with chronic loss of awareness of hypoglycaemic warning symptoms
- Patients with clinically overt macrovascular disease

Intensive insulin therapy is contraindicated in certain groups of patients.

It is important to note that intensive insulin therapy does not reverse established diabetic complications. Even successful pancreatic transplantation with restoration of normoglycaemia perhaps at best retards their progression (see p. 153).

NB Intensive insulin therapy does not reverse established diabetic complications such as advanced retinopathy.

Thus, it is inappropriate to embark on a quest for (possibly elusive) near-normoglycaemia in a patient with, say, a plasma creatinine of 500 μmol/L. This is not to say that good glycaemic control does not matter in such circumstances. Other important considerations, e.g. slowing the rate of progression of co-existing retinopathy, may be very relevant. However, a careful judgement of the risks and benefits for the individual patient is required. Sometimes this may not be easy and there is perhaps an understandable tendency to err on the side of caution. Factors additional to glycaemic control, e.g. hypertension (see p. 240), should also receive appropriate attention.

NB Glycaemic targets must be appropriate for the individual patient.

Type 2 diabetes
There is convincing evidence from observational and intervention studies that the basic relationship between degree and duration of glycaemia and the specific complications of diabetes are similar for both type 1 and type 2 diabetes. For example, the observational Wisconsin Epidemiologic Study of Diabetic Retinopathy provided important data supporting an association between glycaemia and the risk of diabetic complications. However, appropriate controlled clinical trials were required to evaluate the risks and benefits of intensified therapy specifically in patients with type 2 diabetes. These appeared in the 1990s, first with the randomized Kuanomoto trial, conducted in 110 lean, insulin-treated Japanese patients with type 2 diabetes. The results of this trial suggested that better control was indeed associated with benefits in terms of microvascular complications. However, the applicability of the results of this small trial to other populations was

somewhat uncertain. Subsequently, the results of the long-duration and much larger UKPDS were published. A summary of the main points of this trial, the largest of its kind, is presented in Evidence-Based Medicine 2.2. The Hypertension in Diabetes Study was embedded within the main trial; the design and results of the latter study are outlined in more detail on pages 243–245.

┌─ EVIDENCE-BASED MEDICINE 2.2 ─────────────────────────────

UNITED KINGDOM PROSPECTIVE DIABETES STUDY (UKPDS 33 AND 34)

(Lancet 1998; 352: 837–853; 854–865.)
This was designed with the aim of establishing:

- Whether intensive therapy of type 2 diabetes (using oral antidiabetic agents or insulin) reduces the risk of macrovascular and microvascular disease relative to conventional measures (i.e. diet).
- Whether any particular therapy is advantageous (or disadvantageous).

STUDY DESIGN

Between 1977 and 1991, 5102 patients (58% male) with newly diagnosed type 2 diabetes were recruited in 26 centres. Patients were stratified according to ideal body weight, i.e. <120% or >120%. Altogether, 2514 patients were excluded.

- *Non-overweight patients*. If, at the end of a 3-month, dietary run-in period, patients had (a) a fasting plasma glucose <15 mmol/L and (b) no symptoms of hyperglycaemia, they were randomly assigned to either:

a. Conventional treatment – Dietary therapy aiming for fasting glucose <15 mmol/L.
b. Intensive treatment – Aiming for fasting glucose levels <6 mmol/L using either sulphonylureas (chlorpropamide; glibenclamide or glipizide) or insulin (commencing with once-daily ultralente or isophane, with short-acting insulin added if pre-meal glucose levels >7 mmol/L).

- *Overweight patients*. In addition, 753 of 1704 overweight patients whose fasting blood glucose concentration was 6.1–15 mmol/L were randomly assigned to receive (a) metformin as monotherapy (*n*=342) or →

(b) continued treatment with diet alone (*n*=411). The residual 951 overweight patients were allocated to intensive glycaemic control with chlorpropamide (*n*=265), glibenclamide (*n*=277) or insulin (*n*=409).

PROTOCOL AMENDMENTS

During the course of the study, progressive hyperglycaemia was observed in all groups (Fig. 2.4). This led to an amendment allowing the early addition of metformin when, on maximal doses of sulphonylureas, fasting glucose was >6 mmol/L in asymptomatic patients in the intensive treatment group. In this supplementary RCT, 537 non-overweight and overweight patients receiving a maximal dose of sulphonylurea were allocated to (a) continuing with sulphonylurea therapy alone (*n*=269) or (b) the addition of metformin (*n*=268). If marked hyperglycaemia recurred, patients were transferred to insulin.

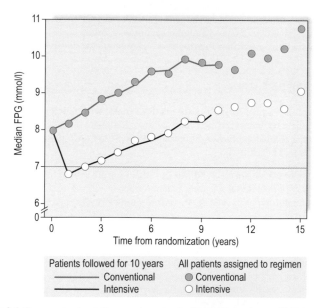

Fig. 2.4 Cross-sectional and 10-year cohort data for fasting plasma glucose (FPG) for patients on intensive (sulphonylureas or insulin) or conventional (diet) therapy in the United Kingdom Prospective Diabetes Study. (Reproduced with permission from UK Prospective Diabetes Study Group. Lancet 1998; 352: 837–853.)

RESULTS

UKPDS 33 EFFECTS OF INTENSIVE CONTROL WITH SULPHONYLUREAS OR INSULIN

Main study

- Over 10 years, the mean HbA_{1c} was 7.0% in the intensive treatment group vs 7.9% for the diet group. There was no difference in HbA_{1c} levels between the different intensive treatment subgroups.
- Compared with the conventional treatment group, there was a 12% reduction in risk of reaching a diabetes-related endpoint with intensive treatment ($P=0.029$), mainly attributable to a 25% reduction in microvascular endpoints ($P=0.0099$; Fig. 2.5). The need for photocoagulation with intensive treatment was reduced ($P=0.0031$). Vibration sense was better preserved at 15 years ($P=0.0052$). Microalbuminuria at 15 years was reduced by 30% ($P=0.033$).
- The reduction in fatal and non-fatal MI (relative risk 0.84) attained borderline statistical significance ($P=0.052$).
- No significant reductions were observed in either diabetes-related deaths or all-cause mortality.

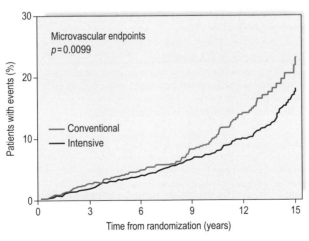

Fig. 2.5 Kaplan–Meier plots of aggregate microvascular endpoints for intensive and conventional treatment groups. (Reproduced with permission from UK Prospective Diabetes Study Group. Lancet 1998; 352: 837–853.)

- No difference was observed between the three intensive agents (chlorpropamide, glibenclamide or insulin) for any of the three aggregate endpoints.
- Hypoglycaemia was more common ($P<0.0001$) in the intensive treatment groups whether analysed by intention to treat and actual therapy. The highest rate was observed for insulin treatment.
- Weight gain was significantly higher in the intensive treatment group (mean 2.9 kg) than in the conventional group ($P<0.001$). Weight gain was highest for insulin-treated patients.

UKPDS 34 EFFECTS OF METFORMIN IN NON-OVERWEIGHT AND OVERWEIGHT PATIENTS

Diet vs metformin in overweight patients
- Mean HbA_{1c} was lower in the metformin-treated group compared with the conventional treatment group (7.4% vs 8.0%).
- Risk reductions were observed for diabetes-related endpoints ($P=0.0023$), diabetes-related death ($P=0.017$) and all-cause mortality ($P=0.011$). For all macrovascular diseases together, the metformin group had a 30% lower risk than those on conventional treatment ($P=0.02$) with a 39% lower risk of MI ($P=0.01$).
- The reduction in diabetes-related endpoints, mortality and stroke was greater than that observed in UKPDS 33 for intensive therapy with sulphonylureas and insulin.

Addition of metformin to sulphonylureas:
- The addition of metformin to sulphonylurea-treated non-overweight and overweight patients was associated with an unexpected 96% increased risk ($P=0.039$) of a diabetes-related death and a 60% increased risk of death from any cause ($P=0.041$).

Combined analysis of the metformin studies:
- A combined analysis of the two metformin studies showed that addition of metformin had an effect comparable to that observed with intensive therapy (sulphonylurea or insulin) in UKPDS 33 with a net reduction in any diabetes-related endpoint of 19% ($P=0.033$). However, the beneficial effect on cardiovascular outcomes observed in the first study was not substantiated.
- Metformin improved glycaemic control without inducing weight gain and was associated with fewer episodes of hypoglycaemia than the other intensive therapies.
  The effects of acarbose are considered on page 125.
  The Hypertension in Diabetes Study is discussed on pages 243–245.

KEY POINTS FROM UKPDS

The key messages to emerge from this complex and lengthy study may be summarized as follows:

1. Improved glycaemic control with either sulphonylureas or insulin is associated with beneficial, long-term effects, principally on microvascular complications.
2. Only a minority of patients with type 2 diabetes are able to achieve and maintain excellent metabolic control with dietary modification alone.
3. Glycaemic control tends to deteriorate with duration of diabetes even when treated with sulphonylureas or insulin.
4. Intensive therapy with sulphonylureas or insulin carries a risk of hypoglycaemia and weight gain. The risks and benefits of therapy must be carefully considered for each patient.

The results point to the potential for major health benefits from better control of glycaemia (and vigorous treatment of hypertension, see p. 240) in patients with type 2 diabetes; a combined approach targeting hyperglycaemia and hypertension is particularly beneficial. In addition, the UKPDS produced some surprises, particularly in relation to metformin (see p. 120). Conventionally, insulin treatment is reserved for patients with type 2 diabetes who fail to respond adequately to diet and oral antidiabetic agents (see p. 131). This effect was also observed in the UKPDS; antidiabetic therapy had to be increased or additional therapy introduced (a new agent every 4–5 years, on average), insulin ultimately being required in a substantial proportion of patients allocated to oral agents. The small but sustained difference in glycaemic control between the conventional and intensive treatment groups was associated with clinically relevant reductions in microvascular endpoints. The risks and benefits of insulin, including higher rate of hypoglycaemia (~2% per annum for major episodes) and weight gain, require that the circumstances of the individual patient are taken into account. Both sulphonylureas and insulin treatment produced increases in plasma insulin concentrations.

MACROVASCULAR DISEASE

In both type 1 and type 2 diabetes there is evidence, albeit inconsistent, suggesting a link between glycaemia and the risk of atherosclerotic vascular disease. However, neither the DCCT nor the UKPDS were able to demonstrate significant reductions in macrovascular events; this may reflect the design, size and patient selection in these trials. Importantly, a favourable trend for a reduction in macrovascular events was observed in each trial (41% in the DCCT; 16% for MI in the UKPDS). Thus, limited data from interventional studies support the notion that good metabolic control is a modifiable factor which deserves attention. This area, which remains the subject of controversy, is discussed on pages 228–240.

Contrary to theoretical concerns, no adverse cardiovascular effects were observed with either sulphonylureas or insulin in the UKPDS. It is generally accepted that reduction in macrovascular disease – the principal cause of mortality in type 2 diabetes – also requires attention to other major modifiable cardiovascular risk factors such as dyslipidaemia, elevated BP and smoking. Controversy about the cardiovascular safety of biguanides dates from the University Group Diabetes Program in the 1970s. This trial, which attracted considerable criticism, suggested an increased mortality rate with phenformin.

The results of the UKPDS have introduced new uncertainties concerning the optimal use of metformin. There is evidence for a powerful beneficial effect on macrovascular complications when the drug is used as initial monotherapy in overweight patients. The efficacy of the drug, combined with the absence of weight gain and beneficial effects on diabetes-related endpoints, recommend its use as first-line treatment in overweight patients. Better glycaemic control did not explain the more favourable outcomes with metformin leading the investigators to speculate about other mechanisms such as improved fibrinolysis. However, this benefit contrasts with the adverse effects on mortality observed when metformin was given to the more heterogeneous group of patients receiving maximal doses of sulphonylureas. The reasons for this discrepancy are uncertain but are widely regarded as a statistical aberration rather than a real effect. The clinical pharmacology of metformin is described on pages 120–125.

ASSESSMENT OF GLYCAEMIC CONTROL

URINALYSIS

GLYCOSURIA

Semi-quantitative testing for the presence of glucose using reagent-impregnated test strips is of limited value. Urinalysis provides retrospective information about glucose levels over a variable period of time. Other limitations of urinalysis include effects of:

● *Renal threshold*. The renal threshold for the reabsorption of glucose in the proximal convoluted tubule – approximately 10 mmol/L on average – varies between individuals. Thus, patients with a low renal threshold will tend to show glycosuria more readily than patients with a high threshold. In fact, some individuals with a low renal threshold may have glycosuria with normal glucose tolerance; this is termed 'renal glycosuria'. Children are particularly liable to test positive for glucose. Conversely, a high threshold, which is common among the elderly, may give a misleading impression of apparently satisfactory control. The renal threshold for glucose may alter with time in an individual according to circumstances. For example, the renal threshold is effectively lowered in pregnancy (see p. 279).

● *Urinary concentration*. Fluid intake and urine concentration may affect glycosuria. Renal impairment may elevate the threshold for glucose reabsorption.

● *Neuropathic bladder*. Delayed bladder emptying, e.g. as a result of diabetic autonomic neuropathy (see p. 209) will reduce the accuracy of the measurements through dilution.

● *Hypoglycaemia*. This cannot be detected by urinalysis.

Good long-term metabolic control requires more accurate information about blood glucose levels in the range generally below the levels reflected in urinary glucose measurements. For elderly patients with type 2 diabetes, urinalysis may provide the patient with reassuring information that diabetes is at least under moderate control. However, the tendency for renal threshold to be elevated in the elderly means that this may be unreliable; pathological degrees of hyperglycaemia may go undetected. Thus, for patients in whom more than avoidance of osmotic symptoms is the therapeutic objective, urinalysis must be supplemented by additional tests.

NB Urinalysis alone is an inadequate means of assessing metabolic control in the majority of diabetic patients.

URINARY KETONES

Semi-quantitative test strips for acetoacetate (e.g. Ketostix) are also available for patients with ketosis-prone diabetes (i.e. type 1 diabetes). These are useful when intercurrent illness leads to disturbance of metabolic control (see intercurrent illness, p. 283). Testing for ketonuria (and, in the laboratory, for ketonaemia) is considered further in Section 4. Neither Ketostix nor Acetest tablets (Bayer Diagnostics) detect 3-hydroxybutyrate (although acetone is detected by Acetest). Occasional underestimation of the degree of ketonaemia using these tests is a well-recognized caveat (see DKA, p. 168). Some blood glucose meters will display text suggesting urinary ketone testing when a high reading is obtained. A blood test for the principal ketone body, 3-hydroxybutyrate, has recently been developed.

GLYCATED HAEMOGLOBIN

HbA_{1c} is formed by the post-translational, non-enzymatic glycation of the N-terminal valine residue of the β chain of red cell haemoglobin. This process, which in other tissues is implicated in the pathogenesis of the long-term complications of diabetes, is discussed on page 8. The proportion of HbA_{1c} to total haemoglobin (normal, non-diabetic, reference range approximately 4–6%) provides a clinically useful index of average glycaemia over the preceding 6–8 weeks. Average HbA_{1c} levels collected over a longer period (i.e. years) provide an estimate of the risk of microvascular complications. Sustained high concentrations identify patients in whom efforts should be made to improve long-term glycaemic control.

● *Glycaemic targets.* Although the DCCT did not identify a threshold of HbA_{1c} below which complications were minimized, consensus panels in the USA and Europe have suggested targets of approximately 7–8%. Clearly, targets must be adjusted appropriately to the circumstances of the individual. As discussed above, a patient with advanced complications would not be expected to benefit from tight glycaemic control; indeed, such an approach might carry unacceptable risks of severe hypoglycaemia. However, for a young, well-motivated patient with type 1 diabetes, the best attainable control should be the general aim, if circumstances and frequency of hypoglycaemia allow. For a fuller discussion on the principles of insulin therapy, see page 131, and on the problems of hypoglycaemia see page 156.

● *Frequency of measurement.* It is generally recommended that HbA_{1c} should be measured every 6 months (or more frequently if indicated) in younger patients with type 1 diabetes. Pregnancy requires monthly monitoring of HbA_{1c} concentrations.

● *Prior sample collection.* The blood can be collected by venesection ahead of the clinic visit (in primary care, by the hospital phlebotomy service or even by the district nurse if necessary). Alternatives include rapid assays for use in the clinic, or self-collection in advance of a fingerprick sample (in a capillary tube or on filter paper) which is mailed to the laboratory.

● *Limitations of HBA_{1c} measurements.* Although glycated haemoglobin levels are a reliable indicator of recent average glycaemic control, they do not provide information about the daily pattern of blood glucose levels; this is required for logical adjustment of insulin doses. This complementary information is obtained from the patient's home blood glucose results (see below). There is, however, a correlation between daily blood glucose concentrations and HbA_{1c} levels. For example, an HbA_{1c} of 8% will reflect mean blood glucose levels of approximately 7 mmol/L; however, lack of standardization of HbA_{1c} assays cautions against firm extrapolations. More recent changes in glycaemia (i.e. within the preceding 4 weeks or so) will influence HbA_{1c} levels more than glucose levels 6 or more weeks ago. Spurious HbA_{1c} levels may arise in states of:

● Blood loss/haemolysis/reduced red cell survival (low HbA_{1c}).

- Haemoglobinopathy
  — Elevated levels of HbS (low HbA_{1c}).
  — Elevated levels of HbF (high HbA_{1c}).

For example, uraemia caused by advanced diabetic nephropathy (see p. 219) is associated with anaemia and reduced erythrocyte survival, thereby falsely lowering HbA_{1c} levels. In parentheses, it is claimed that there is usually a good level of correlation between fasting plasma glucose concentrations and glycated haemoglobin levels in diet- or tablet-treated patients. However, clinically significant discrepancies are frequently encountered.

FRUCTOSAMINE

The generic term 'fructosamine' refers to protein–ketoamine products resulting from the glycation of plasma proteins. The fructosamine assay measures glycated plasma proteins (mainly albumin), reflecting average glycaemia over the preceding 2–3 weeks. This is a shorter period than that assessed using glycated haemoglobin measurements and may be particularly useful when rapid changes in control need to be assessed, e.g. during pregnancy (see p. 270). Levels can be misleading in hypoalbuminaemic states, e.g. nephrotic syndrome (see p. 222).

Some fructosamine assays are subject to interference by hyperuricaemia or hyperlipidaemia. Measurements of fructosamine are less expensive than glycated haemoglobin assays; this may be an important consideration for some laboratory services. The methodology is suitable for automation and rapid results can be obtained for use within a clinic attendance obviating the requirement for a prior blood test.

HOME BLOOD GLUCOSE MONITORING

Self-testing of capillary blood glucose obtained by fingerprick has become an established method for monitoring glycaemic control. Enzyme-impregnated dry strip methods are available which can be used in conjunction with meter devices to improve accuracy.

GLUCOSE OXIDASE REACTION

Most strip methods are based on the glucose oxidase reaction:

$$\text{Glucose} + O_2 \xrightarrow{\text{Glucose oxidase}} \text{Gluconic acid} + H_2O_2$$

The hydrogen peroxide generated by the reaction then reacts with a reduced dye in the test strip producing an oxidized colour proportional to the amount of H_2O_2 formed. This, in turn, reflects the amount of glucose that was oxidized.

PRACTICAL CONSIDERATIONS

Selection of testing system

Many different strips and dedicated meters are available; more than a dozen different meters are currently available in the UK alone. Prices vary considerably; higher prices bring additional facilities such as storage and retrieval of multiple test results within a memory facility and the ability to download results into a personal computer. Special offers by retail outlets may tempt patients who have limited information about the complete range into purchasing machines which are not well suited to their needs. Meters with large digital displays or audio output are available to aid the visually impaired patient. Guidance from trained personnel with up-to-date knowledge of testing systems ensures that patients acquire the most appropriate device for their particular requirements. In addition, supervised instruction of patients (or their carers) in the use of the system should be provided. Non-invasive glucose sensors may be available in the near future.

> **NB** Guidance from the diabetes care team is helpful in the selection of an appropriate home blood glucose testing system.

Instructions and training

The manufacturers' instructions must be followed meticulously if reliable measurements are to be obtained. Some systems utilize light reflectance meters to provide a reading potentially accurate to 0.1 mmol/L. Early systems required that capillary blood be left in contact with the reagent for a specified amount of time; removal by wiping or blotting the blood sample requires careful technique and accurate timing. Most modern meters are not operator time-dependent; however, factors such as the adequacy of the capillary sample and calibration of the meter require attention.

Test strip containers may have a barcode strip or number which is programmed into the meter. Control solutions of specified concentration are available from manufacturers; their telephone helplines are useful sources of customer support. Sub-optimal storage of test strips (e.g. not in their air-tight container) is another potential source of erroneous results.

Adequate training and a system of quality control are vital; even when trained health professionals use such systems, misleading results are possible, particularly in the lower range of blood glucose results. Fingerprick devices are not considered sufficiently reliable to be used routinely in the diagnosis of diabetes (see p. 45).

Practical limitations to self-testing include:
- Inadequate manual dexterity, e.g. deforming rheumatoid arthritis or advanced neuropathy; post-stroke.
- Intellectual inability or incapacity.
- Visual handicap.

When to test?

- *Type 1 diabetes.* Single readings are of relatively limited value, except to confirm or, sometimes importantly, to exclude the possibility of acute hypoglycaemia (see p. 156). More useful is a 'profile' of tests performed at different times of the day, usually in close relation to meals, typically:

  — Before breakfast.
  — Before lunch.
  — Before evening meal.
  — Before retiring to bed.

In addition, a test at 0200–0300 h, although inconvenient, may be important for patients in whom nocturnal hypoglycaemia (which may be asymptomatic) is suspected (see p. 162). Tests pre- and post-exercise can be used to guide reductions in insulin dose or need for additional carbohydrate (see p. 93).

Performance of four or more tests daily is not often sustainable outside of special situations such as pregnancy, although patients on q.d.s. insulin may utilize the results to adjust insulin doses. For patients using the short-acting insulin analogues, lispro or insulin aspart (see p. 135), monitoring of post-prandial glucose levels may also be of relevance.

> **NB** Knowledge of post-prandial glucose levels may be useful in patients receiving rapid-acting insulin analogues.

A reasonable approach for many patients is to perform the equivalent of two or three daily profiles by varying the time of testing from day to day. In this way, an appreciation of the average blood glucose level before breakfast, for example, should become clear. In addition, an indication of the degree of variability and the influence of diet or other factors, e.g. vigorous or sustained exercise the preceding evening may be obtained. More frequent home testing is a prerequisite to attaining very tight glycaemic control safely.

The frequency and accuracy of testing vary considerably between patients; records vary from non-existent to meticulously charted profiles from dedicated (and sometimes obsessional) individuals. Fabricated results are well recognized. Discomfort and inconvenience are the main factors which discourage regular testing in many patients; expense is another consideration for patients in some countries. There is evidence that many patients simply do not test regularly. However, indirect data suggest that, on average, regular self-monitoring is associated with improved glycaemic control in patients with type 1 diabetes.

> **NB** Regular self-monitoring of blood glucose is associated with improved glycaemic control in patients with type 1 diabetes.

Clearly, any therapeutic decisions based on home glucose readings, whether acted upon by the patient or suggested by the supervising nurse or doctor, must depend on the reliability of the readings. However, it can be dispiriting to observe how abnormal results sometimes fail to prompt appropriate changes in insulin doses (even when patients are being closely monitored in hospital). Sometimes major discrepancies between the patient's readings (all apparently very satisfactory, for instance) and the corresponding glycated haemoglobin result (inexplicably high, see above) are encountered. The numerous potential sources of error (see above, including the possibility of erroneous HbA_{1c} results) must be excluded before alternative conclusions are drawn. Collection of dried fingerprick samples on impregnated filter paper which is then sent to the laboratory for analysis is an alternative means of obtaining a daily glucose profile.

• *Type 2 diabetes*. Elderly patients often cope remarkably well with home blood glucose testing; many feel the ability to self-test provides reassurance. For the majority of patients with type 2 diabetes who ultimately require insulin to maintain satisfactory glycaemic control, the initiation of home blood glucose testing is an important preliminary step. However, for patients treated with diet or oral agents, frequent home blood glucose monitoring has relatively little value; testing every few days before breakfast and occasionally at other times of the day (including 1–2 h post-prandially) will usually provide appropriate information since glycaemia is less variable (c.f. type 1 diabetes).

FINGERPRICK DEVICES

Sterile, disposable, single-use lancets may be used in conjunction with simple, hand-held, mechanical devices by which a fingerprick sample is obtained with a minimum of discomfort. This may aid compliance and help to ensure that an adequate sample is obtained. The depth of the puncture can be adjusted. Used lancets must be disposed of appropriately. In the UK, automated fingerprick devices must be purchased by the patient. Laser devices are under trial.

PRINCIPLES OF EDUCATION IN DIABETES

Education of patients is a vitally important component of diabetes care. The complexity and heterogeneity of diabetes, allied to its chronic non-curable nature and emphasis on self-care, demand that some knowledge is acquired by the patient.

KEY GUIDING PRINCIPLES OF EDUCATION

- It must be tailored to the patient's requirements.
- Education per se does not necessarily translate into action.
- It is an ongoing process of reinforcement.
- Educators should receive appropriate training.
- It should be centred on the patient.
- It should acknowledge the patient's cultural and religious background.
- Education should take the form of a partnership.
- The patient's agenda should be addressed.

Other points
- Didactic lectures are generally not very effective at modifying behaviour.
- Individualized or group teaching is generally more productive.
- Interactive computer programs may be useful.
- Overload of information can be counterproductive.
- Children and adolescents require special attention.

THE INITIAL DISCUSSION

An initial, face-to-face session with the patient (together with spouse and carer) may be followed by an interactive group teaching session. Educational literature, e.g. footcare leaflet (see p. 213), contact details of diabetes care team, address of national and local patient organizations, should be provided to reinforce the information. Videotapes – which can be tailored to the needs of ethnic minority groups – may also be useful.

Initial topics
- Brief explanation of the syndrome of diabetes.
- Possible underlying causes or contributory factors.
- Lifestyle changes that should be considered.
- Broad aims of treatment.
- The importance of regular follow-up and monitoring of metabolic control.

ONGOING EDUCATION

- Appropriate targets for weight and glycaemia agreed with patient and family.

- Discussion of the importance of self-management.
- Objectives of minimizing risk of chronic complications.
- Allow opportunity for airing patient's concerns.
- Attempt to foster a positive attitude in the patient.

Many patients will not, or perhaps cannot, comply with the demands of a chronic illness such as diabetes; much self-directed care in diabetes depends on self-discipline and behaviour modification. Many factors may be relevant to this failure, some of which are considered above (see psychological impact, p. 56). Education is an established part of the management of diabetes although its impacts have not been easy to assess. It has been shown that education can lead to a reduction in the incidence of serious complications in high-risk groups such as patients with foot disease (see p. 213). However, the limitations of education have to be recognized; the team should be willing to undertake rigorous audit of the effectiveness of education programmes and to explore new strategies.

ORGANIZATION OF DIABETES CARE

DIABETES CENTRES

Patients (and their families) require education backed up by readily available expert assistance from a multidisciplinary diabetes care team. Arrangements for care vary markedly between countries with differing health care systems. Purpose-built, hospital-based diabetes centres have proved to be popular in the UK and elsewhere. Such centres fulfil a multitude of functions:

- Diagnosis and assessment of new patients.
- Long-term follow-up (usually for selected groups where adequate arrangements exist for the provision or sharing of follow-up with primary care teams; see below).
- Continuing education of patients and staff.
- Education for other groups (e.g. community-based nurses).
- Screening for chronic complications (see Section 5).
- Specialist foot care.
- Provision of specialist medical care for special groups (e.g. pre-pregnancy and during pregnancy, young patients).
- Assessment and treatment of erectile dysfunction (see p. 210).
- Provision of telephone advice.

The aim is to provide these services in an accessible and comfortable environment. The active participation of patients, both as individuals and collectively is to be encouraged; more generally, the concept of self-care is important in the management of a chronic disorder such as diabetes for which the patient, suitably educated and supported, is ultimately largely responsible. Diabetes care may be regarded as a cooperative process between the patient and the health care system. Thus, while patients rightly deserve minimum standards of care (e.g. The European Patients' Charter) it is also recognized that they have certain obligations to ensure that appropriate care is delivered by acquiring knowledge to enable self-care on a day-to-day basis and to maintain regular contact with the health care team.

 NB The philosophy of self-management for patients with diabetes should be actively encouraged.

Specialized care

Special clinics (sometimes outside normal office hours) for adolescents and young adults are held in many centres. Care of special groups of patients such as children and pregnant women may be located either in the diabetes resource centre or in another hospital department, according to local circumstances.

Staff

Staffing of the diabetes centre will typically include:

- Consultant diabetologist. Specialist training in diabetes; team leader.
- Specialist nurse. Most health districts in the UK have at least one, and often more. Responsibilities include education and provision of day-to-day practical direction and support for patients, both in hospital and in the community, organization of staff training, development and implementation of local policies, commissioning of new equipment, introduction and evaluation of new treatments and technologies, research and audit. The diabetes specialist nurse should be well versed in counselling and education skills. Nurses may elect to concentrate on special groups such as children.
- Dietician.
- Podiatrist.

In addition, the services of other specialists will also be required as necessary:

- Nephrologist.
- Obstetrician.
- Vascular surgeon.
- Ophthalmic surgeon.
- Cardiologist.
- Psychologist.

Shared clinics, e.g. between a diabetologist and a nephrologist or an obstetrician, are popular and may help to reduce the number of visits while facilitating the sharing of relevant information.

IN-PATIENT CARE

Diabetic patients account for a disproportionate amount of hospital in-patient activity. Hospital admission is now rarely required for initiation of insulin therapy but is necessary for the management of acute metabolic emergencies (see Section 4). Hospitalization is also frequently required for the management of serious acute micro- and macrovascular complications, notably foot ulceration (see p. 215). Other common conditions such as unstable coronary heart disease and cardiac failure usually necessitate emergency or elective admission.

Surgery is required more often by diabetic patients (see above); close liaison between the surgical and diabetes services is obviously desirable. Written protocols for the management of diabetes during surgery or MI (see p. 230), DKA (see p. 168) or labour (see p. 278) should be agreed upon, implemented, audited and refined. This should be a continual process aiming not just to maintain but to elevate standards of care.

DIABETES IN PRIMARY CARE

The long-term management of diabetic patients in the UK is increasingly being supervised in whole or in part in primary care; this is regarded as particularly appropriate for patients with type 2 diabetes who have satisfactory glycaemic control and no significant diabetic complications. Problems with metabolic control or the detection of complications should prompt consideration of specialist advice. Various models of care have been described, for example:

- Miniclinics. Performed in general practice but based on hospital clinics.
- Integrated care systems. Wherein patient management is shared between the primary and secondary sectors to a greater or lesser degree.

Local circumstances will influence the arrangements within a particular health district. This approach requires close cooperation between hospital-based and primary provision to ensure high standards of care. Ready access to the hospital service and diabetes specialist nurses is necessary. An effective patient register and recall system are crucial components of successful diabetes care within a general practice setting. Regular audit of process and outcome is required; this pertains for hospital-based clinics as well as primary care clinics.

> **NB** A dynamic and regular process of audit is necessary to identify deficiencies and ensure improvements in practice.

Some studies have shown that prompted management of diabetes in primary care can result in good rates of attendance and satisfactory performance of BP measurement and retinal examination. Conversely, unstructured care can lead to losses to follow-up, inferior glycaemic control and increased mortality rates.

 A prompted recall system is regarded as a prerequisite for successful care of diabetes in primary care.

Advisory groups and review procedures

In many parts of the UK, Local Diabetes Service Advisory Groups have been established with the aim of coordinating general practice, hospital services and other parties such as optometrists; patients should be represented on such panels. Consensus guidelines may be drawn up with the aim of ensuring consistency and minimum standards of care. For example, this may allow a district-wide policy for high-quality retinal screening or foot care to be established. Central to the care of patients with diabetes in the UK is the concept of annual review (see below); this encompasses an assessment of current management, metabolic control and status of chronic complications; amendments to treatment and arrangements for future review complete the process.

INFORMATION TECHNOLOGY

Information technology is increasingly important in managing the data generated in the course of comprehensive diabetes care; paper records are now effectively obsolete. A district diabetes database is regarded as essential and requires that data can be easily entered from a variety of sources. Electronic transfer of clinical and laboratory information between general practice and the diabetes centre is becoming more established but needs further investment and development. Annual review record systems with built-in data prompts (see below) and risk assessment programs can be readily incorporated into user-friendly software. Digital image-capturing enables photographs of retinal and foot lesions to be incorporated into the electronic record. Decision support may assist appropriate management by practice nurses and GPs. Interactive computer programs are also valuable educational aids. Programs have also been developed with the aim of providing guidance on changing insulin doses (see p. 145).

 Information technology is now an essential component of structured diabetes management.

ANNUAL REVIEW

The following checklist is recommended for annual review in primary care; aspects of the review may be shared between an appropriately-trained practice nurse and a doctor. The review is prompted by the computerized practice register. Further details of each assessment may be found in the appropriate section, e.g. clinical evaluation of chronic complications, see Section 5. The checklist should form the basis of practice audit (see above); this should be supplemented periodically by questionnaire surveys of patient satisfaction.

> **NB** A comprehensive annual review is the cornerstone of structured diabetes management.

Checklist for annual review

Discussion
- General state of health (physical and psychological).
- Review of results of self-monitoring.
- Enquiry about episodes of hypoglycaemia and hyperglycaemia.
- Knowledge about diabetes and aspects of self-management.
- Enquiry about tobacco and alcohol use.
- Discussion of other diabetes-related problems, e.g. erectile dysfunction.

Physical examination
- Body weight; calculation of body mass index.
- Waist circumference.
- BP measurement.
- Assessment of visual acuity.
- Detailed fundal examination.
- Inspection of feet and footwear.
- Injection sites.

Investigation
- Urinalysis – for protein (or albumin/creatinine ratio; glucose and ketones; as appropriate.
- Glycated haemoglobin concentration (or alternative).
- Serum creatinine and electrolyte concentrations – if proteinuria present, known renal impairment or on diuretics.
- Serum lipids – every 3–5 years or more often as indicated.

Management
- Glycaemic control – diet review; antidiabetic medication; exercise.
- Assessment of co-existing conditions.
- Review of all ancillary medication.
- Attention to modifiable cardiovascular risk factors – antihypertensive therapy; lipid-lowering therapy; aspirin.
- Management of long-term complications – consider specialist referral as appropriate.
- Management plan for next 12 months – specialist referrals; contraception; plans for pregnancy.
- Arrange review date – patients with complications, suboptimal glycaemic control and uncontrolled hypertension will require earlier review.

Patients with chronic complications, suboptimal metabolic control or inadequately-treated hypertension require early and continuing review.

ELEVATING STANDARDS OF CARE

Initiatives at local, national and international level are necessary to improve standards of care for patients with diabetes. At national level, the interests of patients with diabetes are served by organizations such as Diabetes UK (formerly known as the British Diabetic Association) and the ADA. These bodies act as advocates for people with diabetes. Generation of funds for research is another important aspect of their activities; both the British and American national diabetes organizations publish peer-reviewed scientific papers in their respective journals. Annual scientific meetings under the auspices of these bodies bring doctors, nurses, scientists and others together to share and evaluate progress in areas ranging from basic science to clinical care. These national meetings are amplified by international gatherings such as that of the European Association for the Study of Diabetes. The International Diabetes Federation (IDF), founded in 1950, organizes triennial international meetings.

The St Vincent Declaration

Inevitably, there is a political dimension to the provision of diabetes care. International collaborations such as the St Vincent Declaration in Europe represent another facet to the quest for improved outcomes for patients. St Vincent was a gathering of representatives of European government health departments and patient organizations under the aegis of the regional offices of WHO and IDP in 1989. The meeting resulted in unanimous agreement on a series of recommendations of general goals and 5-year targets of improved outcomes for patients. The demand for formal recognition by policy makers of the public health problems presented by diabetes was accompanied by recommendations for research and the setting of ambitious targets:

- Reduce new blindness caused by diabetes by one-third or more.
- Reduce the numbers of patients entering end-stage diabetic renal failure by at least one-third.
- Reduce morbidity and mortality from CHD.
- Achieve outcomes for pregnancy for women with diabetes approximating that of non-diabetic women.

The subsequent 1997 Lisbon Statement acknowledged the initiation of diabetes action programmes in most of the countries which were signatories to the St Vincent Declaration. This was coupled with a resolution to continue collaborative efforts to reduce the impact of diabetes in Europe.

ECONOMICS OF DIABETES CARE

Diabetes mellitus is a common and chronic disorder which consumes a considerable proportion of the health care budget in developed countries. In the UK, it has been estimated that diabetes consumes 5% of total health care costs; this may well be an underestimate. Consider the estimated annual costs of foot ulceration alone – £13 million in the UK and $500 million in the USA. Indirect costs, which are particularly difficult to calculate, include those attributable to acute and chronic morbidity and premature mortality leading to loss of productivity.

> **NB** The socio-economic costs of diabetes are considerable and have probably been underestimated.

Cost-effectiveness of new treatments using relatively expensive therapies, e.g. statins for primary and secondary prevention of CHD, is an increasingly important dimension of care. However, evidence from landmark clinical trials such as the DCCT and the UKPDS has underscored the importance of attaining good long-term metabolic control, difficult though this is at present. Other proven therapeutic strategies such as aggressive treatment of hypertension in type 2 diabetes (see p. 242) demand investment in drugs and effective health care delivery systems.

It has been argued that some of this outlay can be expected to be recouped through reduced requirement for interventions such as retinal photocoagulation or renal replacement therapy; however, clinical trial data suggest that the development of chronic complications may be postponed by several years by better treatment rather than by being completely prevented. The availability of high-cost therapies such as pancreatic transplantation are still limited in some countries such as the UK and this seems likely to continue to be the case.

Analyses of the cost-effectiveness of treatment pose considerable difficulties for health economists; this is still a relatively imprecise discipline and further research is required to improve estimates. The projected increase in the number of patients with diabetes globally points to even greater expenditure in the future; this will undoubtedly present major challenges, particularly for less economically-developed countries.

MANAGEMENT OF DIABETES

NUTRITION THERAPY

PRINCIPLES OF NUTRITION THERAPY

Modification of eating habits forms an important component of management of all forms of diabetes. This is widely appreciated by health professionals and patients alike but is often diminished into a vague notion of the 'diabetic diet'. For the majority of patients, prescribed nutritional modifications mean dietary restriction, the principal objective being to reduce body weight. The strong association between obesity, insulin resistance and type 2 diabetes is considered in more detail in Section 1.

> **NB**   Nutrition therapy is an important cornerstone of management for all forms of diabetes.

Translation of the reports of expert committees into an individualized and detailed dietary prescription requires the input of trained dieticians. However, the general principles that underpin this objective are straightforward and do not require detailed knowledge of clinical nutrition to implement (Table 3.1). Indeed, the diet for the diabetic patient differs little in terms of macronutrient composition from what is currently promulgated as a healthy diet for the population in general. More complex physiological concepts such as the so-called *glycaemic index* of different carbohydrate foods (e.g. carbohydrates in beans cause less elevation of blood glucose than those in potatoes) are of limited value in clinical practice and are not considered further. Much more relevant to success in an individual patient is a realistic approach bolstered by adequate practical training for the patient (and relatives) and an ability to communicate the objectives effectively and sympathetically. At the outset, simple, easy-to-follow guidelines are appropriate at diagnosis (Table 3.1). These act as a prelude to more detailed, personalized advice, ideally from a trained dietician.

GENERAL AIMS OF NUTRITION THERAPY IN DIABETES

The general aims of medical nutrition therapy in diabetes are as follows:

- Improvement in carbohydrate and lipid metabolism to as close to normal as possible.
- Attainment of appropriate body weight and habitus for age and stage of growth and development.
- Avoidance of iatrogenic hypoglycaemia (primarily in insulin-treated patients).
- Attenuation of the progression of complications of diabetes.
- Reduction in the risk of atherosclerosis.

TABLE 3.1 Initial dietary advice for newly-diagnosed patients with diabetes

1. Quench thirst with water or low-calorie, carbonated drinks
2. Avoid sugar and obviously sugary foods
3. Use artificial sweeteners in beverages
4. Cereal, bread, pasta or potatoes should form the main part of each meal
5. Meat, grilled rather than fried, and cheese should be a small part of each meal
6. Fish and pulses are good alternatives to meat
7. Eat plenty of fresh fruit and vegetables
8. Use cooking fats and spreads low in saturated and trans-fatty acids – olive oil or reduced fat spreads are preferable
9. Moderate your alcohol consumption
10. Avoid adding salt to food at the table if hypertensive

The diet must contain the necessary balance of constituents to ensure good general health. The special circumstances pertaining to childhood, pregnancy and lactation require appropriate modification of diet.

Challenges in nutrition therapy for diabetes

The history of dietary modification in diabetes has been summarized in terms of failure. Although this is perhaps too pessimistic, prescribed changes in diet are notoriously difficult to implement; it is not an understatement to say that success is usually limited in the long term. This is especially so for the middle-aged or elderly patient with type 2 diabetes, 75% of whom are overweight or obese (see p. 88). Although few would not intuitively recognize the link between excessive food consumption and adiposity there can be no illusions about the gulf that exists between the objective of weight reduction and chances of success. Dietary modifications often run contrary to a lifetime's habits and preferences which have usually been reinforced by powerful social and cultural influences.

NB Management of obesity is a major challenge in type 2 diabetes.

There is evidence that obese individuals may significantly underestimate their daily calorie consumption. The oft-heard protests from patients about their supposedly miniscule daily food intake (usually detailing the apparently meagre portions consumed that morning!) therefore has to be gently but firmly repudiated if progress is to be made; recognition of the problem is a step forwards. The difficulty here lies in not alienating the patient in the process; a judgemental approach is unlikely to be successful and patients may vote with their feet if they perceive that they are being treated unfairly or unsympathetically. Increased levels of habitual physical exercise should also be encouraged.

The brief outline that follows summarizes the principles upon which modern dietary recommendations are founded. Certain dietary practices are now considered obsolete. Of historical interest only, the severe calorie restriction of the pre-insulin era serves as a reminder of the effects (albeit temporary) that dietary modification can have when the situation is desperate. The emphasis has moved towards increasing the proportion of calories consumed as carbohydrate – even sucrose is permitted. A number of practices are unhelpful or controversial:

● *Unrealistic targets*. The prescription of diets with hopelessly unrealistic targets such as a '1000 kcal daily reducing diet' is a recipe for failure, disillusionment and loss of faith in the dietician.

● *Special foodstuffs*. The purchase of products such as cakes aimed specifically at diabetic patients should be discouraged. These are often more expensive and contain calories in the form of sorbitol or fructose.

● *Very-low calorie diets*. Diets containing as little as 700 kcal/day are not generally recommended; they are useful only for short-term, rapid weight loss which is seldom indicated and may be hazardous in the presence of CHD (see p. 228).

● *Appetite-suppressant drugs*. The combination of the appetite-suppressant drugs, fenfluramine and phenteramine, was particularly popular in the USA in the 1990s (so-called fen-phen therapy). However, primary pulmonary hypertension was reported with this combination. In 1996, the *d*-isomer of the former drug – dexfenfluramine – was introduced; however, it was withdrawn in 1997 following reports of cardiac valvular lesions.

● *Other weight-reducing drugs*. Agents such as diuretics or thyroxine should not be used to achieve weight loss and should be prescribed only when there is a clear medical indication. Recently introduced (and apparently safer) anti-obesity agents are considered below.

Initial dietary assessment
The initial interview with the dietician will focus on the patient's preferences and habits. This should include enquiry about the amount of food eaten outside the home, e.g. by the business traveller, who takes responsibility for cooking at home and whether pre-packaged convenience foods form a substantial part of the diet. Ethnic and social influences are of obvious importance, e.g. the high saturated fat content of traditional South Asian cuisine or the teenager's predilection for fast food.

OBESITY

ASSESSMENT AND MANAGEMENT
Total calorie intake is of primary importance for most patients.

The starting point for discussions about modifying dietary habits must be the simple question:

● Is the patient presently of normal weight, overweight or underweight?

If normal weight, an isocaloric diet is appropriate. If underweight, a temporary gain in weight is required, thereafter levelling off at normality. For the majority of patients with obesity, however, it will be clear that a reduction in total calorie consumption is necessary. The latter principle is founded firmly in the second law of thermodynamics; if energy expenditure is unchanged, then a reduction in intake is necessary to achieve weight loss. The crucial practical questions are:

1. By how much must daily calorie intake be reduced on average?
2. How can this reduction be initiated and subsequently sustained in the majority of patients?

Definitions of overweight and obesity

WHO (1995) defined overweight and obesity in terms of body mass index (BMI) as presented in Table 3.2. BMI is calculated from the formula:

Body weight (kg) *divided* by Height^2 (m)

TABLE 3.2 Definitions of overweight and obesity (WHO, 1995)

Range	Body mass index (kg/m^2)
Normal	19–25
Overweight	25–30
Obesity	30–40
Extreme obesity	40 and over

Tables expressing body weight in terms of percentage above the ideal for height may be used as an alternative; these are widely available (e.g. Metropolitan Life Insurance charts). The maximum upper limit is defined as 20% above the recommended weight. For children, growth charts are required (see p. 262).

REGIONAL ADIPOSITY

Waist-to-hip ratio may also be easily calculated using a flexible tape measure, taking measurements at the point of maximal girth and around the gluteal region. Elevation of waist-to-hip ratio (>0.9 for men, >0.85 for women), which indicates visceral obesity, has come to be regarded as a component of the metabolic syndrome (see Section 1). Measurement of abdominal circumference alone has also been evaluated as a marker for increased risk of type 2 diabetes and cardiovascular disease.

IMPLICATIONS OF OBESITY IN DIABETES

The adverse effects of obesity are demonstrated by epidemiological studies and life insurance data. In addition to increasing the risk of developing type 2 diabetes, obesity is associated with a number of other diseases (Table 3.3) which frequently cause comorbidity in patients with type 2 diabetes. Compared with a body mass index of 21 kg/m^2, the relative risk of developing type 2 diabetes with body mass index of 35 kg/m^2 or over is 100.

TABLE 3.3 Co-morbid conditions associated with or aggravated by the presence of obesity

- Dyslipidaemia
  - Increased total cholesterol
  - Increased LDL-cholesterol
  - Increased plasma triglycerides
  - Reduced HDL-cholesterol
- Hypertension
  - Systolic
  - Diastolic
  - Left ventricular hypertrophy
- Cardiovascular disease
  - CHD
  - Cerebrovascular disease
- Hyperuricaemia
  - Gout
- Osteoarthritis
  - Large weight-bearing joints
- Cholelithiasis
- Reproductive
  - Menstrual irregularity and anovulation
  - Polycystic ovary syndrome
- Respiratory
  - Obstructive sleep apnoea
  - Alveolar hypoventilation syndrome
- Risks of surgery

NB Type 2 diabetes is three times more common among the obese than the non-obese.

Certain forms of cancer – endometrium, breast, colorectal, prostate – are also related to obesity. When type 2 diabetes has developed, the additional effect of obesity in impairing insulin action is held to be relatively minor. Nonetheless, weight loss of 5–10% may produce clinically useful improvements in glycaemia and circulating lipids. There is some evidence that patient survival may be increased by weight loss, possibly independently of glycaemic control.

> **NB** Weight loss of 5–10% may be associated with improvements in carbohydrate and lipid metabolism.

Weight reduction, ideally towards normality but tempered with realistic expectations, is therefore regarded as the cornerstone of managing type 2 diabetes. However, even with intensive personal dietetic support in the setting of a clinical trial, it is the minority of patients (approximately 20%) with type 2 diabetes who are able to normalize their fasting plasma glucose concentrations. In the UKPDS (see p. 65), weight loss during the initial, intensive, 3-month, dietary phase averaged 5 kg; this was associated with a rapid but temporary improvement in fasting plasma glucose concentration (Fig. 2.4, p. 66).

ANTI-OBESITY DRUGS

Drugs can only be an adjunct to lifestyle measures and some have been associated with significant unwanted effects. Anti-obesity agents have only a limited role in the management of obesity and have become somewhat discredited again following a recent resurgence of interest in their use. Nonetheless, the potentially lucrative and expanding market continues to stimulate new developments. Recent developments include:

● *Sibutramine*. This is a serotonin and noradrenaline neuronal reuptake inhibitor licensed currently in the USA and some other countries. Sibutramine is a more selective serotonin re-uptake inhibitor than fenfluramine and dexfenfluramine. It reduces appetite while also producing small increases in energy expenditure via increased thermogenesis. Small increases in BP (an effect also observed with phenteramine) and heart rate have been reported indicating the need for careful monitoring. However, there have been no reports of cardiac valvular lesions to date (c.f. dexfenfluramine).

● *Orlistat*. This drug is a pancreatic lipase inhibitor which inhibits triglyceride digestion by approximately 30%. Undigested fat is excreted unchanged leading to a moderately high incidence of predictable side effects including abdominal pains, flatulence, oily spotting, diarrhoea and urgency. It has been suggested that these side effects may actually encourage compliance with a reduced-fat diet. The use of orlistat in conjunction with diet doubles the weight loss (~10% body weight) compared with diet alone (approximately 5%) after 12 months of treatment. Improvements in glycaemia, total- and LDL-cholesterol concentrations have been reported. In the UK, orlistat is licensed for use in patients with obesity (defined as a BMI

>30 kg/m^2) or in overweight patients (>28 kg/m^2) with additional cardiovascular risk factors. However, patients should have achieved a weight loss of 2.5 kg prior to introduction of the drug; if subsequent weight loss is less than 5% of body weight, therapy should be withdrawn.

The cloning of the adipocyte-derived peptide, leptin, in 1994 brought rapid realization of potential applications in the management of human obesity. However, far from being deficient in leptin, as in the obese *ob/ob* mouse, obese humans tend to have high circulating leptin levels implying hypothalamic insensitivity to the peptide (see Section 1).

Several other drugs are under consideration as satiety factors but the redundancy of mechanisms by which appetite is sustained argues against a major therapeutic application for any single agent.

SURGICAL APPROACHES TO OBESITY

The history of surgery in the management of severe degrees of obesity is also rather chequered:

● *Ileal bypass*. Although effective, it has been largely abandoned because of serious long-term side effects.

● *Jaw-wiring*. This is useful only as a temporary measure in most patients and is not recommended; subsequent re-gain of weight is common and so-called 'cycling' of weight may be disadvantageous.

● *Vertical gastric banding*. This reduces the physical capacity of the stomach, and is perhaps the only surgical treatment which is both effective and relatively safe. However, its application mandates careful selection of patients and expertise in both anaesthetic and surgical technique. It should be considered only for patients with morbid obesity in whom determined attempts using other options have failed.

Thus, the mainstay of treatment remains calorie restriction, ideally coupled with regular exercise leading to increased energy expenditure. These strategies are, of course, by far the cheapest, of known efficacy and, in general, are safe.

CALORIE RESTRICTION

Daily energy requirements may be calculated from the patient's height, age and physical activity using published tables. Adipose tissue contains about 7000 kcal/kg. Sustained weight loss in the obese will occur at a rate of around 0.5 kg/week with a reduction in daily calorie intake of 500 kcal (1.2 MJ). This represents a reduction of around 20% for most patients.

NB A daily reduction of 500 kcal will produce weight loss averaging 0.5 kg per week.

More rapid rates of weight loss will include structural protein, i.e. muscle, as well as fat; this is undesirable since resting energy expenditure, which is determined largely by fat-free mass, will decline as an adaptive response. Resting energy expenditure, which normally accounts for the majority of daily calorie consumption, represents the energy requirements for essential metabolic processes maintaining cell membrane potentials and body temperature. The observation that, on average, the obese have higher resting energy expenditures than the non-obese means that maintenance of body weight requires a proportionately greater calorie intake. Physical exercise, in conjunction with calorie restriction, will help preserve fat-free tissues thereby maintaining resting energy expenditure; this combination offers advantages over calorie reduction alone.

MACRONUTRIENTS

Once the daily total calories are known, the dietary prescription can be discussed in terms of its macronutrient composition, i.e. the proportion eaten as carbohydrate, fat and protein. Current recommendations are presented in Figure 3.1. These are broadly appropriate for both type 1 and type 2 diabetes; important considerations specific to these subtypes require additional comments.

CARBOHYDRATES (3.8 KCAL/G)

Approximately 45% of calories of the UK diet in general are derived from carbohydrate, around 10–20% coming from sucrose. For diabetic patients, it

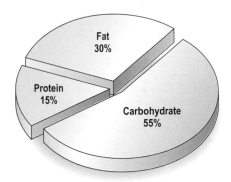

Fig. 3.1 Recommended dietary components as a proportion of total daily calorie consumption.

is recommended that carbohydrates comprise 50–55% of daily calorie allowance. This should be mainly in the form of complex rather than simple carbohydrates, i.e. less rapidly digested starches rather than mono- or disaccharides. Higher intakes of carbohydrate, in the absence of a sufficient increase in fibre, may aggravate hypertriglyceridaemia and are not recommended. Sucrose or fructose (the latter having a lesser effect on plasma glucose) are permitted in limited quantities, i.e. up to a daily maximum of 25 g and should replace other carbohydrates. Artificial sweetening agents, e.g. aspartame, may be used ad libitum.

Dietary fibre has received much attention in recent years. Both cereal fibre and soluble plant fibre reportedly improve glycaemia and lipid profiles; fibre is therefore generally encouraged. However, the chemical composition of the fibre is an important determinant of metabolic effects; cereal fibre supplements, e.g. bran, are of negligible benefit to diabetic patients.

For patients with type 1 diabetes, avoidance of hypoglycaemia is a major objective. Emergency treatment of hypoglycaemia requires rapidly available carbohydrate, glucose or sucrose, often taken as 15 g tablets.

 NB Carbohydrate should contribute >50% of total daily calories.

FATS (9 KCAL/G)

Because of their high energy content, fats represent a major source of excess calorie consumption, particularly in convenience and junk foods. Limit to less than 35% of total calorie consumption. Circulating total and LDL-cholesterol concentrations are modifiable, albeit to a relatively minor extent, principally by reducing saturated fat intake. Saturated fat consumption has also been linked to insulin resistance (see p. 28). It is recommended that saturated fats, mainly derived from meat and dairy products, should comprise less than 10% of total energy intake. Use poly- or mono-unsaturated fatty acids (e.g. olive oil, rapeseed oil) in preference but not in excess. Recently, concern has been expressed that consumption of trans-unsaturated fatty acids in excessive amounts may increase the risk of cardiovascular disease via alterations in lipoproteins. Marine oil supplements, which carry a high calorie load, are not recommended for routine use although consumption of oily fish is encouraged. It is important to bear in mind that these recommendations are founded largely on theoretical considerations and observations in selected populations.

PROTEIN (4 KCAL/G)

This comprises the remainder of the daily caloric intake and should amount to 50–60 g/day by current recommendations, i.e. approximately 0.8 g/kg body weight. Average daily protein intake in many European countries tends to be higher than this at 1.5 g/kg body weight. However, major restriction of protein consumption is instituted only in the context of advanced diabetic nephropathy (see p. 219). There is debate about the potential effects of the source of dietary protein, i.e. animal vs vegetable, on renal function, the suggestion being that substituting the latter for the former may be protective; further study is required.

MICRONUTRIENTS

ANTIOXIDANTS AND TRACE ELEMENTS

Increased oxidant damage mediated by free radicals has been implicated in the promotion of atheroma. Diets in UK populations may be low in the antioxidant β-carotene and vitamins C and E, and consumption of fresh fruit and vegetables is regarded as a sensible recommendation, albeit founded largely on theoretical considerations at present. There are currently no data supporting routine pharmacological supplementation with antioxidants in diabetes. However, some institutions recommend increased antioxidant intake as part of an overall management strategy (see Diabetic nephropathy – Steno type 2 study, p. 226). Similarly, no recommendations exist concerning routine supplementation of the diet with trace elements such as chromium or magnesium.

MINERALS

Salt should be restricted to a maximum of 3 g/day. Diabetic patients have increased exchangeable body sodium. In patients with hypertension, particularly if difficult to control, salt intake should be reduced to less than 2.5 g/day. The BP-lowering role of dietary potassium supplements is uncertain; special care should be used in patients with renal impairment or in those taking potassium-retaining medications. Hyporeninaemic hypoaldosteronism, a feature of diabetic nephropathy, may warrant dietary restriction of potassium.

NB Dietary salt restriction may be beneficial in hypertensive patients.

ALCOHOL

Alcoholic beverages are a variable and potentially important component of diet which may have a bearing on aspects of diabetes (Table 3.4). Calorie load, if excessive, and risk of hypoglycaemia are the principal concerns. Alcohol provides 7 kcal/g of energy – almost twice that of carbohydrates and approaching the energy value of fats.

> **NB** Alcohol can be a significant source of dietary calories.

TABLE 3.4 Potential relevance of excessive alcohol consumption to patients with diabetes

- Calorie burden
  — Obesity

- Hypertension
  — Restriction of alcohol may improve control of hypertension

- Dyslipidaemia
  — Hypertriglyceridaemia

- Hypoglycaemia
  — Exacerbation of insulin or sulphonylurea-induced hypoglycaemia – may occur several hours after consumption
  — Recognition of symptoms of hypoglycaemia may be impaired

- Alcoholic ketoacidosis
  — Even in non-diabetics; rare

- Liver disease
  — Alcoholic steatosis, hepatitis and cirrhosis

- Pancreatitis
  — Risk of secondary diabetes with recurrent or chronic pancreatitis
  — Risk of chronic malabsorption

- Chlorpropamide–alcohol flush syndrome
  — Inhibition of acetaldehyde dehydrogenase

- Neuropathy
  — Exacerbation of chronic diabetic neuropathic syndromes
  — Exacerbation of erectile dysfunction

Hepatic metabolism of alcohol

More than 90% of alcohol is metabolized by the liver. Briefly, the metabolism of alcohol alters the redox state of the liver. The ratio of reduced to oxidized nicotinamide adenine dinucleotide (NAD) is increased, thereby inhibiting gluconeogenesis, i.e. the formation of glucose from 3-carbon precursors.

$$\text{Ethanol} + \text{NAD}^+ \xrightarrow[\substack{\text{Alcohol} \\ \text{dehydrogenase}}]{} \text{Acetaldehyde} + \text{NADH} + \text{H}^+$$

$$\text{Acetaldehyde} + \text{H}_2\text{O} + \text{NAD}^+ \xrightarrow[\substack{\text{Acetaldehyde} \\ \text{dehydrogenase}}]{} \text{Acetate} + \text{NADH} + \text{H}^+$$

Alcohol consumption can predispose to hypoglycaemia even in the absence of intoxication.

Thus, the risk of hypoglycaemia is increased by the reduction in endogenous glucose production from the liver resulting from inhibition of gluconeogenesis. Importantly, hypoglycaemia may occur even at blood alcohol levels not usually associated with intoxication. Hypoglycaemia may occur even in non-diabetics if alcohol is consumed in the absence of sufficient carbohydrate although this tendency may be offset to some extent by an acute reduction in sensitivity of non-hepatic tissues to insulin.

The risk of hypoglycaemia is highest when hepatic glycogen stores are depleted by fasting since glycogenolysis can sustain hepatic glucose production. Particular caution is required in diabetic patients, especially those at high risk of hypoglycaemia. Conversely, the features of hypoglycaemia are sometimes mistaken as those of alcoholic intoxication; this might lead to serious consequences if the correct metabolic disturbance is not recognized and the appropriate treatment denied. The carrying of a card or wearing of a bracelet which identifies the patient as being diabetic should always be encouraged.

 Hypoglycaemia may occur many hours after alcohol consumption – even the following morning.

Alcohol may significantly increase the depth and duration of iatrogenic hypoglycaemia and has been implicated in fatalities. It has been suggested that alcohol may be an underappreciated risk factor for severe sulphonylurea-induced hypoglycaemia.

NB Alcohol can increase the severity and duration of hypoglycaemia.

Late hypoglycaemia occurring after many hours may necessitate extra carbohydrate or a temporary reduction in insulin dose. There may also be a risk of early reactive hypoglycaemia if mixers with high sugar content stimulate insulin release in patients with sufficient endogenous reserve. It is important that patients appreciate that the symptoms of hypoglycaemia may be masked by alcohol.

NB The symptoms of hypoglycaemia may be masked by alcohol.

Alcohol dependence

Alcohol dependence represents a potentially fatal risk to the patient reliant on insulin or treated with sulphonylureas; regular meals should be encouraged. In addition, chronic alcoholism is regarded as a contraindication to metformin therapy since the risk of lactic acidosis may be enhanced by the alterations in redox state (see p. 188). In fact, this caution derives from adverse experience with the related drug phenformin. Alcoholic ketoacidosis is an uncommon but serious metabolic disturbance which may develop in diabetic or non-diabetic alcoholics (see p. 176).

Recommended daily consumption

The recommended maximum daily consumption of alcohol in the UK is:

- 30 g (3 units) for men.
- 20 g (2 units) for women.

In the UK, depending on the strength and volume of the measure, one unit approximates to a half-pint (375 mL) of beer, a single measure (44 mL) of spirits or a glass (120 mL) of wine. Recommendations to patients should include the following advice:

- Never drink and drive.
- Do not substitute alcohol for regular meals or snacks.
- Avoid alcoholic drinks with high sugar content, e.g. sweet wine.
- Avoid lower carbohydrate drinks – tend to be high in alcohol.
- Avoid drinking on an empty stomach.
- Avoid alcohol if there is hypertriglyceridaemia, symptomatic neuropathy or refractory hypertension.
- Carry diabetes identification card in case of emergency.

Beneficial aspects of alcohol

More positively, the regular consumption of moderate quantities of alcohol is associated with favourable effects on cardiovascular risk factors including lower circulating insulin levels, increased HDL-cholesterol levels and reduced coagulability. Recent observational data from the USA suggest that diabetic patients share the benefits of moderate habitual alcohol consumption on mortality from CHD observed in non-diabetics. Low-to-moderate chronic alcohol intake is associated with lower circulating insulin concentrations and improved insulin sensitivity. There is some evidence from epidemiological studies that the risk of developing type 2 diabetes is inversely associated with alcohol intake; moderate alcohol consumption may decrease the risk of type 2 diabetes.

TOBACCO

In contrast to alcohol, smoking has only deleterious effects and should be strongly discouraged. Cigarette smoking has been implicated as an independent, modifiable risk factor for the development of type 2 diabetes (see p. 19).

 NB Cigarette smoking is an independent risk factor for type 2 diabetes.

When glucose intolerance or diabetes has developed, cigarette smoking represents an important and potentially modifiable risk factor for cardiovascular disease and certain microvascular complications (see Section 5). The risk for an individual increases with the accumulation of multiple risk factors greater than can be explained by a simple additive effect. Thus, it becomes particularly important for patients who have a multiplicity of cardiovascular risk factors to cease smoking. Other potentially deleterious adverse effects of smoking are presented in Table 3.5.

TABLE 3.5 Deleterious effects in which cigarette smoking has been implicated in diabetic patients

- Systemic BP
  — Acute elevation
- Insulin sensitivity
  — Reduced in chronic smokers
- Retinopathy
  — Increased risk of development and progression
- Nephropathy
  — Increased risk of development and progression
- Neuropathy
  — Increased risk of chronic distal sensory neuropathy
- Connective tissues
  — Increased risk of limited joint mobility
  — Increased risk of Dupuytren's contracture
- Dermatological
  — Increased risk of necrobiosis lipoidica

Cross-sectional studies indicate that the age-adjusted prevalence of smoking is similar between non-diabetic and diabetic populations. There is evidence that, as for non-diabetics, cardiovascular risk declines when the habit is broken. Behavioural therapy or substitution of cigarettes with nicotine patches or gum may be useful strategies in assisting patients with efforts directed at smoking cessation. Fear of weight gain is often cited by patients. However, this is not inevitable and may be transitory. Limited success in stopping smoking points to the importance of discouraging the acquisition of the habit.

Young patients and certain ethnic groups, who may also have a higher risk of diabetic complications, have been targeted by tobacco companies. Suggested approaches to reduction in tobacco use include:

- Regular reiteration of the adverse effects of cigarettes by all health care professionals.
- Availability of written information in clinic or office, e.g. health education leaflets and posters.
- Encouragement of use of nicotine supplements.
- Designated smoking-cessation clinics.

National campaigns to discourage tobacco consumption should be strongly supported by health care professionals and patient support organizations.

> **NB** Cigarette smoking should be strongly discouraged in diabetic patients.

PHYSICAL EXERCISE

The potential health benefits of regular physical activity remain underappreciated. It has been claimed that inactive adults have approximately twice the risk of premature death and serious medical illness as active individuals, the relative risk associated with a sedentary lifestyle being similar to that associated with hypertension or hypercholesterolaemia. Such observations, if confirmed, would appear to be of particular relevance to patients with diabetes.

The general benefits of exercise argue in favour of its promotion for the population as a whole. However, this provides another striking example of disparity between theoretical considerations and practical implementation. People may realize they should be more active but changing deeply ingrained habits often proves very difficult.

> **NB** A sedentary lifestyle is a major risk factor for coronary heart disease.

Regular physical exercise is therefore regarded as potentially beneficial to the majority of diabetic patients; it should be encouraged wherever possible as an integral component of other lifestyle changes which include nutritional modifications, avoidance of cigarettes and moderate alcohol consumption.

Ideally exercise is performed daily. For the diabetic patient, benefits of regular exercise of sufficient intensity and duration include:

● *Weight control.* This has a synergistic effect on body weight in conjunction with calorie restriction; the two should be combined wherever feasible.

● *Improved metabolic control.* Mediated in part via increased insulin sensitivity. Glucose uptake and glycogen synthesis in skeletal muscle is improved.

● *Improved cardiovascular risk factor profile.* Included are lower total cholesterol, lower triglycerides, increased HDL-cholesterol, lower BP and improved fibrinolysis.

● *Improved cardiovascular conditioning and functional capacity.* This may be associated with psychological benefits including improved sense of well-being and self-confidence.

 Regular physical exercise should be encouraged for diabetic patients wherever possible.

THE METABOLIC (INSULIN RESISTANCE) SYNDROME

In addition to increased calorie consumption, it has been suggested that the parallel decrease in physical activity has contributed significantly to the increasing prevalence of obesity and type 2 diabetes in many populations (see p. 15). Exercise has the capacity to ameliorate several components of the metabolic syndrome (see p. 19) and it is therefore of interest that regular exercise is associated with a reduced risk of developing type 2 diabetes in observational and intervention studies. Moreover, the decrease in risk may be greatest for those most susceptible, i.e. those with obesity, a positive family history and hypertension.

The impact of supervised exercise programmes, in conjunction with dietary modification, is being evaluated in multicentre controlled clinical trials (The US Diabetes Prevention Program and the Finnish Diabetes Prevention Study) in patients with pre-existing impaired glucose tolerance. The hypothesis being tested is that the transition from impaired glucose tolerance to type 2 diabetes may be prevented or delayed. Improvements in blood glucose, BP and lipids have been reported in the intervention group in the Diabetes Prevention Study.

Recent studies have also demonstrated improvement in insulin action not only in patients with type 2 diabetes but also in non-diabetic offspring; this may be of long-term benefit in reducing the risk of developing diabetes in such individuals. However, the design and execution of trials which might confirm this possibility present enormous practical difficulties. Of practical importance, the improvements observed in insulin sensitivity dissipate rapidly when the exercise programme ceases. This underpins the desirability of a daily exercise routine. Conversely, a rapid impairment in insulin sensitivity is observed with immobilization, e.g. enforced bed rest.

There is intriguing evidence that regular exercise is associated with a reduced risk of microvascular complications in patients with type 1 diabetes; increased survival has also been reported. While these results point to important beneficial effects, it should be noted that there may have been an element of self-selection amongst the participants since these were observational rather than randomized prospective studies. Nonetheless, the evidence favours encouragement of regular physical exercise in patients with diabetes. As for other lifestyle modifications, this view is in accordance with current recommendations for the population in general.

 NB Exercise has beneficial effects on multiple aspects of the metabolic (insulin resistance) syndrome.

Motivation and compliance

Not only is the proportion of diabetic patients involved in regular exercise relatively low but the drop-out rate for supervised exercise programmes is high; finding an activity which the patient enjoys is therefore of considerable importance. This might be 20–30 min brisk walking several times per week, mowing the lawn, golf or even household activities. The intensity, frequency and duration of activity are more relevant than the precise form of exercise. Simple measures such as always using the stairs at work rather than the lift are a start. Formal links with a leisure club may be useful. Other strategies to enhance uptake and compliance include:

- Identifying activities which are pleasurable.
- Exercising with family or friends.
- Avoiding unrealistic exercise targets.

The emphasis should be on aerobic, physiologically-sound exercise with a minimal risk of injury. Extreme activity such as marathon running is not appropriate; however, the determined patient should not be put off such pursuits without good reason. Competitive sports represent a major challenge to the insulin-treated patient. However, individuals who surmount the difficulties and reach the pinnacle of their sport serve as important and deserving role models for young patients.

Cautions

A number of problems may serve to limit the exercise capacity of patients with type 2 diabetes including:

- Obesity and associated comorbidity – particularly cardiovascular disease, degenerative joint disease.
- Advanced age and reduced mobility.
- Personal attitudes and (dis)inclinations.

The clinical evaluation of CHD presents a particular difficulty for the middle-aged or elderly patient with type 2 diabetes. The absence of typical symptoms cannot be relied upon (see p. 228) and the question is therefore how rigorously an individual patient should be assessed. In large part, this will be determined by the particular activity that is envisioned. Clearly, it is not necessary to put all patients through exercise ECG if their objective is only to walk a couple of miles each day. More vigorous exercise patterns might require more detailed evaluation and the threshold for requesting exercise ECG should be appropriately low. A slow start to exercise, incrementally building up to higher levels of activity, is prudent. A checklist for patients embarking on an exercise programme is presented in Table 3.6); this should be modified according to individual circumstances.

Table 3.6 Precautions for diabetic patients embarking on an exercise programme

- Discuss intentions in detail with your physician
- Avoid unduly strenuous exercise initially – high risk of CHD events
- Include warm-up and cool-off periods
- Monitor blood glucose levels before and after exercise
- Take extra care in extreme climatic conditions
- Report any symptoms such as chest pain, undue breathlessness
- Use appropriate footwear if evidence of neuropathy
- Inspect feet after running, prolonged walking
- Avoid exercise during periods of poor metabolic control
- Avoid exercise during intercurrent illnesses

 Subclinical CHD represents a potential danger to diabetic patients embarking on an exercise programme.

In addition, care should be taken to avoid situations which might be dangerous for insulin-treated patients, or for individuals in their charge, if hypoglycaemia should occur, e.g. sub-aqua diving, rock climbing, parachuting.

Patients at risk of hypoglycaemia should indulge in high-risk sports with care.

Tissue damage may ensue in patients with chronic complications; for example, an ill-advised walking holiday may result in foot ulceration in a patient with neuropathy (see p. 214). Unfortunately, even well-educated and intelligent patients are sometimes undeterred, with unfortunate consequences. Much less commonly, straining (i.e. Valsalva) activities risk vitreous haemorrhage in patients with neovascularization. The major risk in insulin-treated patients is hypoglycaemia which may be delayed for up to 15 hours post-exercise.

 Exercise may cause late hypoglycaemia in insulin-treated patients.

NORMAL PHYSIOLOGY OF ACUTE EXERCISE

The breakdown of intrinsic stores of glycogen provides the initial energy for exercising skeletal muscle. As intensive exercise continues beyond a few minutes, muscle glycogen becomes depleted and the increased demand for glucose, which may multiply many-fold over pre-exercise levels, is normally matched by an appropriate increase in hepatic glucose production. However, circulating glucose levels may start to fall if exercise is prolonged for several hours in the absence of extra oral consumption of carbohydrate.

During this period, mobilization of non-esterified fatty acids from adipose tissue increases substantially. Fatty acids provide the major source of energy for continuing muscular contraction at this stage; plasma levels of fatty acids may remain elevated for several hours following major exertion such as a marathon. The metabolic changes associated with exercise result primarily from acute changes in circulating levels of insulin and counter-regulatory hormones, notably catecholamines.

The normal fall in plasma insulin levels allows mobilization of glucose from the liver. Reduced endogenous insulin secretion also permits adipocyte lipolysis to accelerate; this is augmented by the lipolytic action of the sympatho-adrenal system (see pp. 159–160). Thus, there is a close match of substrate provision to muscular consumption in non-diabetics. However, for patients treated with exogenous insulin and, to a lesser extent, those treated with sulphonylureas, the inability to acutely lower plasma insulin levels requires strategies to enable exercise to continue without the rapid development of hypoglycaemia.

Type 2 diabetes

For diet-treated diabetic patients these physiological changes will be operative during exercise, although quantitatively their magnitude and effect will be altered by the diabetic state. Patients treated with metformin as monotherapy will not usually need any particular advice about avoiding hypoglycaemia: this should not be a risk. Patients receiving sulphonylureas may find that they need to reduce or omit tablets depending on the intensity and duration of the exercise. This is usually preferable to increasing carbohydrate intake.

Type 1 diabetes

The degree of insulinization at the start of exercise is an important factor which will determine whether plasma glucose rises or falls with exercise:

● *Relative insulin deficiency.* The result is likely to be a rise in plasma glucose level – ketosis may also develop.

● *Good insulinization.* There is a risk of hypoglycaemia since the compensatory rise in hepatic glucose production will be restrained.

An insufficient insulin dose will limit the uptake of glucose by the exercising muscle groups. In addition, the mobilization of fatty acids will be enhanced by the relative insulinopenia and the hormonal balance will tend to favour hepatic ketogenesis (see p. 16). Thus, ketonuria may develop with prolonged exertion.

Striking the balance between too little and too much insulin poses considerable difficulties and in practice careful self-monitoring and experimentation usually prove necessary. Once a dose of exogenous insulin has been injected subcutaneously it will be absorbed into the circulation according to its pharmacokinetic characteristics. Physical exercise per se will tend to enhance the absorption of insulin, regardless of whether it was injected into an exercising limb. To avoid hypoglycaemia during exercise patients may need to:

● Reduce the appropriate insulin dose sufficiently prior to exercise – a 30–50% reduction may be required.

● Consume extra carbohydrate sufficient to sustain blood glucose levels – an extra 20–40 g per hour.

In practice, a combination of these manoeuvres is often used. The insulin dose which will be maximally operative during the period of exercise should be reduced by 30–50%. Capillary blood glucose is checked by the patient and extra carbohydrate, conveniently consumed in the form of mini chocolate bars, taken prior to the exercise if necessary. On average, an hourly boost of 20–40 g carbohydrate will also be required for prolonged exertion. Avoidance of late hypoglycaemia presents an additional challenge. This is best managed by taking additional carbohydrate.

All of this dictates that exercise should be a planned activity for which considerable self-discipline is required. Many factors will influence the response and these recommendations can only serve as a broad guide.

TYPE AND FREQUENCY OF ACTIVITIES

Activities which raise the pulse moderately from its resting rate to submaximal levels are appropriate; discussions of maximal aerobic activity (i.e. Vo_2 max) are not usually clinically relevant. It is considered that the best modalities of exercise, ideally taken in combination, are:

- *Aerobic endurance activities* – walking, running, cycling, swimming, aerobics.
- *Resistance training* – low-intensity, high volume, e.g. circuit training.

It is recommended that a warm-up period of 5–10 min prefaces more vigorous exercise with an appropriate cooling-off period afterwards. Heart rates of 60–80% of maximal (calculated as 220 minus the patient's age) have been suggested for periods of 20–30 min 3–4 times per week. More practical still is to aim for:

- 30 min sustained exercise of moderate degree, e.g. brisk walking or similar, 5–6 days per week.

ORAL ANTIDIABETIC AGENTS

Modifications to diet and lifestyle are seldom sufficient to produce good, long-term, metabolic control in patients with type 2 diabetes, as demonstrated by the UKPDS (see p. 65). Thus, pharmacological adjuncts are required in the majority of patients. Orally-active agents are usually employed in the first instance; insulin is reserved for patients in whom tablets prove insufficient.

> **NB** The majority of patients with type 2 diabetes will require oral antidiabetic agents or insulin in order to attain glycaemic targets.

The choice of drug depends on both clinical and biochemical factors; as with all pharmacological agents, antidiabetic therapy should only be initiated following careful consideration of the possible benefits and risks of treatment for the individual patient. Although the oral antidiabetic agents are generally safe when used appropriately, the most commonly used drugs, sulphonylureas and biguanides, are associated with rare but potentially lethal adverse effects (Table 3.7).

TABLE 3.7 Summary of principal adverse effects of oral antidiabetic agents

Drug	Adverse effects	Comments
Sulphonylureas	*Minor*	
	Weight gain	Common
	Idiosyncratic reactions	More common with first-generation agents
	Major	
	Hypoglycaemia	Mild: fairly common
		Major: rare but high case-fatality rate
Metformin	*Minor*	
	GI symptoms	~10% patients cannot tolerate drug
	Major	
	Lactic acidosis	Rare: almost always in patients with contraindications, especially renal impairment
Acarbose	*Minor*	
	GI symptoms	Common; dose-dependent
	Major	
	Hepatic dysfunction	Rare; idiosyncratic and reversible
Troglitazone*	*Major*	
	Risk of severe hepatotoxicity	Uncommon; monitoring of liver function tests required
Rosiglitazone† Pioglitazone†	*Minor* Weight gain, oedema	No reports of major hepatotoxicity

*No longer available in the UK.
†Expected to be licensed in UK in 2000.

 Selection of oral antidiabetic agents should be based on the potential benefits and risks to the patient.

The first insulin-sensitizing thiazolidinedione drug to reach the market, troglitazone, was withdrawn by its UK distributors shortly after launch in 1997 following reports of severe hepatotoxicity, including fatalities. In 1999, the UK Medicines Control Agency rejected an application for its re-introduction. However, troglitazone remains available in the USA where the overall risk:benefit ratio was judged to be favourable by the Food and Drug Administration; the drug is also available in Japan and 11 other countries. Careful monitoring of liver function tests is required (see p. 130). Two more potent drugs – rosiglitazone and pioglitazone – were launched in the USA in 1999. Whether the latter drugs will prove to be free of serious hepatotoxic effects remains undetermined; the problems with troglitazone did not become apparent until the drug was widely prescribed. However, to date there have been no reports of hepatotoxicity. Guar gum, which although safe has not established a useful therapeutic role because of low-efficacy, unpalatability and gastrointestinal (GI) side effects, is not considered further.

Classification
Oral antidiabetic drugs may usefully be classified by their actions as being either:

- Hypoglycaemic agents.
- Anti-hyperglycaemic agents.

This distinction, which reflects differences in chemistry and hence mode of action, is clinically relevant. Drugs in the latter category do not usually cause hypoglycaemia when used as monotherapy. It should also be noted that other drugs, not used primarily as antidiabetic agents, may also lower plasma glucose concentrations (Table 3.8). The latter agents may potentiate glucose-lowering effects of other drugs.

TABLE 3.8 Hypoglycaemic and anti-hyperglycaemic drugs used to treat type 2 diabetes

Hypoglycaemic drugs	Anti-hyperglycaemic drugs
Sulphonylureas	Biguanides
Repaglinide	α-Glucosidase inhibitors
	Thiazolidinediones
	Guar gum

Anti-hyperglycaemic agents may potentiate the hypoglycaemic actions of other drugs.

Sulphonylureas and biguanides are used extensively in patients with type 2 diabetes. In addition to alleviating osmotic symptoms these agents may also avert acute metabolic states such as hyperosmolar non-ketotic coma (see p. 185) when used appropriately (however their use is contraindicated in such states). However, time-honoured conventions concerning the clinical use of oral antidiabetic agents have attracted criticism and the optimal selection of therapy for patients with type 2 diabetes remains uncertain. The UKPDS did not provide a clear answer to this question (see p. 65). However, the benefits of improved glycaemic control with either oral antidiabetic agents or insulin, particularly on microvascular complications, were clearly demonstrated by this study. Moreover, metformin emerged as the drug of choice for overweight patients.

Use of insulin in type 2 diabetes
The question of when to abandon oral agents in favour of insulin is a particularly vexed one, especially in the obese patient who continues to have inadequate glycaemic control despite strenuous nutritional and lifestyle

advice (see pp. 86–99 and 100–106). Therapeutic failure with oral antidiabetic agents is a well-recognized, if incompletely understood, phenomenon and is conventionally subdivided into two categories:

● *Primary failure.* Approximately 15% of patients (depending on arbitrary and variable definitions) do not show an adequate initial metabolic response to sulphonylureas.

● *Secondary failure.* An additional 5–10% of patients per annum, who initially respond, show a subsequent deterioration in glycaemic control.

In part, the waning of response to oral agents reflects the gradual attrition of endogenous insulin secretion that characterizes type 2 diabetes (see p. 87); dietary factors are also likely to be important in some cases. Patients exhibiting so-called primary failure may have insufficient B-cell reserve at diagnosis to have a satisfactory response to oral agents. A proportion of non-obese, middle-aged patients have autoimmune markers associated with type 1 diabetes; these patients may represent a subgroup that is progressing inevitably to insulin dependence.

> **NB** Failure of a rapid and adequate therapeutic response to oral antidiabetic agents supports the case for insulin treatment.

Failure of response to a sulphonylurea is usually indicative of:

● Marked insulin deficiency.
● Non-compliance with dietary advice.
● Antagonism of insulin action, e.g. corticosteroid therapy.

Degrees of primary failure (i.e. partial but suboptimal responses) are common if strict criteria are applied. Combination therapy or early use of insulin treatment should be considered, especially in younger patients.

Combination oral agent therapy
For patients inadequately controlled by monotherapy sulphonylureas and biguanides may be usefully combined; the effect may be synergistic, i.e. greater than a simple additive effect.

> **NB** Sulphonylureas and metformin may be usefully combined in selected patients with type 2 diabetes.

However, the UKPDS reported an increase in diabetes-related deaths when metformin was added to patients already receiving maximal doses of a sulphonylurea (see below). This finding was not substantiated on a subsequent combined analysis of the entire data and neither the BDA (now Diabetes UK) nor the ADA have recommended changes to the practice of combining these agents. Combination therapy is more likely to be effective in patients with less severe degrees of fasting hyperglycaemia. However, many patients will still not attain adequate glycaemic control. In these circumstances, the addition of a third agent, e.g. an α-glucosidase inhibitor, will usually result in only a minor further improvement at best. The role of thiazolidinediones in this situation requires further study. Insulin therapy then becomes the only alternative, either as monotherapy or in combination with one or more oral agents. The high insulin doses required to achieve satisfactory glycaemic control, particularly in the morbidly obese patient, may prove daunting to all concerned.

> **NB** Additional benefit from oral antidiabetic agents is rarely obtained by escalating doses; consider adding an agent from another class or transfer to insulin treatment.

Contraindications to oral antidiabetic agents

There are a number of acute or temporary clinical situations where oral antidiabetic agents are contraindicated in patients with type 2 diabetes; insulin therapy should be instituted in these circumstances (Table 3.9). After resolution or recovery a satisfactory therapeutic response may be attained following the re-introduction of oral agents.

TABLE 3.9 Indications for insulin in type 2 diabetes

Clinical indication	Rationale for insulin therapy
Major acute intercurrent illness, e.g. septicaemia, MI	Deterioration in metabolic control with sulphonylureas and risk of lactic acidosis with biguanides
Pregnancy	Inadequate metabolic control with oral antidiabetic agents; safety concerns
Surgery	Risk of peri-operative hypoglycaemia (especially with long-acting sulphonylureas); risk of lactic acidosis with biguanides
Acute major metabolic decompensation, i.e. DKA or hyperosmolar nonketosis	Absolute or marked relative insulin deficiency in concert with insulin resistance mandates insulin therapy

SULPHONYLUREAS

Sulphonylureas have been extensively employed in the treatment of type 2 diabetes since their introduction in the 1950s. The first generation of drugs has largely been superseded by more potent second-generation agents (Table 3.10). The most recent addition to the list of sulphonylureas in the UK was glimepiride in 1998.

TABLE 3.10 Manufacturers' recommended doses and duration of action of sulphonylureas

	Daily dosage (mg/day)	Doses per day
First-generation agents		
Tolbutamide	500–3000	2–3
Tolazamide	100–1000	1–2
Chlorpropamide	100–500	1
Second-generation agents		
Glipizide	2.5–20	1–2
Gliclazide	40–320	1–2
Glibenclamide	5–20	1–2
Glimepiride	1–6	1
Gliquidone	15–120	2–3

Note that once-daily dosing may be sufficient even for drugs such as glipizide and gliclazide without loss of efficacy.

MODE OF ACTION

The principal mode of action of the sulphonylureas is enhancement of the sensitivity of the islet B-cell to glucose, resulting in increased insulin release for a specified level of glycaemia. This effect is dependent on the degree of B-cell reserve; sulphonylureas are ineffective in the absence of endogenous insulin secretion. Binding of the drugs to specific receptors in the B-cell membrane leads to inhibition of adenosine triphosphate (ATP)-sensitive potassium channels, causing depolarization of the membrane, influx of calcium and hence release of insulin into the circulation. Reported direct metabolic effects of sulphonylureas in extra-pancreatic tissues appear to be of negligible clinical significance with doses used in humans. The mode of action of the sulphonylureas is outlined in Fig. 3.2. Glimepiride binds predominantly to a different part of the sulphonylurea receptor to other sulphonylureas. The benzoic acid derivative repaglinide binds to the ATP-sensitive potassium channel at a site distinct from sulphonylureas such as glibenclamide. Furthermore, repaglinide does not enter the B-cell to stimulate exocytosis of insulin granules. Other classes of insulin secretagogues and agents which potentiate insulin secretion are under development.

CLINICAL PHARMACOLOGY

The second-generation sulphonylureas, e.g. glibenclamide (glyburide), gliclazide and glipizide, are characterized by higher islet B-cell binding

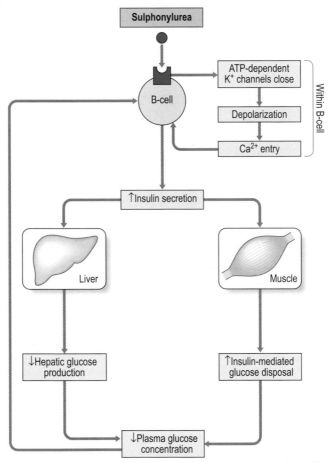

Fig. 3.2 Metabolic actions of sulphonylureas. (Adapted with permission from Krentz AJ. Prescriber 1998; 9: 67–78.)

compared with the older, first-generation drugs such as chlorpropamide and tolbutamide (Table 3.10). This effect, which results from modification of the molecular structure, explains the greater potency of the second-generation agents on a molar basis.

> **NB** Second-generation sulphonylureas are more potent on a molar basis than older agents such as tolbutamide.

Differences in potency are generally not reflected in differences in long-term glycaemic control. However, few controlled prospective studies have compared newer agents with the more established sulphonylureas (see below).

Dose–response relationships

Attention has been drawn to the limited data concerning dose–response relationships for sulphonylureas and their effects on blood glucose. Available evidence suggests that a linear relationship between plasma sulphonylurea concentration and effect on insulin secretion is observed over a relatively narrow range; maximally useful doses may therefore be lower than the manufacturers' recommendations (Table 3.10). However, the lowest dose should always be used when treatment is initiated. Differences in duration of action between sulphonylureas are of relevance to the risk and timing of drug-induced hypoglycaemia (Table 3.10).

 The minimum dosage should always be used when initiating therapy with a sulphonylurea.

Although there are differences in absorption, metabolism and elimination between the various sulphonylureas, these factors do not appear to affect long-term efficacy. However, in the UKPDS, patients assigned to chlorpropamide did not have the same degree of reduction in progression of retinopathy as those assigned to glibenclamide (or insulin); BP was also higher in the chlorpropamide-treated patients.

NB Chlorpropamide is regarded as an obsolete antidiabetic agent.

Moreover, pharmacokinetic differences may have important clinical implications, particularly with respect to the hazard of iatrogenic hypoglycaemia. Absorption of the following drugs is reportedly decreased by food ingestion:

- Tolbutamide.
- Glibenclamide.
- Chlorpropamide.
- Glipizide.

The rate of absorption of glimepiride is also reduced by food. The significance of this effect on long-term metabolic control is uncertain. Intestinal absorption of sulphonylureas may also be reduced in the presence of hyperglycaemia. Plasma half-lives differ considerably between the sulphonylureas (Table 3.11). Absorption of chlorpropamide, glipizide and tolbutamide is delayed by food and it is recommended that these drugs are taken 30 min before a meal. Other factors such as subtle disturbances of upper GI motility owing to autonomic dysfunction may also influence drug absorption but the clinical relevance of these effects is uncertain. It should be noted that the duration of glucose-lowering action generally exceeds the plasma half-life of the drugs; this reflects binding of the drug to B-cells.

There is evidence that the onset of maximal hypoglycaemic effect differs between drugs; this may be modified further by the timing of administration and number of daily doses. For example, glibenclamide suppresses hepatic glucose production more effectively than glipizide. Such differences between drugs have implications for the timing of drug-induced glycaemia, the most serious unwanted effect of these agents.

TABLE 3.11 Plasma half-lives, duration of action and metabolism of the sulphonylureas

	Half-life (h)	Duration of action (h)	Active/inactive metabolites
First-generation agents			
Tolbutamide	4–8	6–12	No
Tolazamide	4–7	12–24	Yes
Chlorpropamide	24–48	24–72	Yes
Second-generation agents			
Glipizide	1–5	≤24	No
Gliclazide	6–15	≤24	No
Glibenclamide	10–16	≤24	Both
Glimepiride	5–8	~24	Both
Gliquidone	12–24	≤24	Yes

In general, hypoglycaemia will be more prolonged if induced by an agent with a longer half-life. Route of elimination is another important factor in evaluating the risk of iatrogenic hypoglycaemia (Table 3.11). The following agents are either excreted unchanged via the kidney or have active metabolites that are cleared renally:

- Chlorpropamide.
- Glibenclamide.
- Tolazamide.
- Gliquidone.

It follows logically that these agents should be avoided in patients with renal impairment. Tolbutamide and glipizide are metabolized to inactive metabolites, whereas gliclazide and gliquidone are excreted renally only to a small extent. The pharmacokinetics of glimepiride appears to be favourable in the presence of mild to moderate renal impairment. These agents are therefore regarded as being better choices in the presence of renal impairment. However, many clinicians would avoid using sulphonylureas altogether, favouring insulin as a safer option. Since all of the sulphonylureas are highly bound to plasma proteins, displacement by other drugs sharing this characteristic may cause hypoglycaemia.

 Renally-eliminated sulphonylureas should not be used in patients with renal impairment.

CLINICAL INDICATIONS

Sulphonylureas are primarily indicated as adjunctive pharmacological therapy in patients with type 2 diabetes who have responded inadequately to appropriate recommendations concerning diet and lifestyle. Non-obese patients are especially suitable for sulphonylurea therapy since these drugs are commonly associated with weight gain. An adequate trial of diet and, where feasible, exercise is indicated in the majority of patients prior to initiation of sulphonylurea therapy.

 Sulphonylureas should in general not be initiated before an adequate trial of diet and lifestyle modifications.

ADVERSE EFFECTS

When used appropriately, sulphonylureas are generally well-tolerated drugs. The range of recognized adverse effects is limited and the effects are usually minor and reversible. Some effects, e.g. weight gain, are probably common to all sulphonylureas (Table 3.12). Other dose-related idiosyncratic reactions such as the alcohol (ethanol) flush are more common with older, first-generation drugs (Table 3.13) such as chlorpropamide (see p. 118). The most serious unwanted effect is hypoglycaemia (see below).

 All sulphonylureas have the capacity to cause severe hypoglycaemia.

Sulphonylurea-induced hypoglycaemia
Few reliable data are available concerning the incidence of hypoglycaemia induced by sulphonylureas, although it is more frequent than is perhaps

TABLE 3.12 Adverse effects associated with sulphonylureas

Effect	Comments
Weight gain	Common; avoid use in overweight or obese patients
Minor hypoglycaemia	More common than perhaps generally appreciated. Patients should be warned of the possibility
Severe hypoglycaemia	Most at risk are elderly patients treated with agents of long duration of action, e.g. chlorpropamide, glibenclamide. Renal impairment, decreased carbohydrate intake, alcohol and drug interactions are important. Prolonged hypoglycaemia may cause permanent neurological impairment or death. Severe hypoglycaemia necessitates hospital treatment
Cardiovascular safety	Controversial

TABLE 3.13 Idiosyncratic adverse effects of sulphonylureas

Adverse effect	Comments
Skin rashes	Uncommon and usually drug-specific; Stevens–Johnson syndrome is rare
Alcohol intolerance	Disulfram-like reaction; particularly common with chlorpropamide
Abnormal liver function	Uncommon and rarely severe; jaundice reported
Blood dyscrasias	Rare
Abnormal water handling	Chlorpropamide sensitizes distal renal tubules to vasopressin causing water retention; co-prescription of thiazide diuretics may cause severe hyponatraemia. Glibenclamide and tolazamide have a mild diuretic action

generally appreciated. Studies suggest that symptomatic hypoglycaemia may occur in up to 20% of patients, but is rarely severe. There are suggestions that the incidence of hypoglycaemia may be lower with glimepiride and the benzoic acid derivative, repaglinide. For glimepiride, the reduced risk of hypoglycaemia may reflect lower plasma insulin levels (see above) whereas the short half-life and close matching of doses to meals may explain, at least in part, the lower rate reported with repaglinide. Data are limited but if confirmed the lower incidence of hypoglycaemia may make the latter drugs particularly suitable for elderly patients. The major recognized risk associated with sulphonylureas is acute severe hypoglycaemia with its risk of death or serious chronic neurological sequelae. The clinical consequences of less severe, recurrent, sulphonylurea-induced hypoglycaemia in patients with type 2 diabetes are unknown. Sulphonylurea-induced hypoglycaemia is discussed more fully on page 166.

Hyperinsulinaemia and weight gain

Insulin has potent anabolic effects; consequently weight gain is a common consequence of therapy with insulin and sulphonylureas. Since the majority of patients with type 2 diabetes are either overweight or obese at diagnosis, this effect runs counter to attempts to reduce body weight through dietary restrictions and lifestyle changes. Obesity increases tissue insulin resistance thereby offsetting gains in B-cell function although the magnitude of this effect is relatively modest in comparison with the inherent insulin resistance associated with type 2 diabetes. Nonetheless, sulphonylureas are usually avoided in obese patients, in whom metformin is considered to be more appropriate. Limited data suggest that glimepiride may be less likely to cause weight gain.

In view of the hypothesized link between elevated plasma insulin levels and atherosclerotic vascular disease, the hyperinsulinaemia induced in the early phase of sulphonylurea treatment has come under renewed scrutiny in recent years. However, with prolonged treatment, plasma insulin levels tend to fall to pretreatment levels, suggesting improvements in tissue sensitivity to insulin, possibly mediated through improved levels of glycaemia. There is some evidence that glimepiride may induce less marked hyperinsulinaemia in comparison to drugs such as glibenclamide despite similar effects on blood glucose.

Hypersensitivity reactions

Skin rashes, including erythema multiforme, are uncommon. In general, these reactions are drug-specific and reversible. Blood dyscrasias are very rare, as is cholestatic jaundice. Chlorpropamide has been associated with attacks of acute intermittent porphyria, and tolbutamide, tolazamide and glymidine (which is actually a sulphapyrimidine) are considered unsafe in susceptible patients. Nausea is sometimes encountered transiently following initiation of sulphonylurea therapy.

Hyponatraemia

Chlorpropamide sensitizes the renal collecting ducts to the actions of vasopressin and, occasionally, excessive water retention leads to hyponatraemia. The hyponatraemia may be exacerbated by certain thiazide diuretics, and elderly patients appear to be particularly susceptible to its development. Glibenclamide and tolazamide, in contrast, have a mild diuretic action.

 Serious hyponatraemia may result from the combination of chlorpropamide and thiazide diuretics.

Chlorpropamide–alcohol flush syndrome

A minority of patients treated with chlorpropamide experience unpleasant symptoms of facial flushing after alcohol. The symptoms are due to an increase in blood acetaldehyde levels caused by inhibition of hepatic acetaldehyde dehydrogenase as in the disulfram reaction (a drug occasionally used to deter consumption in patients with alcohol dependence). This potentially troublesome effect is largely confined to chlorpropamide, although milder symptoms may occasionally be observed with other sulphonylureas.

Cardiovascular safety

Concerns about possible deleterious effects of sulphonylureas on cardiovascular disease, the major cause of mortality in patients with type 2 diabetes, have remained controversial since the 1960s. Animal experiments have implicated a role for deleterious effects on vascular ATP-dependent K^+ channels in ischaemic myocardium. The clinical relevance, if any, of such effects is far from clear. Glimepiride reportedly has no effects on this ion channel in human volunteers and unlike glimenclamide does not impair myocardial ischaemic preconditioning in experimental studies. Data from other clinical studies have suggested that early use of sulphonylureas reduces cardiovascular mortality and the UKPDS found no evidence for a detrimental effect of these agents. However, the Swedish multicentre Diabetes Mellitus Insulin Glucose Infusion in Acute Myocardial Infarction (DIGAMI) study provided evidence favouring preferential use of insulin in patients with type 2 diabetes following MI. This produced a significant reduction in mortality which was sustained for more than 3 years. The DIGAMI trial is discussed in more detail on pages 232–234.

DRUG INTERACTIONS

All sulphonylureas circulate highly bound to plasma proteins, and displacement by other drugs sharing this characteristic may cause hypoglycaemia. Aspirin, sulphonamides and trimethoprim have all been implicated in severe sulphonylurea-induced hypoglycaemia; these cautions should also be observed with the newer agents, glimepiride and repaglinide. Other drugs may potentiate the actions of sulphonylureas via different mechanisms including impaired hepatic metabolism (e.g. monoamine oxidase inhibitors, coumarins, phenylbutazone) and decreased renal excretion (e.g. probenecid) (Table 3.14). Excessive alcohol consumption, particularly in the absence of carbohydrate, may produce severe hypoglycaemia in sulphonylurea-treated patients.

TABLE 3.14 Drugs which may potentiate effects of sulphonylureas

Alcohol
Azapropazone
Chloramphenicol
Cimetidine
Clofibrate
Co-trimoxazole
Cyclophosphamide
Fluconazole
Miconazole
Monoamine-oxidase inhibitors
Phenylbutazone
Probenecid
Ranitidine
Rifampicin
Salicylates
Sulphinpyrazone
Sulphonamides
Tetracyclines
Trimethoprim
Warfarin and other coumarins

NB Mechanisms, multiple for some drugs, include displacement from plasma proteins (e.g. salicylates), decreased hepatic meabolism (e.g. warfarin), intrinsic hypoglycaemic activity (e.g. alcohol) and decreased renal excretion (e.g. probenecid).

MEGLITINIDES

REPAGLINIDE

The carbamolymethyl benzoic acid-derivative, repaglinide, has recently been licensed. This drug is the first of a new group of rapid-acting, insulin secretagogues, the meglitinides (meglitinide being the non-sulphonylurea portion of the glibenclamide molecule).

MODE OF ACTION

Repaglinide binds to a distinct portion of the ATP-dependent K^+ channel in the B-cell membrane. However, unlike sulphonylureas, repaglinide does not stimulate exocytosis of insulin.

PHARMACOKINETICS

Repaglinide is rapidly absorbed, has a short plasma half-life (less than 60 min), is hepatically metabolized and is excreted principally (90%) in the bile.

It is designed for use only when a meal is consumed; if a meal is skipped, no drug is taken. The tablet should ideally be taken 30 min before the meal. This mealtime dosing allows for more flexibility than is possible with once- or twice-daily sulphonylureas which have much longer duration of action (Table 3.11, p. 114). Thus, repaglinide is viewed as a prandial glucose regulator.

CLINICAL EFFICACY

Repaglinide reportedly achieves reductions in post-prandial glucose concentrations of up to 6 mmol/L. Fasting glucose levels also fall and trial data suggest that repaglinide produces reductions in glycated haemoglobin concentrations (approximately 2%) which are slightly greater second generation sulphonylureas such as gliclazide. As with sulphonylureas, selection of patients is important; there should be sufficient B-cell reserve to allow effective stimulation of endogenously-synthesized insulin.

Starting dosage is 0.5 mg (or 1 mg if transferring from another oral agent), titrated upwards at 1–2-week intervals to a maximum single dose of 4 mg with main meals; maximum total daily dose 16 mg. As monotherapy, repaglinide appears to be as effective as metformin. Combining repaglinide with metformin results in control which is superior to that obtained with either agent used alone. Repaglinide is licensed for use in patients inadequately controlled with diet and metformin.

> **NB** Repaglinide allows flexible dosing with meals for patients with type 2 diabetes.

SAFETY AND TOLERABILITY

Repaglinide is generally well tolerated. Contraindications are similar to those for sulphonylureas. Repaglinide appears to be a relatively safe choice in mild-to-moderate renal impairment. However, cautious dose titration is recommended.

• *Hypoglycaemia.* Compared with long-acting sulphonylureas, the risk of severe hypoglycaemia appears to be very low if a meal is missed and the appropriate dose is omitted; in addition, the overall frequency of severe hypoglycaemia may be lower than for sulphonylureas such as glibenclamide.

• *Weight gain.* This has been reported in studies of monotherapy and combination therapy but has generally been modest.

BIGUANIDES

Metformin (dimethylbiguanide) has been the only biguanide available in the UK since the late 1970s; it was introduced into the USA in 1995. To some extent the drug remains in the shadow cast by phenformin which was withdrawn because of an unacceptable incidence of severe, and often fatal, lactic acidosis; this is reflected in the contraindications pertaining to the use of metformin. The metabolic actions of the drug are complex and remain incompletely delineated. It is used either as monotherapy, in combination with sulphonylureas – where the effect on glycaemia is greater than that observed with either drug alone – or less commonly as an adjunct to insulin. Metformin's mode of action, pharmacokinetics and its adverse effects are distinct from those of the sulphonylureas.

MODE OF ACTION

In contrast to the sulphonylureas, metformin does not increase insulin secretion; plasma concentrations of the hormone are either unchanged or decline during treatment. This occurs in concert with a reduction in hyperglycaemia; the drug is therefore regarded as having direct insulin-sensitizing properties. By suppressing gluconeogenesis (the formation of glucose from other 3-carbon intermediates), metformin reduces hepatic glucose output, the principal determinant of fasting plasma glucose levels. In addition, improved insulin action serves to limit post-prandial plasma glucose excursions by promoting tissue glucose uptake with oxidation or storage as glycogen. These effects appear to be mainly due to intracellular actions of the drug distal to the interaction between insulin and its membrane receptor. No convincing effect in reducing GI glucose absorption has been demonstrated although body weight tends to fall on treatment reflecting an anorectic effect. This property makes metformin particularly suitable for overweight or obese patients. The principal metabolic effects of metformin are summarized in Fig. 3.3.

Effects on fatty acid metabolism may contribute to the improvement in glycaemia through decreased activity of the glucose–fatty acid (Randle) cycle in muscle and liver in which these substrates compete for uptake and oxidation (see Section 1, p. 7). Metformin has effects on some other components of the metabolic syndrome (Table 3.15). The clinical implications of these effects are generally only modest and their clinical relevance remains undetermined. However, the beneficial effects of metformin monotherapy in overweight patients in the UKPDS (see p. 65) was not explained entirely by improvement in glycaemia.

NB Metformin has beneficial effects on some components of the metabolic syndrome.

PHARMACOKINETICS

Metformin is absorbed predominantly from the small intestine, attaining high local concentrations. The bioavailability of an oral dose is 50–60%; the

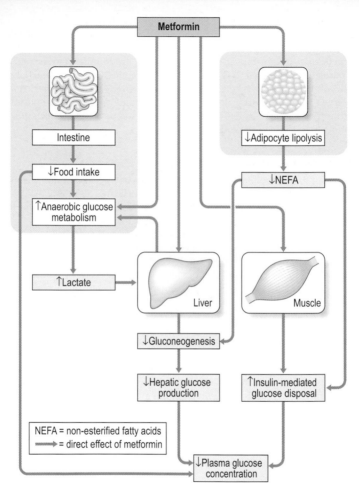

Fig. 3.3 Postulated molecular mechanisms of action of metformin. (Redrawn with permission from: Krentz AJ. Prescriber 1998; 9: 67–78.)

mean plasma half-life is between 2 and 3 hours necessitating 2–3 daily doses. Metformin is not bound to plasma proteins and is therefore not subject to displacement by other drugs such as sulphonylureas. No hepatic metabolism occurs, virtually all of the drug being excreted unchanged in the urine; the drug is secreted by renal tubules.

TABLE 3.15 Effects of metformin on cardiovascular risk factors

Action	Comments
Improved glycaemic control	Hyperglycaemia is linearly associated with CHD in type 2 diabetes
Reduced insulin levels	The role of hyperinsulinaemia in the promotion of atherosclerosis remains controversial
Improved insulin sensitivity	Theoretically of benefit but no clinical evidence of reduced cardiovascular risk
Weight loss	Averages 1–3% during treatment with dietary compliance
Improved lipid profile	Variable reductions in cholesterol and triglycerides; inconsistent reports of increases in HDL-cholesterol
Reduced BP	In obese, non-diabetic women; no convincing evidence in diabetics
Enhanced fibrinolysis	Clinical significance uncertain; relevance to UKPDS results?

ADVERSE EFFECTS

GI disturbances

GI symptoms are perhaps encountered in rather more than the 5–20% of patients suggested by clinical trials. Symptoms include nausea, anorexia, abdominal discomfort and diarrhoea. The last symptom may be troublesome enough to prompt imaging of the lower GI tract; symptoms resolve rapidly on withdrawal. A minority of patients (10% or more) are unable to tolerate these effects and compliance may be reduced in other patients. Introduction of metformin at a low dose – 500 mg daily for the first week – can help reduce the frequency and severity of GI symptoms which may be transient and self-limiting. Other side effects are rare; although reduced serum concentrations of vitamin B_{12} and folate are well documented during metformin treatment, anaemia is virtually never encountered and in practice this risk can be ignored.

Lactate metabolism

Effects of biguanides on other aspects of intermediary metabolism are well documented. Clinically, elevated blood lactate concentrations have been the primary focus of attention because of the association between these drugs and lactic acidosis. For metformin, the risk of fatality from lactic acidosis is estimated to be similar to that from sulphonylurea-induced hypoglycaemia. Unlike phenformin, which inhibits mitochondrial lactate oxidation, metformin has only minor effects on blood lactate unless concentrations of the drug rise to toxic levels. The intrinsic risk of lactic acidosis is considerably lower with metformin than phenformin and the majority of reported cases of metformin-associated lactic acidosis in recent years have been encountered in patients with contraindications to its use (Table 3.16).

Table 3.16 Principal contraindications to metformin

Contraindication	Comments
Renal impairment	Withdraw if plasma creatinine concentration elevated
Cardiac failure	Tissue hypoxia causes increased anaerobic metabolism; hepatic and renal function may also be impaired, failure leading to decreased lactate metabolism and accumulation of metformin, respectively
Ischaemic heart disease	Increased tissue lactate production
Peripheral vascular disease	Increased tissue lactate production during exercise
Hepatic impairment	Decreased lactate clearance
Alcoholism	Decreased lactate clearance
Chronic pulmonary disease	Risk of hypoxaemia
Radiological contrast studies	Withdraw metformin temporarily; maintain adequate hydration

NB The risk of fatality from metformin-associated lactic acidosis is similar to that from sulphonylurea-induced hypoglycaemia.

The principal contraindication is renal impairment since this leads to accumulation of the drug. Particular care should be exercised in patients with proteinuria, the earliest clinical indicator of diabetic nephropathy; renal function should be checked at least annually. An elevated plasma creatinine may denote significant loss of renal function, particularly in elderly patients, mandating withdrawal of the drug. Metformin is generally avoided in clinical conditions in which lactate production is increased (e.g. cardiopulmonary disease) or hepatic clearance impaired (e.g. alcoholism). A cautious approach to prescribing may have contributed to the low rate of reported lactic acidosis in the UK and elsewhere. However, there is evidence that patients with contraindications receive the drug inappropriately.

 Renal impairment is the principal contraindication to metformin therapy.

Hypoglycaemia
A noteworthy aspect of metformin is the virtual absence of risk of hypoglycaemia when used as monotherapy, even when taken in overdose. It has been suggested that this protection is a consequence of continued delivery of lactate (derived from the splanchnic bed) and other gluconeogenic precursors which help to sustain hepatic glucose production as plasma

glucose levels decline). Increased intestinal anaerobic glucose metabolism may also contribute to metformin's anti-hyperglycaemic effects (Fig. 3.3).

DRUG INTERACTIONS

The renal clearance of metformin is reduced by cimetidine and a dosage reduction is appropriate in these circumstances. Metformin may potentiate the hypoglycaemic effects of sulphonylureas.

α-GLUCOSIDASE INHIBITORS

ACARBOSE

Acarbose is the only α-glucosidase inhibitor currently available in the UK; others are in development. The drug, a pseudotetrasaccharide, acts by competitive inhibition of α-glucosidase enzymes (maximal activity against sucrase) in the brush border of the small intestine. The rate of absorption of glucose derived from the enzymatic breakdown of complex dietary carbohydrates is thereby reduced or delayed.

> **NB** Acarbose reduces intestinal absorption of glucose by inhibiting digestive enzyme activities.

For optimal effect, acarbose is taken directly before a meal with a little liquid or chewed with the first mouthful of food. Its main effect is to reduce post-prandial hyperglycaemia although fasting glucose and HbA_{1c} levels may also improve.

Improvement in insulin sensitivity in subjects with impaired glucose tolerance has been reported; postulated mechanisms include reduction of glucose toxicity and hyperinsulinaemia, the latter leading to up-regulation of tissue insulin receptors. Reported stimulation of glucagon-like peptide-1 release from the gut wall may also be relevant. However, acarbose has no direct effects on endogenous insulin release from B-cells and does not affect body weight.

PHARMACOKINETICS

The therapeutic effects of acarbose do not depend on systemic absorption. By contrast, other drugs in this class, e.g. miglitol, are absorbed. Intestinal absorption of acarbose is minimal, a reflection of its molecular size. This may explain the low frequency of side effects such as skin rashes. However, the drug is metabolized by intestinal microorganisms, the inactive metabolites being excreted in the faeces or absorbed and excreted in the urine.

EFFICACY

Acarbose was evaluated in a substudy within the UKPDS (see p. 65). The addition of acarbose to other therapy was associated with an average reduction in median HbA_{1c} of 0.7% at 36 months. A treatment effect was observed in all subgroups. An intention to treat analysis confirmed a small but significant reduction in HbA_{1c} (8.1 vs 8.5%, $P<0.003$).

ADVERSE EFFECTS

GI symptoms

Since the action of acarbose is reduction of glucose absorption in the small intestine, increased carbohydrate is delivered to the large bowel. Fermentation produces intestinal gas resulting in flatulence, abdominal bloating and diarrhoea; these symptoms, which are dose-dependent, occur in 30–75% of patients according to clinical trial reports. Commencing treatment at low doses (50 mg o.d. or b.d.) with slow dose escalation reduces the frequency of symptoms (Table 3.17).

TABLE 3.17 Manufacturer's recommended dosage escalation for acarbose

Week	1	50 mg once daily with main meal
	2	
	3	
	4	
	5	50 mg twice daily
	6	
	7	50 mg three times daily

NB If stomach ache or excessive flatus occurs on increasing the dose, go back one step for another two weeks; then try increasing the dose again.

Advice on avoidance of sucrose in the diet should be reinforced prior to initiating treatment. It is suggested that the decline in frequency of symptoms during the first few weeks of treatment is due to gradual increases in glucosidase activity in the distal small intestine. The drug is contraindicated in intestinal obstruction and in the presence of hepatic dysfunction; the drug has not been assessed in patients with severe renal impairment (Table 3.18). Acarbose is not used during pregnancy or lactation, contraindications which extend to all oral antidiabetic agents.

Hypoglycaemia

When used as monotherapy, acarbose, like metformin, does not cause hypoglycaemia. It may, however, potentiate the hypoglycaemic effects of

TABLE 3.18 Contraindications to acarbose

- Pregnancy and lactation
- Inflammatory bowel disease
- Colonic ulceration
- Intestinal obstruction
- Predisposition to intestinal obstruction
- Hepatic impairment
- Severe renal impairment (<25 ml/min/1.73m^2)
- History of abdominal surgery

sulphonylureas and insulin. Oral treatment should be with glucose since absorption of ingested sucrose will be impaired by the action of the drug.

Hepatic effects
Reversible elevations of plasma concentrations of hepatic transaminases have been reported at high doses. The drug should be avoided in patients with pre-existing hepatic dysfunction. Plasma transaminase levels should be monitored at maximal doses (200 mg t.d.s.). In addition, there have been several reports of more severe but reversible hepatic dysfunction including jaundice. Histologically, an inflammatory cell infiltrate has been observed. This reaction appears to be idiosyncratic.

DRUG INTERACTIONS

The therapeutic effects of acarbose may be reduced by charcoal and pancreatin- and amylase-containing preparations used for pancreatic exocrine insufficiency. Neomycin and cholestyramine may enhance the effects of acarbose on glycaemia; the former drug may also exacerbate its side effects.

THIAZOLIDINEDIONES

The thiazolidinediones represent a new class of drugs which have the effect of enhancing certain metabolic actions of insulin (see p. 3).

MODE OF ACTION

The thiazolidinediones lower glucose by two main mechanisms:

- Increased glucose disposal in peripheral tissues (the principal effect).
- Decreased hepatic glucose production.

These actions are mediated via effects of the drugs with a specific nuclear receptor – the peroxisome proliferator-activated-receptor-gamma (PPAR-γ). Activation of this receptor increases transcription of certain insulin-sensitive genes influencing adipocyte differentiation and function. The active form of

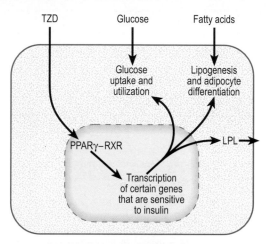

Fig. 3.4 Postulated molecular mechanisms of thiazolidinediones. Key: TZD, thiazolidinedione; PPAR-γ-RXR, peroxisome proliferator-activated receptor-γ-retinoid X receptor complex; LPL, lipoprotein lipase. (Redrawn with permission from Day C. Diabetic Med 1999; 16: 179–192.)

PPAR-γ is a heterodimer with the retinoid-X receptor (Fig. 3.4). Binding of thiazolidinediones to this complex induces a conformational change which ultimately alters the expression of genes involved in the regulation of lipid metabolism including:

- Lipoprotein lipase.
- Fatty acid transporter protein.
- Fatty acyl CoA-synthase.
- Malic enzyme.
- Glucokinase.

Effects on GLUT-4 (see p. 6) and adipocyte leptin expression have also been reported. The combined effect is to increase the uptake of non-esterified fatty acids and increase lipogenesis within adipocytes. However, the precise mechanisms through which these drugs improve insulin sensitivity in glucose metabolism remain to be determined.

Effects on the glucose–fatty acid cycle (see p. 7) are an attractive possibility; amelioration of insulin resistance via reduction in adipocyte-derived, tumour-necrosis factor-α is another (see p. 30). Thiazolidinediones require the presence of a sufficient amount of insulin in order to exert a therapeutic effect. Combining troglitazone with sulphonylureas or metformin is beneficial and may enhance the glucose-lowering effect; insulin doses may be reduced substantially in obese insulin-treated patients with a concomitant improvement in glycaemic control.

TROGLITAZONE
CLINICAL PHARMACOLOGY

Troglitazone is the most-studied drug in the class. It is strongly lipophilic and circulates almost completely bound to plasma proteins. Metabolism occurs in the liver with elimination principally via the bile and faeces. Bioavailability (approximately 50%) is enhanced to some degree by food. Absorption is rapid with peak levels attained in 1–3 hours. Troglitazone produces a lowering of blood glucose levels to a magnitude similar to monotherapy with either a sulphonylurea or metformin (i.e. by approximately 15–25%) in patients with type 2 diabetes; it should be noted that a maximal effect may take 8 weeks to become apparent. In addition to its glucose-lowering action troglitazone causes dose-dependent reductions in plasma concentrations of:

- Insulin.
- C-peptide.
- Non-esterified fatty acids.
- Triglycerides.

Improved insulin action in glucose metabolism has been confirmed using the glucose clamp technique; improvements of up to 50% in insulin-mediated glucose disposal may occur in obese, insulin-resistant individuals (see Section 1). However, it should be noted that 25% or more of trial patients have not shown a therapeutic response to troglitazone; overweight, insulin-resistant patients appear to be the most appropriate candidates for the drug. Effects on other aspects of lipid metabolism include a rise in cardioprotective HDL-cholesterol; however, LDL-cholesterol may also increase, offsetting the beneficial effect. Apolipoprotein B levels are unaffected.

The effects on fatty acids and triglycerides appear to be less dependent on the presence of circulating insulin than the effect on blood glucose. There have been reports of a BP-lowering effect although such an effect has not been evident in all studies. In view of the putative relationship between insulin resistance and hypertension, both of which are prominent features of type 2 diabetes, this observation is of interest. The relevance of the antioxidant effects of troglitazone (which contains a vitamin E moiety) is uncertain (see micronutrients, p. 95).

ADVERSE EFFECTS

Hepatotoxicity
This is the major issue with troglitazone. More than 20 fatalities have been linked to exposure to the drug. Troglitazone is contraindicated in patients with elevations of hepatic transaminases >1.5 of the upper limit of the reference range. A history of liver disease serves as another contraindication.

Hepatic disease is a contraindication to troglitazone.

Monthly measurements of alanine aminotransferase are required during the initial 12 months of therapy, the frequency of testing being reduced thereafter to 3-monthly. Hepatotoxicity appears to be reversible with prompt withdrawal of the drug. Therapy should be discontinued if transaminase levels rise >3 times the upper limit of normal; lesser increases (1.5–2.0) are an indication for weekly monitoring until they return to normal. Troglitazone is no longer licensed for use as initial monotherapy in the USA.

 Careful monitoring of liver function tests is required especially during the early stages of treatment with troglitazone.

Weight gain

Increases of several kilograms in body weight have been reported in clinical trials. This appears to be predictable from the insulin-sensitizing and lipogenic effects of the drug; improved glycaemic control may also reduce urinary glucose losses. There are reports that troglitazone preferentially increases subcutaneous fat deposits whereas visceral adiposity (see p. 19) is simultaneously reduced.

Hypoglycaemia

Although troglitazone is classed as an anti-hyperglycaemic rather than hypoglycaemic drug (Table 3.8, p. 108), the possibility of hypoglycaemia exists when the drug is combined with other agents such as sulphonylureas or insulin; careful monitoring of blood glucose is required and insulin doses may have to be reduced, sometimes substantially.

Cardiovascular effects

Fluid retention with oedema (possibly related to a vasodilator effect), haemodilution and minor decreases in haematocrit have also been reported with troglitazone and rosiglitazone. However, concerns about cardiac hypertrophy in animal studies have not been apparent in humans.

ROSIGLITAZONE

Rosiglitazone is a more potent and more efficacious drug (in terms of glucose-lowering) than troglitazone. The daily recommended dose is 2–4 mg b.d. (or

4–8 mg o.d.). As monotherapy, rosiglitazone 4 mg b.d. produces a reduction in HbA$_{1c}$ of 1.5%; this exceeds the average fall observed with troglitazone.

ADVERSE EFFECTS

Most importantly, there is no evidence to date that rosiglitazone shares the hepatotoxic potential of troglitazone. Nonetheless, baseline and 2-monthly monitoring of plasma alanine aminotransferase is recommended during the first year of treatment. Dose reduction is required in patients with impaired hepatic function; the drug should not be used at all in patients with pre-existing transaminase levels >2.5 times the normal upper limit.

Rosiglitazone monotherapy appears to be associated with a low risk (<2%) of hypoglycaemia. However, as for troglitazone, combination therapy with other agents such as sulphonylureas or insulin may increase the risk of hypoglycaemia. In contrast with troglitazone, rosiglitazone does not induce cytochrome P4503A4 metabolism. Rosiglitazone does not interact significantly with drugs such as nifedipine, oral contraceptives, metformin or acarbose.

PIOGLITAZONE

Pioglitazone is administered once daily in a dose of 30–45 mg. No significant alterations in plasma LDL-cholesterol have been observed in clinical trials to date. This contrasts with the increases in LDL-cholesterol levels reported with troglitazone and rosiglitazone. Pioglitazone, in common with the other thiazolidinediones, may be usefully combined with sulphonylureas, metformin or insulin.

INSULIN THERAPY

Insulin is life sustaining in patients with type 1 diabetes (see Sections 1 and 2). In addition, insulin is often used to improve metabolic control in patients with type 2 diabetes. Technological developments in insulin manufacture have led to welcome refinements, initially with improvements in purity then with the mass production of insulin identical with the human molecule. These have been coupled with easier and more comfortable methods for injection making the practicalities much less daunting.

However, after more than 60 years' experience, the optimal use of insulin and avoidance of the major effect of excess insulin action – hypoglycaemia – remain incompletely determined (see p. 156). Moreover, the widespread transfer to human sequence insulin was associated with difficulties on a scale unforeseen by most diabetologists in the UK. However, it might be argued that this experience has provided insights into the beliefs of at least some patients (and their doctors) about insulin therapy. Subcutaneous insulin can provide only an approximation of the exquisitely-tuned response of the islet B-cells to secretagogues (see p. 3).

Fundamental problems associated with the use of exogenous insulin include:

- Delivery into the systemic rather than portal circulation. This means that plasma insulin concentrations are equally high in the systemic circulation rather than the physiological situation in which portal levels are higher than systemic levels. Thus, hyperinsulinaemia is common.
- Pharmacokinetic differences – delayed onset of action, relative prolongation of effect compared with endogenously secreted insulin, i.e. impaired matching of rise and fall in relation to meals.
- Inability to reduce plasma insulin levels in response to fasting or exercise once insulin has been injected.
- Difficulty in controlling fasting plasma glucose concentration – via suppression of hepatic glucose production – without inducing hypoglycaemia during the night.
- Day-to-day variability in absorption in individual patients; this is higher than is generally appreciated.
- Dietary constraints which include consuming approximately similar quantities of carbohydrate for meals each day and the frequent need for between-meal snacks to prevent pre-prandial hypoglycaemia.

Other difficulties may be presented by certain clinical situations:

- High insulin requirements in obese patients with type 2 diabetes (common) or those with additional causes for insulin resistance (see p. 28).
- Impairment of insulin clearance by complications such as uraemia (relatively common) or the presence of hepatic cirrhosis with risk of hypoglycaemia (see p. 156).
- Increased sensitivity to exogenous insulin in patients with chronic pancreatitis, hypoadrenalism (rare), hypopituitarism (rare).
- Alteration of distribution of circulating insulin by high titres of anti-insulin antibodies (rare, and usually in patients treated for many years with older, unpurified insulins).
- Lower insulin requirements when changing from bovine to porcine or human sequence insulins.
- Propensity for weight gain following the institution of insulin treatment for type 2 diabetes.

When the disparities between normal physiology and exogenous insulin therapy are considered, it is perhaps all the more surprising that so many patients achieve such satisfactory results. The complexity of multiple insulin formulations, delivery devices and regimens has increased recently with the introduction of the rapid-acting insulin analogues, lispro (Humalog®, Eli Lilly) and insulin aspart (Rapitard®, Novo Nordisk). There are currently more than 30 insulin preparations available in the UK. A comprehensive account of all the options would rapidly become outdated by developments.

TYPE 1 DIABETES

Insulin therapy is mandatory for patients with type 1 diabetes (see pp. 14 and 52). Uninterrupted therapy is necessary to avoid potentially life-threatening metabolic decompensation. Occasionally, insulin therapy may be successfully discontinued in a patient who presented with apparent ketosis-prone diabetes. However, this requires careful judgement by an experienced clinician and the general advice to the patient must be to <u>never</u> discontinue insulin.

 Patients with type 1 diabetes should never discontinue their insulin treatment without expert approval.

It is vital that insulin therapy is accompanied by self-monitoring of capillary glucose by the patient (see p. 73) wherever possible.

INITIATION OF INSULIN TREATMENT

The ill patient

The newly-presenting patient with type 1 diabetes who is ill with hyperglycaemia, particularly in concert with heavy ketonuria, should be admitted to hospital promptly for assessment and treatment (see p. 38). Intravenous fluids and insulin may be necessary if there is significant decompensation. When the diabetes has been brought under control, the patient can be transferred to a suitable subcutaneous regimen prior to discharge. The initial treatment of children with diabetes is considered on pages 262–268.

The well patient

For patients not clinically unwell at presentation, insulin treatment may be started on an out-patient basis; this should not usually be delayed more than a few days from diagnosis. Early treatment will:

- Remove the risk of serious metabolic decompensation.
- Relieve the patient of distressing osmotic symptoms.

The basic rules for starting insulin are:

- Relatively small doses initially; avoid hypoglycaemia.
- Patient (or parent if a child) to administer first injection if possible.
- Start treatment as out-patient in most cases.
- Close supervision or assistance from an appropriately-trained professional.

It is difficult to give precise recommendations on the first dose since there is a paucity of data in the literature. However, a daily dose of 16–24 units is appropriate for the majority of adult patients. Larger doses carry the risk of inducing hypoglycaemia thereby denting the patient's faith in the clinician. There is no justification for deliberately inducing an episode of hypoglycaemia (as was once the norm in some centres).

> **NB** Care should be taken to avoid symptomatic hypoglycaemia when insulin is initiated.

This is best administered as two injections of insulin with a medium-duration of action (including biphasic insulins, e.g. 30/70 or 50/50 short-to-medium duration mixtures).

Conventionally, the insulin dose is divided as follows:

- Approximately 70% of the total dose pre-breakfast.
- The remaining 30% before the evening meal.

Alternatively, pre-meal injections of small doses (4–6 units) pre-meals can be given. This allows the patient more practice of giving injections under supervision; transfer to twice-daily insulin would then be appropriate for many patients after the first day or two rather than continuing with a q.d.s. regimen indefinitely.

Close supervision is essential as is readily-obtainable advice, in person or by telephone, from the diabetes care team. Most patients will be started on insulin under the guidance of the local hospital diabetes resource centre or clinic. Some patients, be they elderly, senile or infirm, may be unable to self-administer insulin. Reliance is then placed on a responsible relative or district nurse.

Insulin preparations

The plethora of insulin preparations can be daunting. However, the types of insulin and methods of delivery can be summarized relatively succinctly. On a practical level, it is sensible to acquire familiarity with a few examples in each category. Insulin is one of the few drugs which are prescribed by brand rather than generically in the UK. However, insulin preparations can be classified into relatively few categories according to:

- Species and method of manufacture – animal-derived, semi-synthetic or synthetic.
- Modifications which prolong duration of action.
- Designated mode of delivery (via syringe, pen injector, doser).
- Strength – in the UK all insulin preparations contain 100 units per mL (U100). Other strengths (U40, U80) are still available in some countries.

In addition, the type of preservative is usually manufacturer-specific.

Insulin species

There are three species options:

● *Bovine*. Extracted from cattle pancreas; effectively obsolete but still available for patients who have been on this species for many years. Long-term use often associated with presence of anti-insulin antibodies. Bovine insulin differs from human insulin (Fig. 1.1, p. 3) in three aminoacids (A8, A10 and B30).

● *Porcine*. Differs from human insulin by a single aminoacid (alanine replaces threonine at B30; Fig. 1.1, p. 3). Reserved mainly for patients who have experienced a perceived decrease in warning symptoms of hypoglycaemia with human insulin (see p. 159).

● *Human*. By far the most commonly used and now manufactured predominantly using recombinant DNA technology. Chemical modification of porcine insulin (emp) also still used by one major manufacturer (Novo Nordisk) – so-called 'semi-synthetic' insulin. Method of manufacture is stated on the insulin bottle:
  — *prb* – produced from the precursor molecule proinsulin synthesized by bacteria containing the human proinsulin gene.
  — *pyr* – produced from a precursor synthesized by yeast.
  — *ge* – a more generic abbreviation, i.e. genetically engineered.

  In addition, the insulin analogues – insulin lispro and insulin aspart – have recently been introduced. These are novel molecules not found in nature (Fig. 1.1, p. 3); they are products of genetic engineering:

● *Insulin lispro*. This differs from human insulin in the positions of the aminoacids, B28 proline and B29 lysine (lys-pro becoming lispro), on the B-chain of the molecule.

● *Insulin aspart*. At position B28, proline is replaced by aspartic acid.

  In the UK, bovine insulin is now reserved for the relatively small group of patients who have been treated with this species for many years. Because it differs from human sequence insulin by two aminoacids, it is more antigenic. In addition, earlier insulin preparations had appreciable non-insulin impurities. These patients often have high titres of anti-insulin antibodies which can modify the pharmacokinetics of exogenous insulin, basically prolonging the action of short-acting insulins. Patients being transferred from bovine to human insulins may require a reduction in dose; a 20% initial reduction is recommended to avoid hypoglycaemia. The risk is generally much lower for patients previously treated with porcine insulin unless they have been exposed to older less purified preparations.

> **Patients being transferred from animal to human insulin may require dose reductions.**

Porcine insulin is less immunogenic than bovine insulin. The majority of patients previously treated with porcine insulins have been transferred to human sequence insulin uneventfully. A significant minority, however, insist that they find their diabetes easier to control using porcine insulin, particularly with regard to recognition of hypoglycaemia; the continued availability of this species – in vials only – is in recognition of these often strongly-held views; porcine insulin otherwise offers no advantage over human insulin. The contentious issue of insulin species and hypoglycaemia is discussed on page 162. Note that animal insulins are unacceptable to devout followers of Islam and Judaism and to strict vegans.

Duration of action

● *Short-acting insulins.* First, it should be noted that short-acting insulins (synonyms: soluble, clear, regular, neutral, unmodified) differ slightly in their pharmacokinetics according to species; onset of action following subcutaneous injection is fastest for human, followed by porcine and finally bovine.

> **NB** Human sequence short-acting insulins have a slightly faster onset and shorter duration of action than animal insulins.

These differences, which may reflect lipophilic properties, are small but may be noticeable in some circumstances, particularly when control is already good. For insulin to exert its effects in target tissues it must be absorbed from the subcutaneous injection site and diffuse from the interstitial space into the circulation. The rate at which this occurs is the principal determinant of the speed of onset of the insulin.

Other factors influencing pharmacokinetics include:

● Site of injection – absorption from abdominal wall is faster than from thigh.
● Volume of insulin injected – smaller volumes are more rapidly absorbed.
● Local mechanical factors – massage of injection site increases absorption.

Note that insulin can become denatured with loss of activity if exposed to extremes of high or low temperature; storage at 4°C in a domestic refrigerator is usually recommended; do not freeze. For human short-acting insulin preparations, following subcutaneous injection, the approximate duration of action is as follows:

- Onset – 30 min.
- Peak – 1–3 hours.
- Duration – 4–8 hours.

When injected intravenously, the plasma half-life is less than 5 min; a continuous infusion is therefore required to maintain plasma levels since the insulin will dissipate too rapidly for a sustained therapeutic effect. The only notable exceptions are when an intravenous bolus is required in a diagnostic endocrine test, i.e. the insulin tolerance test, in the assessment of possible severe insulin resistance, or for research purposes. It should be noted that these are the only insulins suitable for intravenous administration – modified insulins must only be injected subcutaneously.

 NB Only unmodified soluble insulins are suitable for intravenous use.

Intramuscular injections last longer but are rarely indicated except as a less attractive alternative to intravenous infusion in the management of DKA (see p. 168). However, inadvertent intramuscular injection is common in thinner patients with little subcutaneous adipose tissue; this may lead to more rapid absorption. This is a particular hazard for the rare patient with lipoatrophic diabetes who requires insulin.

 NB Unintentional intramuscular insulin injection may occur in thin patients with little subcutaneous adipose tissue.

The pharmacokinetics dictate the use of these insulins which should ideally be injected 30–45 min before meals. However, this recommendation is often flouted for obvious practical reasons; a compromise of 10–30 min may be reasonable. The aim is to have plasma insulin levels rising in order to control the increase in plasma glucose that follows the meal; avoidance of hypoglycaemia before the subsequent meal completes the therapeutic objective. If a meal is delayed, there is a risk of hypoglycaemia, particularly if pre-prandial blood glucose is already low. For an elderly patient, possibly senile, reliant on a third party for insulin administration it may be safer to ensure that the meal has been eaten first.

NB Conventional short-acting insulins ideally should be injected 30–45 min pre-meals; in practice, this is often ignored.

• *Rapid-acting insulin analogues*. These are characterized by more rapid absorption, earlier peak and reduced duration of action compared with human soluble insulin:

- Onset – 10–20 min.
- Peak – 1 hour.
- Duration – 3–5 hours.

The analogues represent alternatives to soluble insulin, being designed for use immediately before (or even just after) meals. There is some evidence that their use may be advantageous in the management of some patients with symptomatic unawareness of hypoglycaemia (see p. 159) or nocturnal hypoglycaemia. Studies with insulin aspart demonstrate improved overall glycaemic control and a reduced risk of major nocturnal hypoglycaemia, compared with conventional soluble insulin in patients with type 1 diabetes; patient satisfaction is also improved. However, there are certain situations, e.g. brittle diabetes (see pp. 165 and 266), in which the shorter duration of action of these analogues may be a disadvantage. For patients poorly compliant with their insulin, the rapid dissipation of the analogues might predispose to DKA (see p.168). If adequate basal insulin is administered, e.g. ultralente or b.d. isophane, this risk is diminished and may also facilitate better long-term glycaemic control. Pregnancy is another area where caution with analogues is recommended.

• *Twice-daily mixtures*. Short-acting insulins may be mixed with longer-acting preparations (isophane or less commonly lente) by the patient and are also available in fixed pre-mixed combinations which vary from 10/90 (e.g. Humulin M1, Human Mixtard 10) to 50/50 ratios of short to isophane (e.g. Humulin M5, Human Mixtard 50). A 30/70 mixture is most favoured in the UK and provides a reasonable degree of insulinization throughout the 24-hour period. Although the ratio of insulins is fixed, it is of course possible to use different preparations for the morning and evening injections if the glucose profile suggests that this would be advantageous. Pre-mixed insulins incorporating the insulin analogue lispro and lispro protamine (25/75) have also been introduced in some countries; these are designed to be administered immediately before or even just after meals. Fixed ratios of unmodified insulin aspart to longer-acting insulin are under investigation.

• *Multiple daily insulin injections*. Alternatively, short-acting insulins can be injected pre-breakfast, pre-lunch and pre-dinner; a longer-acting insulin is usually required at 2200 h to provide control through to the following morning. Coupled with frequent blood glucose testing, this regimen forms the basis for so-called intensified insulin therapy when near-normoglycaemia is the aim. It is noteworthy that when transferring from once- or twice-daily to multiple injections, increasing the number of injections may bring improved control with a similar or even lower total daily insulin dose. In part, this may reflect the greater efficiency of closer matching of insulin action to meals.

> **NB** Metabolic control may be obtained with a similar total daily insulin dose if delivered as multiple injections.

Conversely, once-daily insulin will rarely prove sufficient, at least with modern insulin preparations; this would certainly be unsuitable for patients requiring moderate-to-good glycaemic control but may be justified in the occasional elderly or infirm patient in whom good glycaemic control is not being sought.

> **NB** Once-daily insulin regimens generally provide inadequate control and are rarely indicated.

Nonetheless, increasing the dose to reduce fasting hyperglycaemia runs the risk of hypoglycaemia at other times of the day. A general rule of thumb is that a total daily dose of 30–40 units or greater is best given as two or more injections. The exception is when insulin is administered at bedtime in patients with type 2 diabetes, the principal aim being to control fasting plasma glucose concentrations.

Although the DCCT (see p. 60) gave impetus to better glycaemic control, intensified insulin therapy is not suitable for all patients with type 1 diabetes, nor can it be provided routinely and safely by busy hospital clinics. Prerequisites include a commitment to the rigours required in terms of self-monitoring. Contraindications to intensive insulin therapy are presented in Table 3.1 (p. 87). As originally conceived, the aim of pre-meal injections of short-acting insulin, coupled with an injection of longer-acting insulin, was to mimic the major physiological components of daily insulin secretion (see Section 1). Approximately 50% of endogenously-derived insulin is secreted to provide a background or base upon which are superimposed discrete peri-meal boluses of secreted insulin. Long-acting bovine crystalline insulin preparations were often used to provide the basal component. This insulin was considered to be difficult to use in practice since accumulation would occur with successive daily doses; a change in dose would not become evident for several days.

The newer ultralente preparation, Human Ultratard (Novo Nordisk), has a shorter duration of action and is perhaps more appropriately considered a twice-daily insulin. In fact, many UK clinics use isophane preparations accepting that true 24-hour cover is unlikely; reliance is placed on the short-acting insulin component to maintain pre-prandial insulinization. Some centres combine pre-prandial soluble with b.d. protaphane insulin. It should be noted that transfer to a multiple injection regimen does not guarantee improved glycaemic control. The matching of pre-prandial insulin injections to meals, particularly when timing is irregular from day to day, provides greater flexibility, and overall glycaemic control is similar to that observed with twice-daily insulins unless determined efforts are directed at improving control. Indeed, it might be thought that the scope for abusing the regimen by omitting meals and insulin could be greater with multiple injection regimens.

Careful consideration is therefore required for each patient; multiple injections should not be a reflex response to attainment of inadequate control with more conventional regimens.

> **NB** Multiple daily insulin injection regimens do not necessarily result in improved overall glycaemic control.

● *Intermediate-duration insulins: isophane.* Complexing insulin with protamine produces cloudy isophane preparations with slower onset and longer durations of action; these are known generically as isophane or neutral protamine Hagedorn (NPH). These well-established and widely-used preparations have the following pharmacokinetic properties:

● Onset – 1–2 hours.
● Peak – 4–8 hours.
● Duration – 12–18 hours.

Such preparations (e.g. Humulin I, Human Insulatard) may be used either as twice-daily preparations as monotherapy or, more commonly, in conjunction with short-acting insulins – nowadays often as pre-mixed biphasic preparations. Patients with type 1 diabetes may find that control is satisfactory initially with twice-daily isophane insulin but that pre-lunch and pre-bed hyperglycaemia subsequently necessitates the introduction of a short-acting component. This may reflect the waning of residual insulin secretion recognized as the 'honeymoon' period (see p. 14). Alternatively, isophane insulins are injected at around 2200 h as the longer-acting, overnight component of a multiple daily injection regimen.

● *Longer-acting insulins: PZI and lente preparations.* Protamine zinc insulin (Hypurin bovine PZI, CP Pharmaceuticals) is now little used although there are some patients who have been maintained on this preparation for many years. It is a long-acting (over 24 hours) insulin which presents potential problems when mixed with short-acting insulin. This arises because an excess of protamine in the preparation effectively converts a variable and unpredictable proportion of the short-acting insulin into a longer-acting insulin. However, patients maintained on this preparation need not be transferred to alternative insulins in the absence of any difficulties. This general principle may be applied to other occasionally-encountered patients whose insulin regimens do not conform to conventional prescribing recommendations; as long as both patient and supervising clinician are satisfied there seems little to be gained for changes based on theoretical considerations.

> **NB** Unconventional insulin regimens may occasionally prove to be effective and safe in individual patients.

Increasing the zinc content of the insulin preparation results in amorphous and ultimately crystalline insulins with prolonged actions:

- Amorphous – with the shortest duration of action.
- Semilente – 30% amorphous, 70% crystalline.
- Crystalline – longest duration of action.

Examples of semilente insulins include Human Monotard (Novo Nordisk) and Humulin Lente (Eli Lilly); these are most appropriately used twice daily. Lente insulins contain an excess of zinc ions which also modify the action of short-acting insulin to some extent if mixed in the same syringe. This delays the rise in plasma insulin concentrations but in practice, this seems to be of minor clinical importance as long as the mixture is injected without delay. However, the combination of lente and short-acting insulins is not suitable for use in biphasic insulin preparations which contain isophane insulins exclusively. Lente insulins have become less popular with the emergence of the biphasic insulins.

- *Long-acting insulin analogues.* Long-acting insulin analogues are now under investigation. The first of these, HOE 901 (Hoechst Marion Roussel) should be available in 2000. This reportedly avoids the peak concentrations associated with conventional longer-acting insulins. NN 304 (Novo Nordisk) represents a different approach; a fatty acyl group is attached to the B chain of the insulin molecule which results in binding to albumin in the circulation.

Free mixing of insulins
When mixing short-acting and longer-duration insulins in the same syringe, the practical rules should be followed to avoid cross-contamination of the two vials; the short-acting insulin should always be drawn up first:

1. Draw up volume of air equivalent to required dose of isophane (cloudy) insulin into the syringe.
2. Inject this air into isophane insulin vial.
3. Draw up volume of air equivalent to required dose of short-acting (clear) insulin into syringe.
4. Inject this air into short-acting insulin vial.
5. Draw up the dose of short-acting insulin, expelling air bubbles by gentle tapping of syringe.
6. Carefully draw up the dose of isophane from the cloudy vial, avoiding injecting any of the syringe contents back into this vial.

INSULIN DELIVERY SYSTEMS

Subcutaneous insulin injections

Self-administered subcutaneous injection using a syringe has been the mainstay of insulin therapy since its first clinical application in 1922. Advances in design have made insulin injection in the modern era more convenient and much less unpleasant. No longer must reusable glass syringes and needles be sterilized and stored in surgical spirit. Injection site abscesses, rare even in those days, are today virtually unheard of. Disposable, plastic insulin syringes with integral fine, lubricated needles are the norm. These can be reused for a week or more and are simply stored in a domestic refrigerator between injections. The safety of this practice is undisputed and local sepsis is most unlikely.

> **NB** Disposable, plastic insulin syringes may be reused several times by an individual patient.

Blunting of the needle, which nowadays is of narrower Gauge (28 or 29) than those used with the old glass syringes (17), tends to be the limiting factor. There are several U100 syringes available in the following sizes:

- 1.0 mL – 100 unit maximum capacity.
- 0.5 mL – 50 unit maximum capacity.
- 0.3 mL – 30 unit maximum capacity.

Care should be taken to note whether gradations are marked in 1 or 2 unit increments. Technical problems with modern syringes are very uncommon. Cloudy insulins should be inverted a few times to ensure adequate suspension.

Injection technique

The insulin is drawn up as previously outlined taking particular care to expel bubbles of air. It is no longer considered necessary to prepare the injection site with an alcohol swab although the skin should at least be clean. The following steps are routinely recommended:

- Raise a thick pinch of skin between forefinger and thumb at the intended injection site.
- Insert the needle decisively up to the hilt at an angle between 45 and 90°.
- Depress the plunger firmly with sustained, smooth pressure.
- Withdraw the needle.

Drawing back on the plunger before injecting to check that a vein has not been entered is regarded as redundant advice. Too shallow an injection will be delivered intradermally; this can be painful and may cause local atrophy evident as pitting. Too deep, and the insulin may be delivered intramuscularly. Routine compression of the injection site is regarded as unnecessary.

Anatomical injection sites

Traditionally, patients are advised to rotate the location of their injection sites (Fig. 3.5). This helps to avoid local reactions to insulin, which are, principally:

● *Allergy.* Local allergic reactions are uncommon with modern insulin preparations; reactions to diluent or preservatives are sometimes thought to be of relevance; a change of brand may help but many cases resolve spontaneously. Transient tender nodules developing at the injection site are suggestive; generalized allergic reactions are exceedingly uncommon. Testing kits are available from insulin manufacturers. Major insulin resistance due to high titres of anti-insulin antibodies which cause antigen–antibody complexes is very uncommon; corticosteroids may be useful.

● *Lipohypertrophy.* Localized areas of lipohypertrophy (Plate 3), although comfortable to inject into, are thought to cause erratic absorption of insulin from the site. The hypertrophy is attributed to the trophic effects of insulin on fat metabolism. Avoidance of the area may lead to regression; liposuction has been used.

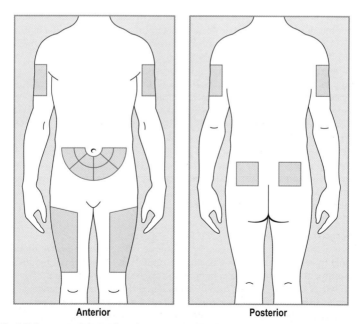

Anterior   **Posterior**

Fig. 3.5 Recommended sites for subcutaneous insulin injection.

● *Lipoatrophy*. This has become rare since the introduction of highly-purified, and more recently human sequence, insulins. It may be improved by the injection of highly-purified soluble insulin around the edge of the lesion.

Patients occasionally complain of recurrent minor local bleeding or bruising which rarely presents any real cause for concern.

Disposal of needles
Clipper devices are available for the safe disposal of used syringe needles. Boxes designed to contain used sharps should be disposed of appropriately. Local authorities may offer a needle disposal service.

Pen injector devices and insulin dosers
These have gained considerable popularity in recent years and are suitable for the majority of insulin-treated patients. Pen injectors are self-contained devices which obviate the need to draw insulin into a syringe from the vial. Errors arising from air bubbles are also eliminated as long as the needle is cleared by expelling 2–4 units before use. The required dose is dialled up and then injected by depressing a plunger. This can be useful for the visually impaired (magnifiers are available) and patients with arthritis or other physical problems interfering with manual dexterity. Compliance with treatment may be improved, especially in children and adolescents, by the use of a pen; few would opt for a conventional syringe. However, overall glycaemic control is not necessarily improved.

A range of designs with different features are available. The patient should be allowed to choose from the range. Options range from preloaded, entirely disposable, one-piece pens containing 300 units insulin and an integral needle to reusable pens which take cartridges of insulin (containing 150 units). For the latter devices, disposable needles are required. The maximum single dose that can be delivered ranges from 36 to 100 units; the lowest dose that can be delivered is 2 units. A pen may be used to give boluses of short-acting or analogue insulin more conveniently before meals. Premixed insulins can also be delivered twice-daily using pens. However, animal insulins are not available for use in pen injectors. More sophisticated insulin dosers have recently been introduced.

Continuous subcutaneous insulin infusion
This is a specialized insulin delivery technique suitable for intensive therapy offered by a few centres with a particular interest in the system; it requires commitment on the part of the patient and back-up from a diabetes care team with expertise. Briefly, insulin is delivered through a subcutaneous cannula sited in the lower abdominal wall from a programmable, battery-powered syringe driver worn on the belt. A basal rate is set upon which boluses of insulin are triggered by the patient to cover meals. The technique

requires frequent home blood glucose testing for safe use. There is a risk of mechanical failure which may lead to the rapid development of DKA (see p. 168). Skin infections are more common than with conventional injection therapy. The use of this mode of delivery has declined in recent years, and multiple daily insulin injection regimens are now preferred by most centres in the UK.

 NB Rapid development of DKA has been reported with continuous subcutaneous insulin infusion.

OTHER MODES OF INSULIN DELIVERY

These are either infrequently-used or experimental and include:

● *Jet injectors.* These are designed to eject high-pressure droplets of insulin which penetrate the skin. May be uncomfortable; insulin delivery is erratic. In any case, true needle phobia, the principal indication, is rare.

● *Implantable insulin pumps.* These are largely experimental and confined to a few enthusiastic centres. Insulin is released into the peritoneal cavity via a cannula running from the subcutaneous pump. The insulin enters the portal vein maintaining the portal:systemic ratio that pertains in normal physiology. Basal rates and bolus delivery can be programmed externally. The insulin is refilled every 1–3 months by injection. However, the technique is invasive and there is ample scope for technical difficulties; catheter blockage and insulin precipitation within the pump predominate.

● *Nasal insulin.* Bioavailability is low although absorption is rapid; experimental.

● *Pulmonary insulin.* In phase III clinical trials. The lungs have a large surface area making them an attractive site for insulin delivery by aerosol. Pre-prandial doses administered by a breath-activated device are under evaluation.

ALTERING INSULIN DOSES

Patients vary in their capacity and willingness to adjust their own insulin doses. Some will never make an adjustment; the advice of the specialist nurse can be helpful in such cases and close telephone contact is reassuring. Other patients will alter doses too frequently according to their latest home capillary readings – this can lead to a 'roller-coaster' effect with glycaemic instability and is best avoided. Although there are some general principles to be followed, there are no hard and fast rules; caution and common sense are guiding principles.

- Alter one insulin dose at a time.
- Alter the appropriate insulin based on knowledge of the pharmacokinetics of the insulin preparations being used. For example, on twice-daily mixtures of short- and medium-acting insulin:

Time of hyperglycaemia	Insulin dose to increase
Pre-breakfast	Pre-dinner (or pre-bed)
Pre-lunch	Pre-breakfast short-acting
Pre-dinner	Pre-breakfast medium-acting
Pre-bed	Pre-dinner short-acting

- Allow a few days to observe the effect of the change; daily fluctuations must be taken into account.
- A relatively small change – 2–4 units – is generally safe; larger changes may be indicated in some instances but care should be taken to avoid inducing hypoglycaemia. Such small alterations are not always appropriate; the magnitude of the increase or decrease should reflect the overall insulin dose. For example, for a patient stabilized on a daily dose of 40 units a change of 4 units is 10% of the total; for a patient on 100 units, a proportionately similar change would be 10 units. Moreover, when insulin has just been initiated, tiny daily increases in dose may be too cautious. However, experience is required in judging whether larger increases are indicated.
- If recurrent hypoglycaemia occurs at the higher dose, the patient should drop back to the previous dose pending review.
- Remember that increasing the dose of a pre-mixed insulin preparation will increase both the short- and the longer-acting components.
- Be prepared for discrepancies between theory based on insulin pharmacokinetics and the realities of clinical practice.

UNWANTED EFFECTS OF INSULIN THERAPY

Weight gain

This is a common consequence of insulin (and sulphonylurea) treatment. In patients with type 1 diabetes, some regain of lost body weight is appropriate; this reflects the physiological anabolic effects of insulin. However, in patients with type 2 diabetes, the initiation of insulin therapy because of inadequate glycaemic control with oral agents is often associated with unwelcome weight gain. Over the course of the UKPDS the gain in additional weight (above that observed in patients treated with diet alone) in the insulin-treated group was twice as large (4.0 vs 1.7 kg) than that observed with glibenclamide. Reduced urinary glucose loss has been identified as an important factor in other studies. Dietary counter-measures may be partially effective, particularly when combined with an exercise programme. Weight gain is not inevitable but it can detract from the sense of achievement for some patients. It tends to plateau after a few months possibly reflecting the resetting of a physiological homeostatic mechanism.

Insulin oedema

This is a rare complication of insulin therapy. Oedema of the feet and legs develops shortly after the initiation of insulin which resolves with continued therapy. The aetiology is uncertain but insulin-mediated sodium and water retention by the kidney has been postulated.

Transient deterioration of retinopathy

A rapid and sometimes marked transient deterioration in pre-existing retinopathy may follow the institution of improved glycaemic control, e.g. when insulin is commenced after tablet failure.

Insulin neuritis

An analogous complication is so-called insulin neuritis wherein acute symptomatic neuropathy, which may be very unpleasant, develops following the institution of insulin treatment. Histological studies in acute painful neuropathies have demonstrated actively regenerating neurones which are thought to be the origin of the symptoms. Rapid alterations in osmotically-active intraneural molecules, e.g. sorbitol (see Section 1) are thought to be relevant. The prognosis appears to be generally favourable with continued good glycaemic control. Symptomatic treatment may be required until recovery which may not always be complete; subclinical neuropathy pre-dating the improved control may have been present in some cases. The condition is uncommon.

Postural hypotension

A clinically significant fall in BP shortly after insulin injection is very rare. The vasodilator effects of insulin have been implicated but the pathophysiology remains uncertain.

Severe insulin resistance

The definition is ultimately arbitrary and time-honoured conventions such as daily insulin doses in excess of 100–200 units to control glycaemia are largely of historical interest. The concept of insulin resistance is discussed on pages 28–35.

● *Severe insulin resistance syndromes.* Specific causes of severe insulin resistance, congenital or acquired, are very rare (see Section 1, p. 28).

● *Brittle diabetes.* Apparently high insulin requirements are a feature of some patients with idiopathic brittle diabetes (see pages 165 and 266).

● *Hormonal stress response to intercurrent illness.* Transient insulin resistance may arise in the course of intercurrent illnesses, e.g. sepsis; temporary increases in insulin doses, sometimes necessitating a change to intravenous or multiple subcutaneous doses of short-acting insulin, are required (see p. 283). Insulin may be required during the course of such an illness in patients previously well maintained on oral antidiabetic agents; this will usually be done in hospital. With resolution of the acute episode, re-introduction of oral therapy may be possible.

● *Anti-insulin antibodies.* The role of acquired anti-insulin antibodies, once thought to be an important mechanism of insulin resistance, has faded with modern, less antigenic insulin preparations.

● *Obesity.* Clinical insulin resistance is now largely confined to patients with type 2 diabetes whose obesity limits attainment of glycaemic targets despite large doses of insulin.

Renal failure

Care is required with insulin treatment in patients with progressive renal impairment. Decreased insulin degradation by the failing kidneys, reduced renal gluconeogenesis and anorexia with decreased caloric intake may all contribute. Reductions in insulin dose, sometimes substantial, may be required.

Progressive renal failure may necessitate reductions in insulin dose.

Some patients with end-stage renal failure on continuous ambulatory peritoneal dialysis (CAPD) (see p. 226) inject their insulin into the dialysate bags thereby delivering insulin intraperitoneally. Insulin requirements vary enormously between patients and are in part dependent on the strength of dialysate used; hypertonic solutions contain high concentrations of glucose.

TYPE 2 DIABETES

Insulin is the treatment of choice for certain clinical situations (Table 3.9, p. 110). Often this will be because oral agents are contraindicated; in other situations, glycaemic control will be inadequate or there is evidence for benefit from use of insulin preferentially (e.g. following MI, see p. 230). In many instances, insulin will be a temporary measure. Success when restarting oral agents can usually be predicted by excellent glycaemic control with relatively small insulin doses (less than 20 units daily being an approximate guide). Safety considerations will also point to the preferential use of insulin in other circumstances, e.g. in patients with significant renal impairment (see Section 5, pp. 219–228); here risk to benefit considerations favour insulin as renal function deteriorates. In addition, however, a significant proportion of patients with type 2 diabetes will ultimately require insulin therapy in the long term because of failure of oral agents to provide adequate glycaemic control – so-called secondary failure (see above).

Reservations about insulin therapy in patients with type 2 diabetes, particularly elderly patients with cardiovascular complications, have focused on the risks of hypoglycaemia and weight gain. Hypoglycaemia occurs with considerably lower frequency than in patients with type 1 diabetes (see p. 156); however, this may be of paramount importance in the elderly, socially isolated, demented or otherwise infirm patient. In the UKPDS (see p. 65), insulin treatment was associated with an average of 1.8 episodes of severe hypoglycaemia per annum.

> **NB** Hypoglycaemia among insulin-treated patients with type 2 diabetes is much less common than in patients with type 1 diabetes.

INSULIN THERAPY AND MACROVASCULAR DISEASE

To date, no clear evidence has emerged implicating exogenous insulin therapy in the promotion of cardiovascular disease with recent evidence including that from the UKPDS data (see p. 65). Epidemiological and clinical trial data provide evidence for a beneficial effect of good glycaemic control on the appearance and progression of microvascular complications in patients with type 2 diabetes; such data provide a logical basis for intensive insulin therapy, particularly in younger patients and in ethnic groups characterized by earlier onset of diabetes who are at higher risk of developing serious complications. Since cardiovascular disease accounts for approximately 70% of deaths in patients with type 2 diabetes reducing this risk is a major therapeutic objective. Insulin therapy has several advantageous effects including improved glycaemic control, circulating lipids and fibrinolysis.

PATIENT ACCEPTABILITY

Clinical studies suggest that insulin therapy can be successful if patients are selected and prepared carefully. Twice-daily isophane or pre-mixed insulins are used routinely in many centres; pen injectors or dosers are suitable for most patients and may increase acceptability by increasing convenience. Morbidly obese patients inadequately controlled with oral agents remain a particularly difficult therapeutic problem. Some centres use a combination of oral antidiabetic agents and bedtime insulin; this may prove to be more expensive than using insulin as monotherapy. Patient acceptance of insulin may be facilitated by a positive attitude from the diabetes care team and discussion of the possibility early in the course of type 2 diabetes. Studies suggest that quality of life is not necessarily impaired by the additional rigours of life on insulin. Indeed, the improvement in well-being experienced by the patient whose glycaemic control is improved after months or years of hyperglycaemia is rewarding for patient and professional alike. Adequate support from a multidisciplinary diabetes care team is an important component of safe and effective insulin therapy for patients with type 2 diabetes.

COMBINATION THERAPY WITH INSULIN AND ORAL AGENTS

• *Sulphonylureas with insulin.* No clear long-term benefits of such combined therapy has yet emerged; nonetheless this approach has enthusiastic proponents and is gaining popularity. Several studies (generally relatively small sample sizes and of limited duration) have suggested that concomitant treatment using insulin and sulphonylureas may allow reduction in insulin doses of up to 50%. Isophane insulin may be administered at bedtime, with sulphonylureas being taken during the day. This aims to control fasting plasma glucose concentrations with the bedtime insulin by suppressing hepatic glucose production (see Section 1). Clearly, given the mode of action of sulphonylureas (see p. 111), this approach is dependent on partial residual B-cell function. The usefulness of combination therapy in the longer term is less certain. Since B-cell function deteriorates inexorably in the majority of patients with type 2 diabetes, it seems likely that sulphonylureas would ultimately lose their effect; full replacement therapy with insulin would then be required.

• *Metformin with insulin.* There is increasing evidence that concomitant use of metformin may help to avert weight gain when patients with type 2 diabetes are transferred to insulin. A recent RCT also suggested that metformin and insulin (at bedtime) when compared with other regimens (including twice-daily insulin) was associated with the better glycaemic control and lowest risk of hypoglycaemia during the first year of therapy. Patients assigned to this combination used more insulin to attain fasting blood glucose targets. Some centres are now routinely continuing metformin in overweight patients when insulin is introduced; further studies are required to determine the optimal regimens for subgroups of patients with different clinical and biochemical characteristics.

NB Metformin may avert weight gain associated with insulin treatment in patients with type 2 diabetes.

● *Thiazolidinediones with insulin.* There is accumulating evidence that the insulin-sensitizing drugs, troglitazone, rosiglitazone and pioglitazone, may allow insulin doses to be reduced; reductions >50% have been reported in some trials of obese, insulin-treated patients after the addition of troglitazone. Dose reductions with concomitant improvements in glycaemic control have been observed in studies of rosiglitazone. However, the potential for weight gain is not eliminated by this approach.

> **NB** Combination therapy with insulin and a thiazolidinedione may allow reductions in insulin dose.

DISCONTINUATION OF INSULIN THERAPY

In some situations it may be appropriate to consider whether insulin treatment may be safely discontinued. This may be particularly advantageous for the occasional elderly or infirm patient. The assumption must be that the patient has type 2 diabetes that can be adequately controlled with oral agents. To a large extent this will depend on the clinical evidence:

- There should usually be no history of ketosis.
- The patient must not have been underweight at diagnosis.
- Humoral markers of autoimmune diabetes (see p. 11) should be absent.

The need for only small doses of insulin is not a reliable guide to lack of dependence upon insulin; insulin requirements vary considerably between patients.

> **NB** Insulin dose cannot be reliably equated with the need for insulin treatment.

A trial of a sulphonylurea, e.g. following a presentation with hyperosmolar non-ketotic state (see p. 185), requires careful judgement. Similarly, transfer back to oral agents when insulin treatment has been initiated because of a myocardial infarction (see p. 230) requires an analysis of potential risks and benefits, both in the short and longer term. Similar considerations pertain to reversion to tablets following delivery in female patients whose diabetes has been temporarily controlled with insulin during pregnancy; if control was suboptimal prior to conception, then continuing with insulin (albeit in a lower dose, see p. 277) may be the best option.

Measurement of plasma (or urinary) C-peptide, which is co-secreted with insulin on an equimolar basis, provides a measure of endogenous insulin reserve. Stimulation tests (e.g. peak C-peptide response 6 min following a 1 mg intravenous injection of glucagon) have been used in clinical studies to classify patients. Plasma C-peptide has also been used to assess response to therapies aiming to preserve B-cell function in patients with newly-diagnosed type 1 diabetes (see Section 1). The test is rarely used in clinical practice but may be of use in doubtful cases; an adequate response indicates a high likelihood of being able to discontinue insulin; expertise is required in the interpretation of such tests.

PANCREATIC AND ISLET CELL TRANSPLANTATION

COMBINED KIDNEY AND PANCREAS GRAFTS

Pancreatic allotransplantation, either whole organ or segmental, is most often performed in concert with a renal transplant in selected patients with type 1 diabetes and end-stage nephropathy (see p. 219). More than 9000 pancreatic transplants have been performed worldwide, most in centres in the USA, the procedure being less frequently performed in Europe and elsewhere. Patient and graft survival rates now approach those for other organs being approximately 80% and 70% at 5 years. The advantages of a combined pancreas plus renal transplant must be weighed against increased rates of postoperative morbidity from thrombosis, infection and pancreatitis. However, the need for chronic immunosuppression (with agents such as prednisolone, cyclosporin or tacrolimus which, incidentally, are diabetogenic, see p. 22) is the principal reason which generally precludes pancreatic transplantation in non-uraemic patients. These drugs are associated with a risk of serious side effects including:

- Neoplasia (several-fold increase).
- Infection (especially with cytomegalovirus).
- Nephrotoxicity.

Recurrence of type 1 diabetes in the graft is uncommon with the use of adequate immunosuppression. The benefits of co-transplanting a pancreas with a kidney have now been well documented and include:

- Restoration of insulin-independence.
- Improved recipient survival.
- Protection of renal grafts from re-emergence of diabetic nephropathy.

More than 50% of patients will still be free of the need for exogenous insulin 5 years post-transplant; approximately 20% require a second pancreatic graft. Although insulin (usually delivered systemically via the iliac veins rather than into the portal system) and glucagon secretion and regulation of intermediary metabolism are not entirely normalized, the recipient's quality of life is improved by:

- Abolition of need for insulin injections.
- Dietary relaxation.
- Absence of risk of severe hypoglycaemia (see p. 156).
- Obviation of self-monitoring of glycaemia (see p. 73).

Thus, although the procedure is associated with higher surgical risks, a strong case can be made for considering suitable kidney transplant recipients for a simultaneous or interval pancreas graft, particularly in the light of evidence of protection for renal grafts. The effect on other established complications such as retinopathy (which is often advanced, see p. 194) and neuropathy (which often includes impairment of autonomic reflex tests, see p. 204) is confined to stabilization or minor improvement. It has been suggested, however, that mortality rates among patients with impaired autonomic reflex tests are reduced by a successful pancreatic graft.

LIVING-RELATED DONORS

Most pancreatic grafts are derived from cadavers. A limited number of segmental grafts have been donated by living relatives of the recipient. However, this may not be without risks to the donor, beyond those associated with the surgical procurement. Studies in the USA of living-related donors who have undergone hemi-pancreatectomy have shown degrees of glucose intolerance; the long-term outcome is presently uncertain for these donors, who may be at increased risk of developing diabetes themselves.

SOLITARY PANCREAS TRANSPLANTATION

Although some centres will consider solitary pancreatic transplantation, the indications are somewhat controversial (e.g. recurrent incapacitating hypoglycaemia; overwhelming emotional difficulties detracting from insulin treatment) in the light of the adverse effects of immunosuppression; other less heroic approaches may be successful.

ISLET CELL TRANSPLANTATION

Although more attractive for a number of reasons, technical difficulties continue to relegate this less-invasive procedure to clinical experimentation in a few centres worldwide; prolonged insulin-independence has been achieved in few patients. The longer-term effects on chronic complications have not been evaluated. Efforts directed to obviating the need for immunosuppression continue but the obstacles appear formidable.

ACUTE METABOLIC COMPLICATIONS

HYPOGLYCAEMIA

TYPE 1 DIABETES

Iatrogenic hypoglycaemia is the most serious and feared hazard of treatment. The great majority of episodes occur in patients with type 1 diabetes approximately 10% of whom will, on average, experience one severe episode (i.e. causing coma or convulsions) per year.

> **NB** Hypoglycaemia is the most-feared complication of therapy in insulin-treated patients.

The risk of severe hypoglycaemia increases as glycaemic control is improved; this is the principal factor limiting the attainment of glycaemic targets in intensive insulin therapy (see p. 131).

> **NB** In patients with type 1 diabetes, risk of severe hypoglycaemia is inversely related to glycaemic control.

Hypoglycaemia in type 1 diabetes is particularly common during the night and often goes undetected (see p. 162). Insulin-induced hypoglycaemia is also implicated in occasional sudden death in young patients (see p. 162). The risk of hypoglycaemia bars insulin-treated diabetics from certain occupations (see p. 288).

> **NB** Nocturnal hypoglycaemia is often asymptomatic in insulin-treated patients.

Iatrogenic hypoglycaemia results from either:

- A mismatch between supply of glucose for metabolic requirements (e.g. as a result of a missed meal) and rate of utilization (e.g. an increase due to physical exercise).
- A relative excess of insulin (either exogenous or endogenous, i.e. stimulated by a sulphonylurea) leading to a fall in the circulating glucose concentration.

Other causes of hypoglycaemia in insulin-treated patients are presented in Table 4.1. Their effects in individual patients are variable.

Knowledge of the pathophysiology of hypoglycaemia underpins strategies for avoidance and treatment. Cerebral function is critically

---

TABLE 4.1 Causes of recurrent hypoglycaemia in insulin-treated patients

Changes in insulin pharmacokinetics
— Change of insulin species, e.g. bovine to human
— Change of anatomical injection site
— Development of renal impairment
— Effect of ambient temperature
— Effect of exercise on insulin absorption

Altered insulin sensitivity
— Acute resolution of insulin resistance post-partum
— Hypopituitarism or Addison's disease
— Hypothyroidism
— Weight loss or calorie restriction
— Resolution of drug-induced insulin resistance, e.g. withdrawal of steroid therapy

Others
— Recovery of partial endogenous insulin secretion (honeymoon period)
— Malabsorption syndrome. e.g. coeliac disease
— Gastroparesis due to autonomic neuropathy
— Severe liver disease
— Eating disorders (anorexia/bulimia)

---

dependent on an adequate supply of glucose from the circulation. Glucose is transported into the brain across the blood–brain barrier by a facilitative glucose transporter protein – GLUT 1 (see p. 6). Studies in humans indicate that the rate of glucose transport into the brain can be modified by changes in plasma glucose levels. In particular, antecedent hypoglycaemia causes up-regulation of glucose transport, i.e. more glucose is transported across the blood–brain barrier during subsequent episodes of hypoglycaemia. This adaptive response has important clinical implications (see later). The most serious consequence of acute hypoglycaemia is cerebral dysfunction with the risk of:

- Injury (to self or others).
- Generalized epileptic seizures.
- Coma.

Cognitive impairment progresses ultimately to loss of consciousness as plasma glucose falls. Seizures and transient focal neurological deficits may occur. Prolonged severe hypoglycaemia, often exacerbated by excessive alcohol consumption, may produce cerebral oedema and permanent brain damage. Recurrent severe hypoglycaemia may cause intellectual impairment in young children (see p. 265). Clinically, hypoglycaemia may be usefully graded as follows:

Grade 1 Biochemical hypoglycaemia in the absence of symptoms.
Grade 2 Mild symptomatic – treated successfully by the patient.
Grade 3 Severe – assistance required from another person.
Grade 4 Very severe – causing coma or convulsions.

PATHOPHYSIOLOGY OF HYPOGLYCAEMIA

The physiological response to acute hypoglycaemia comprises:

- Suppression of endogenous insulin secretion (Fig. 4.1).
- Activation of a hierarchy of counter-regulatory responses (Fig. 4.1; see Section 1).

Counter-regulatory hormone responses

As plasma glucose concentration progressively falls, hormones which antagonize the actions of insulin are secreted in the following sequence:

- Glucagon.
- Catecholamines – adrenaline and noradrenaline.
- Cortisol.
- Growth hormone.

Secretion of catecholamines occurs in the setting of generalized sympathetic nervous system activation. Glucagon and catecholamines are the principal hormones which protect against acute hypoglycaemia. These hormones stimulate glycogenolysis and gluconeogenesis, thereby increasing hepatic glucose production (see p. 6); enhanced hormone-stimulated lipolysis may also contribute to recovery from hypoglycaemia through stimulatory effects on gluconeogenesis (see pp. 6–7). If healthy subjects are given carefully-controlled doses of insulin, the secretion of these hormones occurs at arterialized plasma glucose levels of approximately 3.8 mmol/L, the

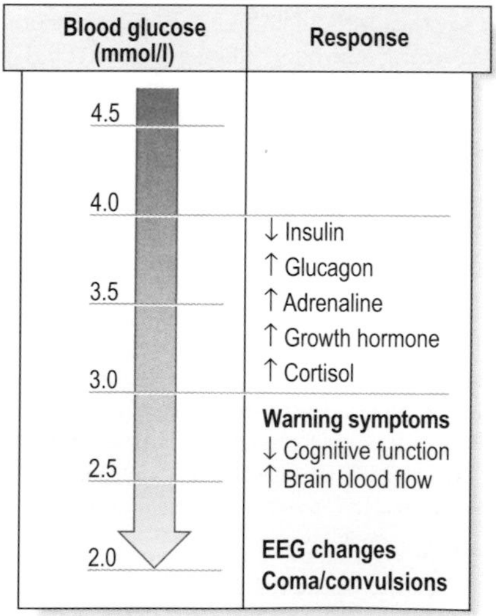

Blood glucose (mmol/l)	Response
4.5	
4.0	
3.5	↓ Insulin ↑ Glucagon ↑ Adrenaline ↑ Growth hormone ↑ Cortisol
3.0	
2.5	**Warning symptoms** ↓ Cognitive function ↑ Brain blood flow
2.0	**EEG changes** **Coma/convulsions**

Fig. 4.1 Heirarchy of hormonal responses to acute hypoglycaemia. NB. Thresholds are modifiable by factors such as antecedent hypoglycaemia.

secretion of cortisol occurring at lower levels. If the response of either glucagon or catecholamines is inadequate, the other will usually compensate. However, deficiency of both will result in severe hypoglycaemia.

 Failure of counter-regulatory hormone responses predisposes to severe recurrent hypoglycaemia.

Cortisol and growth hormone play a less important role during acute hypoglycaemia being more important in later recovery of glucose levels. However, deficiencies of these hormones, e.g. cortisol deficiency in autoimmune Addison's disease (see p. 24) – which is more common in patients with type 1 diabetes – can lead directly to or exacerbate hypoglycaemia. Hypopituitarism may have a similar effect (see p. 25). For example, prior to the introduction of photocoagulation for proliferative diabetic retinopathy (see p. 194), hypophysectomy was sometimes performed in selected patients with type 1 diabetes. Follow-up of these patients showed them to be at high risk of hypoglycaemia, often fatal.

Warning symptoms
The symptoms and signs of acute hypoglycaemia may be divided into two main categories:

- *Autonomic (adrenergic)* – arising from activation of the sympatho-adrenal system (Table 4.2).

- *Neuroglycopenic* – resulting from inadequate cerebral glucose delivery (Table 4.2).

Other features are regarded as belonging to neither category (Table 4.2). Under experimental conditions, adrenergic activation occurs at a higher plasma glucose concentration than that at which cerebral function becomes impaired (2.7 mmol/L). Thus, the patient is alerted to the falling plasma glucose concentration by adrenergic activation and is usually able to take corrective action.

Hypoglycaemia unawareness
If these warning symptoms are deficient or perception of them is impaired, e.g. by certain drugs or alcohol (see pp. 97 and 166), then the patient may become irrational and aggressive as a result of neuroglycopenia. Prompt assistance from another party may then be required to avert loss of consciousness and more serious sequelae.

NB Severe hypoglycaemia carries risks of coma, convulsions, injury and rarely even death.

TABLE 4.2 Autonomic, neuroglycopenic and non-specific symptoms and signs in acute hypoglycaemia

Autonomic (adrenergic)
— Tremor
— Sweating
— Anxiety
— Pallor
— Nausea
— Tachycardia
— Palpitations
— Shivering
— Increased pulse pressure

Neuroglycopenia
— Impaired concentration
— Confusion
— Irrational, uncharacteristic or inappropriate behaviour
— Difficulty in speaking
— Non-cooperation or aggression
— Drowsiness progressing to coma
— Focal neurological signs including transient hemiplegia
— Focal or generalized convulsions
— Permanent neurological damage if prolonged, severe hypoglycaemia

Non-specific
— Hunger
— Weakness
— Blurred vision

Effect of insulin. Insulin treatment of long duration (i.e. 5 years or more) is often associated with defective glucagon responses to hypoglycaemia. In addition, intensive insulin therapy (aiming for sustained near-normoglycaemia) may be associated with loss of autonomic hypoglycaemic warning symptoms, resulting in high risk of recurrent severe hypoglycaemia.

In the DCCT (see p. 60), the overall risk of severe hypoglycaemia was increased approximately 3-fold in the intensively-treated group. This was observed in spite of strenuous efforts to exclude patients who were thought to be at highest risk of hypoglycaemia. The relation between rate of severe hypoglycaemia and mean HbA_{1c} level was inverse and curvilinear (Fig. 2.3, p. 63). Factors predisposing to severe hypoglycaemia are presented in Table 4.3. However, in a significant proportion of instances, a clear predisposing factor could not be identified even with careful scrutiny of the circumstances by experienced investigators.

Antecedent hypoglycaemia can alter the glycaemic threshold for counter-regulatory hormone secretion; scrupulous avoidance of hypoglycaemia may restore symptoms. Clinical studies have shown that intensive insulin therapy leads to symptoms which develop at lower plasma glucose levels. Thus, the patient has less time between the onset of symptoms until the development of severe neuroglycopenia. Recurrent

---

TABLE 4.3 Risk factors for severe hypoglycaemia

- History of severe hypoglycaemia
- History of symptomatic unawareness of hypoglycaemia
- Impaired counter-regulatory hormone responses
- Intensive insulin therapy
- Glycated haemoglobin within the non-diabetic range
- Long-duration type 1 diabetes
- Alcohol consumption

---

hypoglycaemia, even if asymptomatic, is therefore a contraindication to intensive insulin therapy in patients with type 1 diabetes (see p. 131). Of related interest, non-diabetic patients with chronic recurrent hypoglycaemia owing to insulinomas may also lose typical symptoms and signs of hypoglycaemia.

Asymptomatic hypoglycaemia is a contraindication to intensive insulin therapy.

Advice about driving. Patients with loss of warning symptoms of hypoglycaemia should not continue driving motor vehicles. Since hypoglycaemia while driving could have serious consequences this should be conveyed to the patient, preferably in writing; the advice should also be recorded in the patient's casenotes. Fatalities have occurred in this situation, involving innocent bystanders. In the UK patients should also be reminded that it is their legal responsibility to inform the driving licensing authority – the UK Driver and Vehicle Licensing Authority (see p. 288). A hospital specialist's report will usually be requested by the authority. The patient's licence is withdrawn until there is convincing evidence that there is no longer any danger.

Meticulous avoidance of glucose levels – aiming for none below 4.0 mmol/L – may restore warning symptoms; with care, this may not necessarily have to compromise overall glycaemic control. However, many patients with hypoglycaemia unawareness have only moderate glycaemic control as judged by glycated haemoglobin concentrations. The utility of rapid-acting insulin analogues (see below and p. 138) is being explored. However, it may prove difficult to dissect out improvements attributable to altered pharmacokinetics from increased education and input from the diabetes care team. Certainly, adequate expert supervision is required to achieve the objective of breaking the vicious cycle. Although the loss of warning symptoms has been described as a form of acquired autonomic dysfunction, it is generally accepted that classical diabetic autonomic neuropathy per se is not usually responsible (see p. 209).

Patients with loss of warning symptoms of hypoglycaemia must not drive motor vehicles.

NOCTURNAL HYPOGLYCAEMIA

Nocturnal hypoglycaemia has been implicated in the sudden death of some young patients (so-called 'dead in bed' syndrome). Catecholamine-mediated falls in plasma potassium concentration leading to cardiac arrhythmias have been implicated but this remains unproven. The frequent occurrence of nocturnal hypoglycaemia – which may affect more than 50% of patients and often goes unrecognized – may be an important cause of hypoglycaemia unawareness. Conventional strategies to minimize nocturnal hypoglycaemia include:

- Reducing the dose of evening intermediate insulin.
- Moving the time of the evening injection of intermediate insulin to 2200 h.
- Eating a snack containing 10–20 g carbohydrate before bed.
- Avoiding excessive alcohol consumption.

Evidence has emerged suggesting that the contribution of the evening dose of short-acting insulin to the problem of hypoglycaemia at 3 a.m. has hitherto been underestimated. Recent evidence points to a lower rate of nocturnal hypoglycaemia when the insulin analogues lispro or insulin aspart (see p. 135) are used in place of human insulin. Since lispro and aspart have a shorter duration of action, their effects will dissipate earlier in the evening, resulting in lower plasma insulin concentrations in the early hours of the night.

 Evening doses of conventional short-acting insulins may contribute to hypoglycaemia during the night.

In addition, the physiological responses to insulin-induced hypoglycaemia are impaired during stages 3–4 (slow wave) of sleep.

INSULIN SPECIES AND RISK OF HYPOGLYCAEMIA

In the UK, there has been intense debate about the effect of insulin species in relation to warning symptoms of hypoglycaemia. The issue arose from complaints from a minority of patients that, on changing from animal to human sequence insulin, symptoms were reduced in intensity predisposing to recurrent hypoglycaemia. Certainly, it is recognized that a change of species may necessitate changes in insulin dosage (see p. 145). Differences in pharmacokinetics and, in some patients with diabetes of long duration, the presence of high titres of anti-insulin antibodies are sometimes responsible (see

p. 148). This is particularly true for patients changing from bovine to less immunogenic porcine or human insulins. Whether there is any effect of species per se on the symptom complex of hypoglycaemia remains less certain.

Alternative causes of hypoglycaemia must always be excluded. Although experimental studies have, in general, provided no evidence of a species effect on warning symptoms, minor pharmacokinetic differences between species may perhaps be of clinical importance in some circumstances. Small differences in counter-regulatory hormone responses have, in fact, been reported between insulin species. Duration of diabetes and antecedent glycaemic control are important confounding influences. The debate in the UK about human insulin has polarized views on both sides. However, it has been accepted that the patient's views should be respected; a request to change species should be treated sympathetically. Reassuringly, no evidence of an increased mortality rate with human insulin has emerged. The great majority of patients in the UK and elsewhere are now treated with human sequence insulin (see p. 135).

TREATMENT OF INSULIN-INDUCED HYPOGLYCAEMIA

Grade 1–2 hypoglycaemia

Insulin-treated patients are advised to carry dextrose tablets at all times. However, surveys indicate that a high proportion do not comply; periodic reiteration of this advice is required. At the onset of symptoms patients should take either:

- 2–4 dextrose tablets.
- 2 teaspoonfuls of sugar (10 g), honey or jam (ideally in water).
- A small glass of carbonated sugar-containing soft drink.

If there is no improvement within 5–10 min, the treatment should be repeated. If the next meal is not imminent, a snack (e.g. biscuit, sandwich, piece of fruit) should be eaten to maintain blood glucose. Over-treatment should be avoided if possible.

Grade 3–4 hypoglycaemia

Friends, colleagues or relatives may recognize the development of hypoglycaemia before patients themselves. A subtle change in appearance or behaviour may prompt a third party to encourage oral carbohydrate consumption. Unfortunately, cognitive dysfunction may lead to a negative or even hostile response. If the level of consciousness falls, it becomes hazardous to try to forcibly administer carbohydrate by mouth. Alternatives include:

- *Buccal glucose gel.* Proprietary thick glucose gels (e.g. Hypostop) or honey, can be smeared on the buccal mucosa. Variable efficacy.

- *Intravenous glucose.* Administer 25 mL of 50% dextrose (or 100 mL of 20% dextrose) into a large vein, ideally after cannulation; paramedical expertise is required. This will usually lead to restoration of consciousness within a few minutes. Extravasation of hypertonic 50% dextrose can cause tissue necrosis and thrombophlebitis may complicate intravenous delivery.

 Hypertonic (50%) dextrose must be administered into a large vein in order to avoid extravasation.

• *Glucagon.* Parenteral glucagon (1 mg = 1 Unit) can be given by intravenous, subcutaneous or, most reliably and conveniently, intramuscular injection. Glucagon mobilizes glucose from hepatic glucagon stores and so is ineffective in starved patients; it is therefore unsuitable for alcoholics. Relatives or friends can learn how to reconstitute and administer glucagon which is supplied in the form of a kit. This may bolster confidence when dealing with a patient prone to recurrent, severe hypoglycaemia. If glucagon is ineffective within 10–15 minutes, then intravenous dextrose should be administered.

 Intramuscular glucagon may be administered by relatives or friends to hypoglycaemic patients.

Recovery from hypoglycaemia may be delayed if:

• The hypoglycaemia has been very prolonged or severe.
• An alternative cause for impairment of consciousness (e.g. stroke, drug overdose) co-exists.
• The patient is post-ictal (convulsion caused by hypoglycaemia).

If the development of cerebral oedema is suspected, adjunctive treatment, i.e. intravenous dexamethasone (4–6 mg 6-hourly) or mannitol, is usually administered in an intensive care setting. However, evidence for the efficacy of these drugs, or for other measures such as controlled hyperventilation, is sparse. Cranial CT imaging should be obtained.

INSULIN OVERDOSE

Occasionally, a patient presents having deliberately administered an excessive dose of insulin with the intent of self-harm. It is usually possible to treat the resulting hypoglycaemia with a continuous infusion of 5% or 10% dextrose. Extreme measures such as surgical excision of the injection site are rarely, if ever, indicated. Psychiatric assessment may be required after recovery. On occasion, severe, prolonged hypoglycaemia may result in permanent cognitive damage, personality change or chronic behavioural difficulties occasionally reminiscent of a frontal lobe syndrome. The potential for neuronal damage resulting from severe recurrent hypoglycaemia is a particular concern in young children (see p. 265).

BEHAVIOURAL PROBLEMS SPECIFIC TO TYPE 1 DIABETES

(See also pages 56 and 266 for further discussions of psychological problems in relation to diabetes.)

Idiopathic brittle diabetes

This term is well known to most professionals involved with the care of diabetes. Disruptive episodes of hypoglycaemia may alternate with recurrent ketoacidosis leading to repeated hospitalization and the focusing of much attention on the individual concerned. The patients are typically overweight females in their teens or early 20s with psychosocial difficulties and apparently relatively high insulin requirements. Menstrual irregularities are common. No convincing evidence has emerged in favour of an intrinsic difference in the metabolism of these individuals. Convincing anecdotal evidence of at times astonishing degrees of deliberate manipulation is available which has been known to mislead many well-meaning and experienced professionals. The long-term outlook is not good for such patients; some die from acute metabolic emergencies or suicide. Attempts can be made to alter the self-destructive behaviour pattern but the problem often remains resistant to reasoned support.

Factitious remission of type 1 diabetes

The rare occurrence of factitious 'remission' of type 1 diabetes is considered on page 15. In this situation, patients claim that insulin requirements have fallen dramatically and quite spontaneously. Uncommon organic causes of increased insulin sensitivity must be excluded (see Section 1).

Hypoglycaemia by proxy

This is a particularly disturbing but rare situation in which a patient (usually a child) is subjected to deliberate hypoglycaemia by parents or carers; fatalities have been recorded.

TYPE 2 DIABETES

Hypoglycaemia is much less frequently encountered in patients with type 2 diabetes, even when treated with insulin (see p. 131). Severe hypoglycaemia complicating sulphonylurea therapy is relatively uncommon but is important since it usually occurs in the elderly and carries a relatively high risk of fatality. Neither metformin nor acarbose are associated with any risk of hypoglycaemia when used as monotherapy (see pp. 124 and 126). However, these drugs may exacerbate hypoglycaemia caused by other agents.

SULPHONYLUREAS AND HYPOGLYCAEMIA

Few reliable data are available concerning the incidence of hypoglycaemia induced by sulphonylureas, although it is more frequent than is generally appreciated. During the UKPDS's first year (see p. 65), symptoms of mild hypoglycaemia were reported in 31%, 7% and 8% of diet-failed patients receiving glibenclamide, chlorpropamide or insulin, respectively. The major recognized risk associated with sulphonylureas is acute severe hypoglycaemia with the risk of death or serious chronic neurological sequelae.

NB Severe sulphonylurea-induced hypoglycaemia is a medical emergency.

The clinical consequences of less severe recurrent sulphonylurea-induced hypoglycaemia are unknown but are of particular concern in the elderly. Severe hypoglycaemia is the most catastrophic unwanted effect of the sulphonylureas. Although it is an uncommon complication of therapy, it is associated with a high mortality (approximately 10%).

NB Severe sulphonylurea-induced hypoglycaemia has a high case-fatality rate.

While case-fatality rates among insulin-treated patients admitted to hospital with hypoglycaemia are generally low, an average mortality rate of 3–4% has been reported in most series of profound hypoglycaemia in insulin-treated patients.

Risk factors for severe sulphonylurea-induced hypoglycaemia
Longer-acting hypoglycaemia agents (e.g. chlorpropamide, glibenclamide) are most likely to be responsible but any sulphonylurea has the potential to cause severe hypoglycaemia (see p. 115). Long-acting agents should be avoided in the elderly.

 Long-acting sulphonylureas, e.g. chlorpropamide and glibenclamide, are particularly liable to cause severe hypoglycaemia.

Tolbutamide is associated with a reported rate of hypoglycaemia that is approximately one-fifth of that for chlorpropamide and glibenclamide, with glipizide carrying an intermediate risk. Agents predominantly excreted via the kidney (e.g. glibenclamide) should be avoided in renal impairment (see p. 114).

 NB All sulphonylureas have the potential to cause severe hypoglycaemia.

Sulphonylurea-induced suppression of hepatic glucose production may cause profound and protracted hypoglycaemia, especially in elderly patients, in individuals with intercurrent illnesses and reduced caloric intake, or when taken in combination with other compounds with hypoglycaemic potential, e.g. alcohol. The importance of the latter factor may be underestimated in elderly patients. The potential for drug interactions must be borne in mind (see Section 3). Presentation with altered conscious level or focal neurological signs may lead to the erroneous diagnosis of an acute cerebrovascular event, and the possibility of hypoglycaemia should always be excluded in patients presenting with these features.

Management

Recurrent symptoms suggestive of hypoglycaemia should prompt a reduction in dose or withdrawal of the medication responsible. Patients with severe sulphonylurea-induced hypoglycaemia should be admitted promptly to hospital; relapse following initial resuscitation with oral or intravenous glucose may necessitate prolonged infusions of dextrose. Delivery of an intravenous bolus of dextrose – a potent insulin secretagogue – will stimulate further insulin release, especially in patients with relatively well-preserved B-cell function. This predictable consequence of treatment, combined with the long duration of action of drugs such as chlorpropamide and glibenclamide, explains the tendency for hypoglycaemia to recur.

NB Relapse after resuscitation is common in severe sulphonylurea-induced hypoglycaemia.

The antihypertensive agent, diazoxide (see p. 23), and the somatostatin analogue, octreotide (see p. 168), offer a more direct approach by inhibiting stimulated endogenous insulin secretion; these drugs have been used successfully as adjuncts to intravenous dextrose. However, neither is licensed for this indication in the UK.

● *Intravenous dextrose*. This remains the mainstay of therapy; it is well recognized that continuous infusions of 5% or 10% dextrose may be required for several days.

● *Diazoxide*. This drug antagonizes the actions of sulphonylureas by opening ATP-sensitive potassium channels in the membranes of islet B-cells.

However, the drug is associated with adverse cardiovascular effects, including tachycardia and orthostatic hypotension. These may be hazardous particularly in elderly patients with a compromised vasculature or impaired baroreceptor reflexes.

- *Hydrocortisone.* This has been advocated; however, there is scant evidence for efficacy. High doses may cause hypokalaemia.

- *Glucagon.* This also stimulates endogenous insulin release and therefore cannot be recommended.

- *Mannitol.* This is recommended for cerebral oedema; dexamethasone is an alternative (see p. 164).

- *Octreotide.* This has been shown to be an effective and well-tolerated agent for the prevention of sulphonylurea-induced hypoglycaemia under controlled experimental conditions. However, clinical experience for this indication remains very limited.

Serum potassium should be monitored and intravenous supplements administered if hypokalaemia develops – high plasma insulin levels will increase transport of potassium into cells (see Section 1). The renal elimination of chlorpropamide may be greatly enhanced by forced alkaline diuresis.

DIABETIC KETOACIDOSIS

DKA continues to be an important cause of morbidity and mortality in patients with type 1 diabetes. In a recent UK survey of patients diagnosed under the age of 30 years, DKA was identified as the cause of death in 54% of males; only 6% of deaths were attributed to hypoglycaemia (see above). Although younger patients are principally affected, DKA may occasionally be precipitated in patients with type 2 diabetes during severe intercurrent illness. Moreover, DKA can affect patients in any age group. Female patients predominate in some published series; a small subgroup, the majority under the age of 20, may present with multiple episodes. Many episodes of DKA appear to be avoidable with appropriate early action.

DEFINITION
The cardinal biochemical features of DKA are:

- Hyperketonaemia.
- Metabolic acidosis.
- Hyperglycaemia.

Although no universally agreed criteria for diagnosis exist, the following working definition is suggested:

1. Severe uncontrolled diabetes requiring emergency treatment with insulin and intravenous fluids.
2. Urine Ketostix reaction ++ or greater, or plasma Ketostix + or more.
3. An arterial (or capillary) plasma bicarbonate concentration <15 mmol/L.

Notes

— This definition is arbitrary.
— Hyperglycaemia, although usually marked, is not a reliable guide to the severity of acidosis.
— Semi-quantitative methods such as Acetest or Ketostix are used to test urine at the bedside. In the occasional case where urine cannot be obtained, the hospital clinical chemistry laboratory can test serum or plasma for ketones.

 NB The degree of hyperglycaemia is not a reliable guide to the severity of the metabolic disturbance in DKA.

MORTALITY

Prior to the introduction of insulin into clinical practice, DKA was invariably fatal. The average mortality rate for DKA today is approximately 5% although reported rates vary between centres. While definitions of DKA and patient selection account for a proportion of this variation, mortality tends to be higher in less specialized units and in certain groups of patients such as the elderly. Although a number of DKA-related deaths are the inevitable consequence of associated conditions such as overwhelming infection or MI, others are still potentially preventable; delays in presentation or diagnosis and errors in management remain important factors.

PRECIPITATING FACTORS

• *Infection.* This is the commonest identifiable precipitant of DKA in Western countries.

• *New cases of diabetes.* These account for 10% or more of episodes.

• *Management errors.* These contribute a similar percentage to infection. This usually means that insulin treatment has been inappropriately discontinued.

Often no cause can be identified with certainty. Inappropriate changes in insulin dosage initiated either by the patient or following medical advice are included in the latter category; it is therefore crucially important that patients (and health care professionals) understand the risk of metabolic decompensation that may ensue during intercurrent illness (see p. 283). Most importantly, insulin must not be discontinued; indeed, increased doses are often necessary during illness. Perhaps surprisingly, MI is responsible for only 1% of episodes with miscellaneous conditions accounting for the remainder. No definite precipitating cause can be identified in 30–40% of episodes. Patients on continuous subcutaneous insulin infusion (see p. 142) may be at higher risk; this has been attributed to the small subcutaneous depot of insulin providing less protection against metabolic decompensation. Rapid-acting insulin analogues may be inappropriate for non-compliant patients; the shorter duration of action may lead more readily to metabolic decompensation if doses are omitted (see p. 136). Audit evidence points to non-compliance being a major factor in poor long-term glycaemic control and DKA in younger patients with type 1 diabetes.

PATHOGENESIS

DKA is characterized hormonally by:

- Elevated counter-regulatory (catabolic) hormone concentrations (see p. 3).
- An absolute or, more commonly, a relative deficiency of insulin.

Although residual endogenous insulin secretion may protect against DKA in some patients, suppression of B-cell secretion by catecholamines during intercurrent illness may occasionally precipitate DKA in patients with type 2 diabetes.

NB DKA usually reflects a relative rather than an absolute deficiency of insulin.

Insulin deficiency leads to an early rise in plasma glucagon concentration. As hyperglycaemia and DKA develop, dehydration and acidosis stimulate the release of catecholamines (adrenaline and noradrenaline) and cortisol. A vicious circle develops in which worsening metabolic decompensation stimulates further secretion of catabolic hormones. Hepatic overproduction of glucose and ketone bodies in concert with impaired disposal of these substrates by other tissue maintains the metabolic disturbance.

HYPERGLYCAEMIA

Insulin deficiency and elevated plasma levels of catabolic hormones (particularly glucagon and catecholamines) result in increased rates of hepatic glycogenolysis and gluconeogenesis. Renal gluconeogenesis is also enhanced in the presence of acidosis. Glucose disposal by peripheral tissues such as muscle and adipose tissue is reduced by deficiency of insulin while elevated plasma levels of catabolic hormones and fatty acids induce tissue insulin resistance. Thus, blood glucose concentration falls more slowly during treatment in patients with higher levels of catabolic hormones caused by infection. However, it should be stressed that clinically important degrees of insulin resistance are rarely encountered during treatment with modern insulin regimens; 5–10 units insulin per hour usually suffice in adults.

HYPERKETONAEMIA

Plasma ketone body concentrations are often raised 200–300 times normal fasting values. Ketone bodies are strong organic acids which dissociate fully at physiological pH, resulting in equimolar generation of hydrogen ions. Rapid rises in plasma hydrogen ion concentration in DKA outstrip the buffering capacity of the body fluids and tissues. The ensuing metabolic acidosis has a number of serious detrimental physiological effects which account for many of the cardinal features of DKA (Table 4.4). Acidosis may also:

- Exert a negative inotropic effect on cardiac muscle.
- Exacerbate systemic hypotension via peripheral vasodilatation.
- Increase the risk of ventricular arrhythmias.
- Induce respiratory depression with pH <7.0.
- Exacerbate insulin resistance.

TABLE 4.4 Cardinal clinical features of DKA

Clinical feature	Comments
Polyuria, nocturia; thirst	Usually prominent
Nausea, vomiting	Due to hyperketonaemia
Air hunger	Acidotic or Kussmaul respiration
Confusion, drowsiness, coma	Coma is associated with worse prognosis
Acute weight loss	Due to dehydration and tissue catabolism
Generalized muscular weakness	Due to dehydration, hypokalaemia
Visual disturbance	Blurred vision owing to rapid osmotic changes in lens
Abdominal pain	Due to acidosis; rarely severe
Muscular cramps	Usually a minor symptom

Ketogenesis

In DKA, insulin deficiency and catabolic hormone excess promote breakdown of adipocyte triglyceride (lipolysis). Concurrently, re-esterification is impaired; this combination results in the release of non-esterified fatty acids into the circulation (see p. 6). Fatty acids are the principal substrate for hepatic ketogenesis and are converted to coenzyme A

(CoA) derivatives prior to transportation into the mitochondria by an active transport system (the carnitine shuttle). In DKA, the hormonal imbalance strongly favours entry of fatty acids into the mitochondria and the preferential formation of ketone bodies:

- Acetoacetate.
- 3-hydroxybutyrate.

Within the mitochondria, fatty acyl-CoA undergoes β-oxidation resulting in the formation of acetyl-CoA which is then completely oxidized in the tricarboxylic acid cycle, utilized in lipid synthesis, or partially oxidized to ketone bodies. Acetone is formed by the spontaneous decarboxylation of acetoacetate. Although acetone concentration is elevated in ketoacidosis, it does not contribute to the metabolic acidosis. Acetone is highly fat soluble and is excreted slowly via the lungs.

Ketone body disposal

With the exception of the liver, most tissues have the capacity to utilize ketone bodies. Oxidation of ketone anions during treatment neutralizes the acidosis by the generation of equimolar amounts of bicarbonate ions. Excretion of ketone bodies via the kidney and lung is also important. However, urinary ketone excretion exacerbates the loss of cations such as sodium and potassium.

FLUID AND ELECTROLYTE DEPLETION

Hyperglycaemia causes an osmotic diuresis when the renal threshold for glucose is exceeded leading to dehydration and secondary losses of electrolytes (Table 4.5); ketonuria compounds the loss of water. The hormonal imbalance exacerbates renal sodium depletion. Metabolic acidosis leads to displacement of intracellular potassium by hydrogen ions which are subsequently lost in vomit or urine. Hyperventilation, fever and sweating owing to infection may further exacerbate fluid and electrolyte depletion, resulting in average losses of body water in adults of approximately 5 L. Reduced renal blood flow impairs elimination of glucose and ketone bodies.

TABLE 4.5 Average electrolyte deficits in adults with DKA	
Sodium	500 mmol
Chloride	350 mmol
Potassium	300–1000 mmol
Calcium	50–100 mmol
Phosphate	50–100 mmol
Magnesium	25–50 mmol

Potassium depletion

Despite a considerable total body deficit, plasma potassium levels are usually normal or high at presentation. Acidosis, insulin deficiency and renal impairment contribute to hyperkalaemia. Hypokalaemia at presentation signifies a marked deficiency of body potassium which may be enhanced by antecedent diuretic therapy.

Plasma potassium concentration is an unreliable indicator of whole-body potassium status.

Phosphate

Total body phosphate deficiency is a characteristic feature of DKA. The benefits of phosphate replacement have not been substantiated and so this is not recommended as a routine measure. In rare cases in which severe phosphate depletion is thought to be clinically relevant, caution is necessary to avoid iatrogenic hypocalcaemia.

Care must be taken to avoid iatrogenic hypocalcaemia if phosphate replacements are administered.

CLINICAL FEATURES

The cardinal symptoms of DKA (Table 4.4) usually develop over several days; all too often it is the onset of vomiting that finally precipitates emergency admission to hospital.

- *Dehydration.* Signs of dehydration, i.e. decreased skin turgor, postural hypotension and (sinus) tachycardia are usually prominent.

- *Metabolic acidosis.* This stimulates the medullary respiratory centre causing deep and rapid respirations (Kussmaul breathing).
    The odour of acetone may be apparent to those whose olfactory sense permits its detection. Acidosis-induced peripheral vasodilatation exacerbates hypotension and leads to hypothermia; rectal temperature should be taken with a low-reading thermometer if hypothermia is suspected.

- *Impairment of conscious level.* This is common to some degree although frank coma occurs in only about 10% of patients. The mechanism by which ketoacidosis induces coma remains obscure; impairment of consciousness correlates with plasma glucose concentration and osmolarity. Coma at presentation is associated with a worse prognosis and co-existing causes of coma such as stroke, head injury or drug overdose should always be considered and excluded as appropriate (Table 4.6).

TABLE 4.6 Causes of coma or impaired conciousness in diabetic patients

- DKA
- Non-ketotic hyperosmolar coma
- Hypoglycaemia
- Lactic acidosis
- Other causes:
  — Stroke (more common in diabetic patients)
  — Post-ictal (including hypoglycaemia – convulsions may cause a self-correcting lactic acidosis)
  — Cerebral trauma (may follow hypoglycaemia)
  — Ethanol intoxication (may induce or exacerbate hypoglycaemia in diabetic patients)
  — Overdose of drugs (e.g. benzodiazepines, tricyclics)

● *Leukocytosis.* This is common in DKA and does not necessarily indicate infection.

● *Gastric stasis.* A succussion splash may be evident on abdominal examination.

● *Generalized abdominal pain.* This may occur in younger patients with severe acidosis. If pain does not resolve within a few hours of treatment, another cause should be suspected. Plasma amylase may be unhelpful as levels may be elevated non-specifically in DKA.

DIAGNOSIS

Delays in initiating therapy may be disastrous and the diagnosis should be considered in any unconscious or hyperventilating patient. A rapid clinical examination and bedside blood and urine tests should allow a tentative diagnosis to be made on arrival at hospital, or even at home by the GP.

NB DKA should be considered in any unconscious or hyperventilating patient.

Treatment should then be commenced without delay. The initial clinical and biochemical assessment of a patient with suspected DKA is shown in Table 4.7.

NB Performance of routine investigations should not delay initiation of treatment and transfer to a high-dependency or intensive care unit.

TABLE 4.7 Initial management of a patient with suspected DKA

History
Initially, brief and relevant, including:
- Previous episodes of DKA
- Potential precipitating causes
- Comorbid conditions

Physical examination
Rapid but thorough assessment for:
- Signs of dehydration
- Level of consciousness
- Metabolic acidosis (Kussmaul respiration)
- Systemic hypotension
- Hypothermia
- Gastric stasis
- Precipitating conditions (e.g. pneumonia, pyelonephritis)

Biochemical assessment
Confirm diagnosis by bedside measurement of:
- Blood glucose (by glucose–oxidase reagent test strip)
- Urinary ketones (Ketostix)

Venous blood is withdrawn for laboratory measurement of:
- Glucose
- Urea (BUN)
- Electrolytes (sodium, potassium, ± chloride)
- Complete blood count
- Blood cultures

An arterial blood sample (corrected for hypothermia) is taken for:
- pH
- Bicarbonate
- P_{CO_2}
- P_{O_2} (if shocked)

Repeat laboratory measurement of blood glucose, electrolytes, urea, gases at 2 and 6 h

Other investigations
As indicated by the circumstances:
- Chest X-ray
- Microbial culture of urine, sputum
- ECG
- Sickle cell test

BUN = Blood urea nitrogen

• *Capillary blood.* The presence of hyperglycaemia may be rapidly confirmed at the bedside using a glucose–oxidase reagent strip. DKA presenting in the absence of marked hyperglycaemia is recognized. Reduced carbohydrate intake may predispose to the development of DKA with relatively small increments in blood glucose concentration. True euglycaemic DKA is, however, very uncommon.

• *Urine.* If available, should be tested for the presence of glucose and, most importantly, for ketones.

● *Venous blood.* This is withdrawn for laboratory measurement of glucose, urea (BUN), electrolytes and blood count. Plasma creatinine concentration may be falsely elevated in DKA because of assay interference by acetoacetate and this may lead to an erroneous diagnosis of renal failure. Despite a proportionally greater loss of body water, plasma sodium concentrations are usually normal or low, although plasma electrolyte concentrations may be falsely depressed by grossly elevated plasma lipid concentrations in DKA. Plasma should therefore be inspected for turbidity.

Eruptive xanthomata and lipaemia retinalis are recognized complications which respond to treatment of the ketoacidosis. Serum transaminases and creatine phosphokinase may be non-specifically elevated in DKA and may be mistaken for evidence of acute MI. Plasma ketone body concentration can be measured (semi-quantitatively) with a nitroprusside-based reaction. These tests are essentially specific for acetoacetate and do not react with 3-hydroxybutyrate. Acetone reacts only weakly with nitroprusside.

● *Arterial blood.* The acidosis is quantified by measurement of arterial (or capillary) pH, PCO_2 and bicarbonate concentration. Arterial PO_2 should be measured in severely shocked patients.

A severe metabolic acidosis in the absence of hyperglycaemia (or other obvious cause of acidosis such as renal failure) raises the possibility of either:

● *Lactic acidosis (see p. 188).*

● *Alcoholic ketoacidosis.* This occurs in alcoholics following a binge. Reduced carbohydrate intake owing to vomiting (from gastritis or pancreatitis) together with sympathetic activation secondary to alcohol withdrawal stimulates lipolysis and hence ketogenesis. Metabolism of alcohol induces a more reduced, hepatic mitochondrial redox state; the ratio of blood 3-hydroxybutyrate:acetoacetate may be markedly elevated (up to 10:1). Under these circumstances, the Ketostix reaction may give a misleadingly negative or 'trace' reaction. A similar diagnostic caveat may occasionally be encountered when significant lactic acidosis co-exists with ketoacidosis (see below). In the absence of significant hyperglycaemia, treatment of alcoholic ketoacidosis comprises rehydration with intravenous glucose and electrolyte replacement.

> **NB** The degree of ketonaemia may be underestimated in alcoholic ketoacidosis.

● *Anion gap acidosis.* Some causes of an anion gap acidosis are shown in Table 4.8. The anion gap is elevated when plasma:

[sodium] ([chloride] + [bicarbonate]) >15 mmol/L

TABLE 4.8 Causes of an anion gap acidosis

- Ketoacidosis
  — DKA
  — Alcoholic ketoacidosis
- Lactic acidosis
- Chronic renal failure
- Drug toxicity
  — Methanol (metabolized to formic acid)
  — Ethylene glycol (metabolized to oxalic acid)
  — Salicylate poisoning (severe)

Potassium is not included since the plasma level of this ion may be altered significantly by acid–base disturbances. The normal anion gap of about 10–15 mmol/L is accounted for by proteins, phosphate, sulphate and lactate ions. When the anion gap is increased, measurement of the plasma concentration of specific anions (e.g. ketone bodies, lactate) may confirm the aetiology of the acidosis. Although DKA usually presents as an anion gap acidosis (anion gap typically 25–35 mmol/L), a wide variety of acid–base disturbances have been reported.

● *Bacteriological culture.* Samples of urine and blood (prior to antibiotics) are mandatory in all cases and broad-spectrum antibiotics should be given if infection is suspected.

An underlying cause for DKA should be diligently sought in all patients although investigations should not delay the initiation of treatment and transfer to a high-dependency or intensive care unit.

 Severe DKA should be managed in a high-dependency or intensive care unit.

Some of the potential pitfalls in the diagnosis and management of DKA are summarized in Table 4.9.

TREATMENT OF DKA IN ADULTS

For the treatment of DKA in children, see page 264.
In addition to general supportive care and attention to underlying or associated conditions, specific treatment comprises:

- Rehydration with intravenous fluids.
- Replacement of electrolytes.
- Administration of insulin.

TABLE 4.9 Pitfalls in the diagnosis and management of DKA

- *Acetone on breath*
  A useful sign; note that many individuals cannot detect acetone
- *Fever*
  May be absent in the presence of infection (peripheral vasodilatation causes cooling)
- *Blood leukocytosis*
  Neutrophil count may be non-specifically raised
- *Plasma sodium concentration*
  May be falsely lowered initially by high lipid and glucose levels and may appear to rise suddenly after insulin treatment lowers plasma glucose and lipid levels
- *Plasma potassium concentration*
  May be temporarily raised (by acidosis) despite severe total body potassium depletion
- *Plasma creatinine concentration*
  May be falsely elevated (assay interference by ketone bodies)
- *Ketostix testing*
  May show 'negative' or 'trace' result when lactic acidosis or alcoholic ketoacidosis co-exist with DKA (predominance of 3-hydroxybutyrate). Ketostix reaction may become temporarily stronger during succesful treatment of DKA (conversion of 3-hydroxybutyrate to acetoacetate)
- *Plasma transaminases and creatine kinase*
  May be non-specifically raised; may lead to an erroneous suspicion of MI

General medical care and close supervision of the ketoacidotic patient by trained medical and nursing staff in a unit with a high staff-to-patient ratio are vitally important. A treatment flowchart must always be used and updated meticulously. Accurate recording of fluid balance may necessitate a urinary catheter if no urine is passed in the first 4 hours. An initial treatment plan for DKA in adults is shown in Table 4.10.

Rehydration

- *Initial therapy.* Adequate rehydration is a vital aspect of treatment which contributes directly to reductions in hyperglycaemia and counter-regulatory hormone levels.

NB Adequate rehydration is vital in the treatment of DKA.

Considerable variations in fluid and electrolyte disturbances are observed between patients and the following recommendations represent only a guide to therapy. Rehydration is commenced with isotonic saline (150 mmol/L) containing appropriate potassium supplements (see below). Isotonic saline is used in preference to hypotonic saline (unless plasma osmolarity is significantly raised) in order to minimize the rapid movement of extracellular water into cells as blood glucose and osmolarity fall with

TABLE 4.10 Guidelines for the management of severe DKA in adults

Fluids and electrolytes

Volumes
- 1 L/h × 3, thereafter adjusted according to requirements

Fluids
- Isotonic ('normal') saline (150 mmol/L) is routine
- Hypotonic ('half-normal') saline (75 mmol/L) if serum sodium exceeds 150 mmol/L (no more than 1–2 L – consider 5% dextrose with increased insulin if marked hypernatraemia)
- 5% dextrose 1L 4–6 hrly when blood glucose has fallen to 15 mmol/L (severely dehydrated patients may require simultaneous saline infusion)
- Sodium bicarbonate (100 mmol) as 1.26% solution (or 8.4% solution if large vein cannulated) if pH <7.0 (with extra potassium — see text)

Potassium
- No potassium in first 1 L unless initial plasma potassium <3.5 mmol/L
- Thereafter, add dosages below to each 1 L of fluid:

If plasma K[+]
    <4.0 mmol/L, add 40 mmol KCl (severe hypokalaemia may require more aggressive KCl replacement).
    3.5–5.5. mmol/L, add 20 mmol KCl
    >5.5 mmol/L, add no KCl

Insulin

By continuous intravenous infusion:
- A bolus of 20 units intravenously may be given while an insulin infusion is being prepared
- Give 6 units/h initially until blood glucose has fallen to 15 mmol/L. Thereafter, adjust rate (1–4 units/h usually) during dextrose infusion to maintain blood glucose 5–10 mmol/L until patient is eating again

Other points
- Search for and treat precipitating cause (e.g. infection, MI)
- Hypotension usually responds to adequate fluid replacement
- Central venous pressure (CVP) monitoring in elderly patients or if cardiac disease present
- Pass nasogastric tube if conscious level impaired to avoid aspiration of gastric contents
- Urinary catheter if conscious level impaired or no urine passed within 4 h of start of therapy
- Continuous ECG monitoring may warn of hyper- or hypokalaemia (plasma potassium should be measured at 0, 2 and 6 h – or more often as indicated)
- Adult respiratory distress syndrome (ARDS) – mechanical ventilation (100% O_2, IPPV), avoid fluid overload
- Mannitol (up to 1 g/kg intravenously) if cerebral oedema suspected. Dexamethasone as alternative (induces insulin resistance). Consider cranial CT to exclude other pathology (e.g. cerebral haemorrhage, venous sinus thrombosis)
- Treat specific thromboembolic complications if they occur
- Meticulously updated clinical and biochemical record using a purpose-designed flowchart

treatment; such shifts have been implicated in the pathogenesis of the serious complication of cerebral oedema (see p. 184).

Rehydration of the patient must take account of continuing polyuria and approximately 6–10 L of fluid may be required during the first 24 hours. In an average adult, 1 L of saline is infused every hour for the first 3 hours. The rate of infusion is then adjusted according to the clinical state of the patient. Considerable care is required in elderly patients or those with cardiac disease; monitoring of CVP or pulmonary wedge pressure is strongly recommended in these circumstances.

 Fluid overload during treatment is a potential hazard in the elderly, particularly in the presence of cardiovascular disease.

Occasionally, patients with relatively low admission plasma glucose concentrations may require a simultaneous infusion of dextrose to allow administration of sufficient insulin to suppress lipolysis and ketogenesis without inducing hypoglycaemia. A rising sodium (above 150 mmol/L) may necessitate the temporary substitution of hypotonic saline (75 mmol/L) or 5% dextrose (with an appropriate increase in the dose of insulin).

● *Subsequent therapy.* As soon as the plasma glucose has fallen to 15 mmol/L or below, saline is discontinued and an infusion of 5% dextrose is commenced at a rate of around 250 mL/h; this will avoid hypoglycaemia until the patient is eating again since the insulin infusion must be continued, albeit usually at a lower rate. Although the use of hypertonic (10%) dextrose at this stage of treatment produces a slightly faster fall in blood total ketone, bodies, this is not reflected in a more rapid resolution of the acidosis. Alternating infusions between saline and dextrose according to the blood glucose concentration should be avoided at this stage. Use only 5% dextrose, varying the insulin infusion rate to keep the blood glucose level under control.

Electrolyte replacement

Cardiac arrhythmias induced by iatrogenic hypokalaemia represent a major and avoidable cause of death. Hypokalaemia may also induce life-threatening weakness of respiratory muscles.

 Severe hypokalaemia complicating treatment of DKA is potentially fatal and is usually avoidable.

Potassium. Potassium is predominantly (98%) an intracellular ion, and insulin treatment with a rising pH stimulates the entry of extracellular potassium into cells. On average 20 mmol of potassium (administered as 1.5 g potassium chloride) will be required in each litre of fluid following the start of insulin therapy. Continuous ECG monitoring may indicate signs of hyper- or hypokalaemia, but this cannot replace monitoring of the plasma potassium concentration; this should be checked regularly (2-hourly during the initial stages) and potassium supplements adjusted appropriately. Particular care must be exercised in patients with renal failure, anuria or oliguria (less than 40 mL/h). If hypokalaemia is present (plasma potassium <3.5 mmol/L) potassium supplements should be doubled to 40 mmoL/h; if hyperkalaemia develops, potassium should be temporarily withheld, pending the result of further measurements.

Care must be taken to avoid hyperkalaemia in patients with renal impairment or oliguria.

Insulin therapy
The aims of insulin treatment in DKA are:

- Inhibition of lipolysis (and hence ketogenesis).
- Inhibition of hepatic glucose production.
- Enhanced disposal of glucose and ketone bodies by peripheral tissues.

- *Insulin infusion.* Soluble insulin only has a plasma half-life of approximately 5 min; intermittent, intravenous injections therefore lead to unpredictable and fluctuating plasma insulin concentrations. Maximal stimulation of potassium transport into cells occurs with pharmacological plasma insulin concentrations and the risk of hypokalaemia is therefore greater with large doses of insulin.

With modern insulin regimens complications of treatment such as hypokalaemia and late hypoglycaemia are less common than with obsolete, intermittent bolus regimens. Soluble insulin (e.g. Human Actrapid (Novo-Nordisk) or Humulin S (Lilly)) is best administered as a continuous, intravenous infusion at a rate of 5–10 (usually 6) units/h in adults. This produces steady plasma insulin concentrations which should adequately suppress lipolysis, ketogenesis and hepatic glucose production even in the presence of elevated levels of catabolic hormones (see Section 1).

Insulin is diluted to a convenient concentration (usually 1 unit/mL) with isotonic saline in a 50 mL syringe and delivered by a syringe-driver infusion pump connected via a Y connector. The infusion apparatus should be flushed through before connection to the patient in order to prevent adsorption of insulin to the plastic. Alternatively, insulin can be added to 500 mL isotonic saline; the insulin must be injected using a needle long enough to completely clear the injection port.

- *Monitoring of response.* With intravenous regimens, blood glucose is checked at the bedside at hourly intervals and the infusion rate is reduced to 1–4 units/h when blood glucose has fallen to 10–15 mmol/L. The infusion rate should be adjusted to maintain blood glucose concentration at between

5–10 mmol/L until the patient is eating again and subcutaneous insulin is recommenced. The rate required at this stage will vary according to the degree of insulin resistance (see above) and the rate of concomitant dextrose infusion. Both intravenous and intramuscular regimens should produce a steady and predictable fall in plasma glucose concentrations, averaging 4–6 mmol/h.

The commonest causes of failure to respond are mechanical problems such as the pump being inadvertently switched off or set at the wrong rate, and blockage of the delivery line. It is sound practice to cross-check (and record on the flow chart) the prescribed rate of insulin delivery against the volume infused each hour during treatment.

During treatment of DKA, there is increased conversion of 3-hydroxybutyrate to acetoacetate. Nitroprusside-based tests may therefore raise concerns that ketosis is either not resolving or is even worsening. A rising plasma bicarbonate concentration will allay such fears.

NB Ketonuria may increase transiently during successful treatment of DKA.

- *Transfer to subcutaneous insulin.* The first subcutaneous injection should comprise or include an appropriate dose of short-acting insulin. Precise recommendations are difficult to make but an injection of 8–12 units soluble insulin might be required initially by many adult patients, considerably more in some others (previous insulin doses are a useful guide). The subcutaneous insulin should be administered 30–60 min before the intravenous infusion is terminated to allow time for absorption of insulin from the subcutaneous depot thereby avoiding transient insulinopenia.

- *Intramuscular insulin.* If intravenous insulin administration is impracticable for any reason, an intramuscular regimen can be used as a safe alternative. This begins with a bolus of 20 units short-acting insulin, followed by 6 units/h into the deltoid until blood glucose has reached 15 mmol/L. Insufficient rehydration may cause erratic absorption of intramuscular injections, resulting in apparent insulin resistance.

If the plasma glucose concentration has not fallen after 2 hours of treatment, the fluid balance of the patient should be reappraised and intravenous insulin begun. Subcutaneous insulin may subsequently be commenced, with the start of a 5% dextrose infusion, at a dosage of about 8–10 units 4-hourly and continued for about 24 hours, when the patient's usual insulin regimen is reintroduced.

Bicarbonate

- *Indications.* The role of bicarbonate in the management of DKA remains controversial and no large clinical trials in severely acidotic patients with

DKA have been performed. However, blood pH levels 7.0 or below may lead to life-threatening respiratory depression and hypotension. Small doses of bicarbonate (approximately 100 mmol) may be beneficial if the patient is severely acidotic or if cardiorespiratory collapse appears imminent. Transfer to an intensive care unit should be considered.

● *Adverse metabolic effects.* Administration of bicarbonate into the extracellular space may actually exacerbate intracellular acidosis. Bicarbonate ions (which cannot diffuse across cell membranes) combine with H^+ ions extracellularly, producing carbonic acid which dissociates into water and CO_2. The latter readily enters cells where the reverse reaction occurs, generating H^+ (and bicarbonate ions) intracellularly.

Administration of alkali is associated with a number of potentially serious adverse effects, particularly hypokalaemia. Paradoxical acidosis of cerebrospinal fluid (the clinical significance of which is disputed), adverse effects on the oxyhaemoglobin dissociation curve and overshoot alkalosis are other unwanted effects. Concern has also been expressed about the potential for accelerating ketogenesis (and lactate generation) by elevating pH with bicarbonate. The fall in blood ketone body and lactate concentrations is delayed by sodium bicarbonate infusion.

● *Dosage and administration.* Bicarbonate (100 mmol) should be infused at 1.26% solution (or 8.4% solution) over 30 min and repeated if necessary to raise the pH to 7.0–7.2. Complete correction of the acidosis should not be attempted since concurrent metabolism of ketone anions may lead to over-alkalinization. Extra potassium (20 mmol potassium per 100 mmol bicarbonate) must always be administered when bicarbonate is infused and plasma potassium concentration should be re-checked afterwards. A solution of 8.4% sodium bicarbonate is extremely irritant and because of its tendency to cause thrombosis should only be infused into a large (ideally central) vein; extravasated solution often causes extensive local necrosis.

 Bicarbonate therapy is rarely indicated and carries potential hazards.

Other measures

● *Gastric stasis.* The stomach of a patient with DKA may contain 1–2 L of fluid and if the level of consciousness is depressed, there is a danger of inhalation of vomitus. Passing a nasogastric tube carries a risk of precipitating vomiting in an uncooperative patient unless the airway is protected by endotracheal intubation.

● *Hypotension.* It is often advocated that persistent systemic hypotension (<80 mmHg systolic) should be treated with plasma expanders. This is rarely necessary in practice; adequate rehydration usually obviates such measures.

ACUTE COMPLICATIONS

Cerebral oedema
Cerebral oedema is a rare and incompletely understood cause of mortality in DKA which appears to have an unfortunate predilection for affecting children (see p. 264).

Adult respiratory distress syndrome
ARDS has been reported in patients with DKA, usually in patients under 50 years of age. Clinical features include dyspnoea, tachypnoea, central cyanosis and non-specific chest signs. Arterial hypoxia is characteristic and chest X-ray reveals bilateral pulmonary infiltrates (Plate 4). Management involves respiratory support with intermittent positive pressure ventilation and avoidance of fluid overload.

Thromboembolism
Thromboembolic complications can cause mortality in DKA as a consequence of:

● Dehydration.
● Increased blood viscosity.
● Increased coagulability.

Disseminated intravascular coagulation has also been reported as a rare complication. The role of routine anticoagulation has not been clearly established in DKA and in the absence of other risk factors is not generally recommended. However, low-dose subcutaneous heparin (5000 units b.d.) is often administered with the aim of avoiding venous thromboembolism.

Rhinocerebral mucormycosis
Rarely, an aggressive opportunistic fungal infection develops in patients with DKA or other metabolic acidoses. The lesion arises in the paranasal sinuses and rapidly invades adjacent tissues (nose, sinuses, orbit and brain). Treatment comprises correction of acidosis, surgical excision of affected tissue and parenteral antifungal agents. The course is often fulminant and the condition carries a high mortality.

Rhabdomyolysis
Elevation of plasma myoglobin and creatine kinase concentrations may occur in DKA. However, clinically important renal complications of rhabdomyolysis are uncommon. Acute renal failure caused by rhabdomyolysis may be somewhat more common in the diabetic hyperosmolar non-ketotic syndrome (see p. 185) but is nonetheless a rare complication.

COUNSELLING AND FOLLOW-UP

As DKA is a life-threatening condition, it demands a thorough exploration of the circumstances leading to the admission. There is often a need for re-education of the patient (and sometimes of health care professionals). Re-emphasis of sick day rules – in particular the importance of continuing insulin – may be required (see p. 283). The problem of recurrent DKA in young women is more problematic. The elderly patient with type 1 diabetes, particularly if intellectually impaired, or otherwise infirm or socially isolated, is also at risk of recurrent episodes (see Section 6).

> **NB** An episode of DKA should prompt a thorough review of the precipitating events; re-education may be indicated.

DKA usually denotes a clear requirement for continued (and uninterrupted) insulin treatment. However, some patients, particularly if Black, may present in DKA and yet not require insulin in the longer term.

DIABETIC HYPEROSMOLAR NON-KETOTIC SYNDROME

PATHOPHYSIOLOGY

The diabetic hyperosmolar non-ketotic syndrome is characterized by:

- Marked hyperglycaemia (plasma glucose usually in excess of 50 mmol/L).
- Profound dehydration with pre-renal uraemia.
- Depression of the level of consciousness; coma is well recognized.

Note that significant hyperketonaemia, ketonuria and acidosis are usually absent (although there is some overlap between the syndromes of DKA and the hyperosmolar non-ketotic state). Insulin concentrations in peripheral blood similar to those in patients with DKA and the absence of significant ketosis are unexplained. Suppression of lipolysis (see p. 6) by the hyperosmolar state has been suggested and aspects of the catabolic hormone response may be less marked than in patients with DKA.

> **NB** By definition, the hyperosmolar syndrome is not associated with significant ketosis.

INCIDENCE AND MORTALITY

Although less common than DKA (ratio approximately 1:10 in the UK), the mortality rate is considerably higher at 30% or more per episode. The high mortality in part reflects the high incidence of serious associated disorders and complications.

> **NB** The hyperosmolar syndrome carries a high case-fatality rate.

CLINICAL FEATURES

Patients with hyperosmolar non-ketotic decompensation are usually middle aged or elderly. Black patients are more frequently represented in series of hyperosmolar non-ketotic decompensation relative to their contribution to episodes of DKA. Up to two-thirds of cases occur in patients with previously undiagnosed type 2 diabetes. Hypertension and treatment with diuretics are well-recognized features which may be of relevance to the pathophysiology (see Section 1). Characteristic symptoms are:

- Polyuria.
- Intense thirst.
- Gradual clouding of consciousness.

In the absence of vomiting, which is a prominent symptom of DKA, many patients drink large volumes of carbonated, glucose-containing drinks which only exacerbate thirst and hyperglycaemia. The symptoms may develop over several weeks. Coma and severe dehydration with arterial hypotension are common and reversible focal neurological signs or motor seizures may occur. Kussmaul respiration (see p. 173) is not a feature since acidosis is minor or absent. Many patients are in a moribund state when admitted to hospital.

Precipitating factors

Hyperosmolar non-ketosis has many precipitating causes, which may co-exist in individual patients. Infection is frequently present and hyperosmolar decompensation following treatment with antihypertensive drugs such as diuretics and beta-blockers has been reported. Many other drugs have been implicated in the development of the syndrome. However, while some of these drugs (e.g. corticosteroids, non-selective beta-blockers) have measurable effects on glucose tolerance and insulin sensitivity, the relevance of others, e.g. chlorpromazine, remains uncertain.

DIAGNOSIS

The insidious nature of the condition often leads to delays in diagnosis; an erroneous provisional diagnosis of stroke is not uncommon. The hyperosmolar non-ketotic syndrome must therefore enter the differential diagnosis of any patient presenting with otherwise unexplained impairment of consciousness or focal neurological signs, dehydration or shock.

> **NB** The hyperosmolar non-ketotic syndrome may present as impairment of consciousness, focal neurology, dehydration or shock.

● *Urinalysis.* This will reveal heavy glycosuria and a negative or perhaps 'trace' reaction with Ketostix.

● *Blood chemistry.* The diagnosis is confirmed by a markedly raised plasma glucose concentration. Pre-renal uraemia, a raised haematocrit, and a mild leukocytosis are common. Depression of consciousness generally occurs when plasma osmolality exceeds about 340 mosmol/L. Although there is considerable inter-individual variation, alternative causes of an impaired level of consciousness should be considered in patients whose osmolality is less marked.

Plasma osmolality

Plasma osmolality (the osmotic pressure exerted by a fluid across a membrane) can be measured in the laboratory (e.g. by freezing point depression), and can be estimated using the formula:

Plasma osmolality = $2 \times$ (plasma Na^+ + plasma K^+)
(mosmol/L)   + plasma glucose
                  + plasma urea
(where Na^+, K^+, glucose and urea are in mmol/L)

The values for Na^+ and K^+ are doubled to allow for their associated Cl^- anions.

Although total body sodium is reduced, plasma sodium concentration at presentation may be low, normal or high, depending on the degree of concomitant water deficit. The degree of dehydration is generally greater than in DKA. As in DKA, hypertriglyceridaemia and hyperglycaemia may falsely depress the sodium concentration.

> **NB** Plasma sodium concentrations may be depressed by hyperglycaemia or hypertriglyceridaemia.

Plasma bicarbonate is usually above 15 mmol/L although renal impairment may lead to some retention of H^+ ions and hypotension may produce a degree of lactic acidaemia. Non-traumatic rhabdomyolysis may occasionally be severe enough to precipitate acute renal failure (see p. 184).

TREATMENT

Successful management of hyperosmolar non-ketotic coma depends on good general care of the unconscious patient and prompt recognition and treatment of underlying causes.

● *Initial therapy*. Intravenous rehydration, electrolyte replacement and insulin therapy are usually similar to that recommended for DKA. Controversy surrounds the choice of isotonic or hypotonic saline for intitial rehydration and no RCTs have been performed. It is recommended that isotonic saline (150 mmol/L) is used in preference to hypotonic saline (75 mmol/L) unless plasma sodium exceeds 150 mmol/L. A rise in plasma sodium is frequently observed as blood glucose falls with treatment, and water moves back into the intracellular compartment. The rise in sodium may also be partially explained by the reciprocal relationship that exists between plasma glucose and sodium concentrations.

● *Thromboembolic complications*. Despite the high frequency of thromboembolic complications in patients with hyperosmolar non-ketotic coma, the role of routine anticoagulation remains uncertain. Neurological signs usually reverse when hyperglycaemia is controlled; epilepsy also responds to insulin and rehydration, but often not to specific anti-epileptic drugs in the presence of hyperosmolality.

● *Subsequent antidiabetic treatment*. Although insulin treatment is usually recommended for the first few months, these patients generally secrete significant quantities of endogenous insulin, allowing successful long-term treatment with oral hypoglycaemic agents. Possible precipitating factors (e.g. thiazide diuretics, glucose drinks) must be carefully avoided in the future.

LACTIC ACIDOSIS

LACTATE METABOLISM

Lactate and hydrogen ions (H^+) are the products of anaerobic glycolysis, the reaction of which can be summarized as:

$$\text{glucose} \longrightarrow 2 \text{ lactate}^- + 2 \text{ H}^+$$

The principal lactic acid-producing organs are:

● Skeletal muscle.
● Brain.

- Erythrocytes.
- Renal medulla.

The liver, kidneys and heart normally extract lactate but may become net producers of lactic acid under conditions of severe ischaemia. Lactic acid (pK_a 3.8) is almost completely dissociated at body pH. Lactate produced by glycolysis may be completely oxidized to CO_2 and water in the tricarboxylic acid cycle, thereby consuming an equimolar amount of hydrogen ions:

$$lactate^- + 3\,O_2 + H^+ \longrightarrow 3\,CO_2 + 3\,H_2O$$

Alternatively, lactate may enter the gluconeogenesis pathway in the liver and kidney to reform glucose (the Cori cycle), a process which also consumes H^+ ions:

$$2\,lactate^- + 2\,H^+ \longrightarrow glucose$$

LACTIC ACIDOSIS

Pathological degrees of hyperlactataemia accompanied by acidosis may arise as a consequence of overproduction of lactate and hydrogen ions (e.g. with tissue hypoxia), a decrease in their clearance (e.g. reduced hepatic lactate clearance in severe shock, impaired gluconeogenesis in severe acidosis) or a combination of these two processes. Normal fasting blood lactate concentrations range from approximately 0.5–1.5 mmol/L. Severe lactic acidosis (defined arbitrarily as a metabolic acidosis with a blood lactate concentration of greater than 5 mmol/L) is encountered in two main clinical settings (Table 4.11):

- *Type A.* This is primarily associated with states of tissue hypoxia such as shock or cardiac failure.

- *Type B.* This is much less common; it is associated with several systemic diseases including diabetes mellitus, drugs and toxins or inborn errors of metabolism.

Tissue hypoxia is not an obvious feature of type B lactic acidosis although hypotension and hypoxia may supervene as pre-terminal events. The clinical features of lactic acidosis are similar to those of other causes of severe metabolic acidosis; additional features of precipitating or associated conditions may also be observed.

LACTIC ACIDOSIS ASSOCIATED WITH DIABETES MELLITUS

Despite the frequent presence of macrovascular and microvascular complications which favour tissue hypoxia, severe lactic acidosis is only

TABLE 4.11 Classification and causes of lactic acidosis

Type A (Primarily associated with tissue hypoxia)
- Shock
  - Cardiogenic
  - Endotoxic
  - Hypovolaemic
- Cardiac failure
- Asphyxia
- Carbon monoxide poisoning

Type B

1. Systemic disorders
- Diabetes mellitus
- Neoplasia
- Liver disease
- Convulsions

2. Drugs and toxins
- Biguanides (especially phenformin)
- Ethanol
- Methanol
- Salicylates
- Fructose/sorbitol/xylitol (in parenteral nutrition)
- Zidovudine

3. Inborn errors of metabolism
- Type I glycogen storage disease
- Fructose 1,6-diphosphatase deficiency

4. D-lactic acidosis due to abnormal gut flora; rare

rarely associated with diabetes mellitus. Type B lactic acidosis is a well-recognized complication of biguanide therapy (see p. 120) for type 2 diabetes and a degree of hyperlactataemia is relatively common in DKA.

Biguanides and lactic acidosis

The incidence of lactic acidosis in diabetic patients has declined dramatically since the withdrawal of the biguanide phenformin in many countries including the UK and USA during the 1970s. The incidence of lactic acidosis associated with phenformin was approximately 10–15 times that observed with metformin because of differences in chemical structure resulting in binding to the inner mitochondrial membrane and interference with oxidative metabolism (see p. 122). In addition, there is an inherited inability of some individuals to inactivate the drug in the liver by hydroxylation.

Lactic acidosis associated with phenformin treatment carries a poor prognosis with approximately a 50% mortality rate. Lactic acidosis complicating therapy with metformin is, however, rare and occurs almost exclusively in patients in whom biguanide therapy is contraindicated, e.g. patients with renal impairment. Many diabetic patients treated with insulin or phenformin show asymptomatic daily elevations in blood lactate.

Hyperlactataemia in DKA

Significant hyperlactataemia is found in 10–15% of cases of DKA and usually responds to routine treatment of the ketoacidosis. This may reflect the effect of hydrogen ions generated in DKA on cellular redox state. Predictable rises in blood lactate concentration occur when treatment is instituted. Insulin suppresses gluconeogenesis thus reducing hepatic extraction of lactate from the blood, while facilitating peripheral glucose uptake and metabolism with lactate generation. This rise in lactate is generally transient and insignificant although larger increments were observed with outmoded high-dose insulin regimens.

TREATMENT AND PROGNOSIS

The generally poor prognosis associated with severe lactic acidosis is largely determined by the severity of the underlying condition. An exception is lactic acidosis secondary to generalized epileptic convulsions; this is self-limiting and requires no specific treatment.

 Transient lactic acidosis following convulsions does not require bicarbonate therapy.

Despite controversy surrounding the theoretical and clinical benefits of alkali therapy, intravenous bicarbonate remains the mainstay of supportive treatment for cases of severe lactic acidosis.

- *Intravenous bicarbonate.* Massive quantities may be required to elevate arterial pH; simultaneous dialysis has been recommended to avoid sodium overload. Haemodialysis may also be beneficial in removing metformin when accumulation of this drug is associated with lactic acidosis. The concentration of the drug can be measured in plasma but the result is usually available only after treatment. Obtain expert advice.

- *Sodium dichloroacetate.* This has received attention as a potential adjunct in the management of lactic acidosis. By stimulating the activity of pyruvate dehydrogenase, dichloroacetate lowers blood lactate levels in patients with lactic acidosis associated with a variety of conditions. Acid–base status may be improved, but there is no reduction in mortality in patients with type A lactic acidosis.

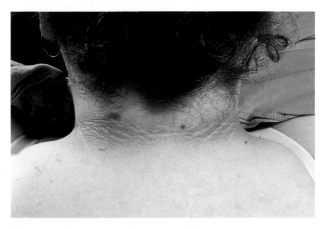

Plate 1 Acanthosis nigricans in a patient with hyperandrogenism and hyperinsulinaemia.

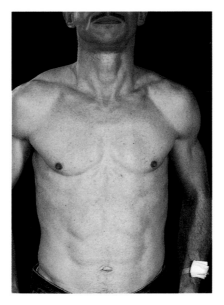

Plate 2 Total acquired lipodystrophy with diabetes and hyperlipidaemia.

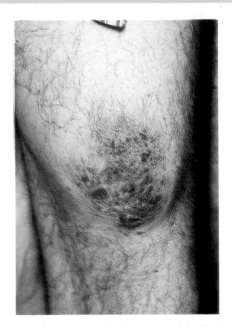

Plate 3 Insulin-induced lipohypertrophy of the thigh.

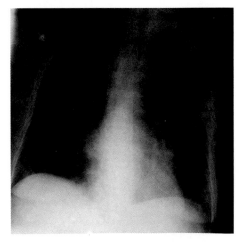

Plate 4 Radiographic appearances of ARDS complicating treatment of DKA.

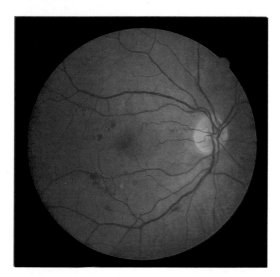

Plate 5 Background retinopathy – microaneurysms and blot haemorrhages.

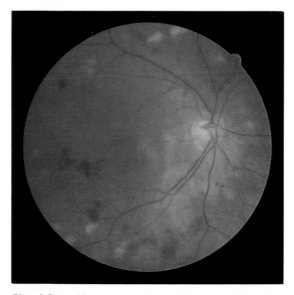

Plate 6 Pre-proliferative retinopathy – multiple haemorrhages and cotton-wool spots.

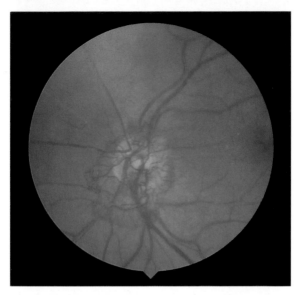

Plate 7 Proliferative retinopathy – new vessels arising from the optic disc.

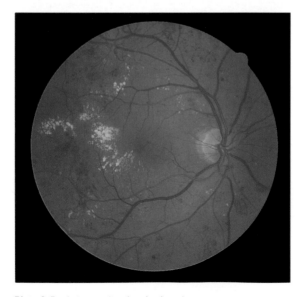

Plate 8 Exudative maculopathy – hard exudates.

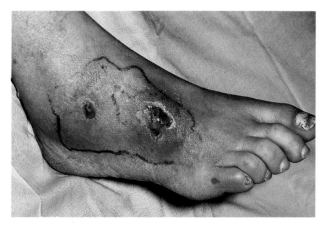

Plate 9 Diabetic polyneuropathy – clawing of toes and burn sustained from sitting in front of an open fire; ink marks indicate area of maximum cellulitis.

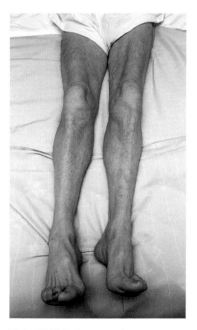

Plate 10 Diabetic amyotrophy – asymmetrical wasting of thighs.

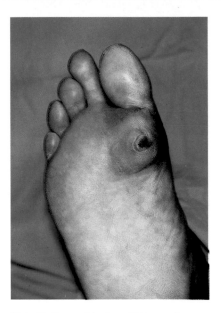

Plate 11 Neuropathic ulcer with haemorrhage over first metatarsal head.

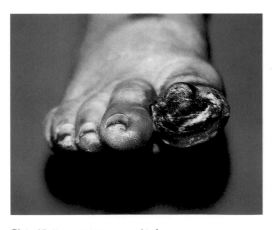

Plate 12 Gangrene in a neuropathic foot.

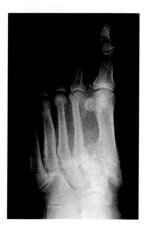

Plate 13 Charcot neuroarthropathy – progression of degenerative changes in bones of feet over 2 years.

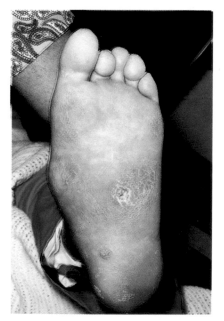

Plate 14 End-stage Charcot neuroarthropathy.

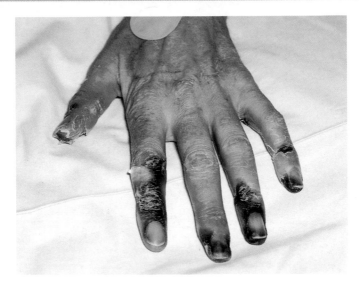

Plate 15 Gangrene in a patient with end-stage renal failure secondary to diabetic nephropathy.

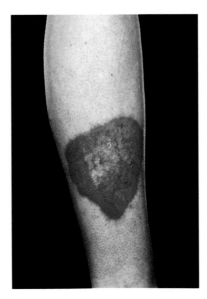

Plate 16 Necrobiosis lipoidica diabeticorum.

COMPLICATIONS

The propensity of patients with diabetes to develop chronic tissue complications, microvascular disease and non-specific macrovascular complications is outlined in Section 1 (see pp. 7–9). A brief discussion of the biochemistry and histology of microvascular disease together with an outline of hypotheses relating to the production of tissue damage may also be found in Section 1. In this section, clinical aspects of these complications, the cause of great morbidity and premature mortality, are considered in more detail.

OCULAR COMPLICATIONS

Clinically significant ocular complications associated with diabetes include:

- Transient visual disturbances secondary to osmotic changes.
- Retinopathy – the cause of >80% blindness in diabetics.
- Cataracts – develop earlier in diabetic patients.
- Glaucoma – primary or secondary to diabetic retinopathy.
- Iritis – associated with autoimmune type 1 diabetes.

DIABETIC RETINOPATHY

KEY POINTS

- Diabetes is the principal cause of partial sight and blind registration in Western or industrialized countries.
- Diabetic retinopathy is asymptomatic until well advanced.
- Effective treatment is available for diabetic retinopathy.
- Laser photocoagulation must be applied before retinopathy is too advanced.
- Patients must be screened regularly using an effective system.

Epidemiological studies indicate that the determinants of diabetic retinopathy are essentially similar for type 1 and type 2 diabetes. The principal factors determining the development and progression of diabetic retinopathy are:

- The duration of diabetes.
- Degree of chronic glycaemic control.

Thus, the prevalence of any degree of retinopathy is highest in younger, insulin-treated patients than in non-insulin-treated, older patients with type 2 diabetes. However, severe retinopathy may develop in both major subtypes of diabetes. Other factors, notably hypertension, also have an important influence. This was demonstrated in the Hypertension in Diabetes study (see p. 243). Studies in the USA show that the risk of retinopathy is higher amongst certain ethnic groups compared with non-Hispanic whites:

- Native Americans.
- Mexican Americans.
- African Americans.

This increased risk does not appear to be attributable to differences in glycaemic control or other risk factors.

TYPE 1 DIABETES

The development of clinically significant retinopathy (as opposed to functional changes, including hyperglycaemic-associated increased retinal blood flow or subtle subclinical perceptual alterations), requires a long period of pathological hyperglycaemia. Thus, retinopathy is absent at diagnosis but after 15–20 years of disease, the prevalence is more than 95%. Proliferative retinopathy is infrequently encountered within 5 years of diagnosis but approximately 40–60% of patients will develop proliferative retinopathy after 20–30 years. Glycaemic control is an important factor, as demonstrated by the DCCT (see p. 60).

> **NB** Retinopathy develops in the majority of type 1 diabetes with long-duration disease.

The DCCT also demonstrated the phenomenon of transient deterioration following acute improvement in glycaemic control. Among patients with pre-existing retinopathy in the intensive treatment group whose control was improved, there was a lag phase in the first few years of the trial during which retinopathy progressed more rapidly. Importantly, however, retinopathy in this group was subsequently significantly reduced overall. Thus, this effect is not an argument for therapeutic nihilism. The benefits of long-term, tight glycaemic control are clear with continued good control. Careful surveillance – with timely laser photocoagulation, if necessary – is required for patients with retinopathy during periods when glycaemic control is acutely improved. The well-recognized risk of sudden deterioration of retinopathy during pregnancy (see pp. 272–273) may, in part, reflect improvements in glycaemic control. Acute reduction in blood flow leading to retinal hypoxia is a postulated mechanism. The contribution of recurrent hypoglycaemia is less certain.

Pre-existing retinopathy may deteriorate transiently when glycaemic control is acutely improved.

TYPE 2 DIABETES

Approximately 20% of patients may have retinopathy at diagnosis, the prevalence increasing with age, and careful fundoscopy is therefore mandatory in newly-presenting patients. As far as retinopathy is concerned, maculopathy is the major cause of visual loss in this group of patients. However, cataract is relatively common (see p. 203). Control of hypertension is important in the prevention of visual impairment owing to maculopathy.

> **NB** Hypertension has a major influence on the progression of diabetic retinopathy.

OCULAR SYMPTOMS IN DIABETES

Unless it has reached a very advanced stage, diabetic eye disease is largely asymptomatic. Ocular symptoms attributable to diabetes include:

- *Transient disturbance of refraction* – usually myopia; may be a presenting symptom of diabetes (see Section 2) or may occur with institution of antidiabetic therapy. Patients are advised to defer eye tests until diabetic control has been stabilized. Osmotic changes within the ocular lens are held to be primarily responsible.

Other less commonly encountered but important symptoms include:

- *Gradual loss of vision* – suggestive of maculopathy or cataract.

- *Sudden painless loss of vision* – vitreous haemorrhage. Retinal arterial and venous thrombosis may also occur in diabetic patients.

- *Appearance of 'floaters'* – possible small or recurrent vitreous haemorrhage.

- *Chronic pain and redness* – rubeosis and secondary glaucoma.

- *Field defects and impaired night vision* – sequelae of extensive laser photocoagulation.

In addition, extraocular cranial nerve palsies may cause diplopia (see p. 205). Hypoglycaemia may cause transient visual disturbance (see p. 160).

> **NB** Diabetic retinopathy and its sequelae are usually asymptomatic until well advanced.

SCREENING FOR DIABETIC RETINOPATHY

Early recognition of diabetic retinopathy is crucial in order that laser therapy can be administered at a stage when useful vision can be preserved. Annual checks of corrected visual acuity combined with expert evaluation of the fundus are required. In the UK, diabetologists, trained GPs or optometrists usually perform direct fundoscopy in the clinic or surgery. In the USA and elsewhere, an ophthalmologist or optometrist will provide this service.

Visual acuity

Corrected best visual acuity is measured at 6 m using a well-illuminated Snellen chart. Patients should wear their long-distance spectacles as required. A pinhole will correct refractive errors to approximately 6/9. Test each eye separately. Visual acuity should be tested before instillation of mydriatic eye drops. Impaired visual acuity, which does not improve with pinhole testing, suggests:

- Maculopathy.
- Cataract.

Retinal examination

If direct ophthalmoscopy is employed, the pupils must be pharmacologically dilated using 1% tropicamide instilled 10–15 min beforehand. This is usually quite safe but the effect of the tropicamide may take several hours to wear off; transient local discomfort is common. The pupils of elderly patients, and particularly patients with overt diabetic neuropathy, may not dilate well; autonomic imbalance is postulated. Cautions and contraindications to mydriasis are few:

- *A history of angle-closure glaucoma.* An acute attack may be provoked by tropicamide (see above).

- *Driving.* This should be avoided, if possible. Dazzle from headlights and impaired visual acuity (which may fall transiently below legal requirements) carry obvious risks after tropicamide; alternative transport should be arranged in advance. Although pilocarpine is sometimes used to reverse the effect of tropicamide the effect may only be partial, the pupil becoming fixed in mid-dilatation. Reading is also affected.

- *History of intraocular surgery.* Rarely a problem but the advice of the ophthalmologist should be sought if there is doubt. Dislocation of some forms of intraocular lens implants may occur with pupillary dilatation.

For clinical trials, seven-field, stereoscopic, fundal photography through dilated pupils is regarded as the most rigorous assessment; the photographs require expertise in interpretation and detailed grading systems have been developed. Clinical assessment may be superior in detecting subtle changes associated with macular oedema.

Non-mydriatic retinal cameras

These cameras can provide colour photographs of the optic disc and macula which have been extensively used in UK screening programmes. The photographs obtained using this technique require expert evaluation; high-resolution video cameras with digital data capture are a more recent development. Studies suggest that cameras may improve the detection rate for maculopathy. Digital data have the additional advantage of being suitable for electronic transfer and incorporation into computer-based record systems.

Frequency of screening

Type 1 diabetes. For children, it is generally agreed that annual examination of the fundi need only commence after the onset of puberty (see p. 267). Examination of all post-pubertal patients at diagnosis and annually thereafter is routine at some centres. Alternatively, patients with classical type 1 diabetes presenting under the age of 30 years may be examined:

— 3–5 years from diagnosis or onset of puberty.
— Annually thereafter.

This reflects the low incidence of sight-threatening retinopathy in the first few years after diagnosis. Chronic, very poor glycaemic control (HbA_{1c} levels >10% or recurrent episodes of ketoacidosis, see p. 156) should prompt more frequent examinations.

> **NB** Annual eye examinations are recommended for all diabetic patients beyond puberty.

Type 2 diabetes. The possibility that retinopathy may have developed prior to diagnosis (see Section 2) and the tendency for maculopathy to develop within a few years require that all patients are examined:

— At diagnosis.
— Annually thereafter.

For all patients, more frequent examination should be considered if retinopathy is detected. Patients who have returned to the clinic having defaulted from follow-up should always have their eyes examined. Eye assessment before and during pregnancy is considered on page 273.

> **NB** Patients who have temporarily defaulted should always have an eye examination.

Cost-effectiveness of screening for diabetic retinopathy

Several studies have assessed the cost-effectiveness of screening for diabetic retinopathy in the UK, USA and elsewhere. Screening by ophthalmoscopy or retinal photography provides a relatively inexpensive means of preserving vision. Moreover, screening has been shown to be cost-effective by avoidance of the economic consequences of disability payments for serious visual impairment. Local circumstances will dictate which method, or combination of methods described above, is used. Coordination between the screening programme and the units providing treatment is required to ensure prompt assessment and appropriate follow-up.

CLASSIFICATION OF DIABETIC RETINOPATHY

For clinical purposes, diabetic retinopathy is classified into several well-defined stages. It is common, but not inevitable for retinopathy to pass from one stage to the next, potentially more serious stage. The clinical importance of this classification derives from the likelihood of successful treatment for the earlier stages (Table 5.1). The benefits of photocoagulation were proven in RCTs initially using the xenon arc and later the argon laser.

TABLE 5.1 Classification of diabetic retinopathy

- Background retinopathy
- Pre-proliferative retinopathy
- Proliferative retinopathy
- Advanced diabetic eye disease
- Maculopathy

Maculopathy denotes the presence of retinopathy concentrated at the macula, i.e. within the temporal vessels, approaching the fovea. Since maculopathy may threaten central vision, particularly in patients with type 2 diabetes, it represents an important category. Advanced diabetic eye disease includes the sequelae of vitreous haemorrhage and secondary rubeotic glaucoma; visual impairment is always present to some degree – often blindness.

> **NB** Proliferative retinopathy and maculopathy are potentially sight-threatening forms of diabetic retinopathy.

Background retinopathy
This is characterized ophthalmoscopically (Plate 5) by:

- Microaneurysms.
- Intraretinal blot or, less often, flame haemorrhages.
- Hard exudates (waxy-looking, lipid deposits from damaged vessels).

In isolation, venous dilatation is not regarded as evidence of retinopathy. All of these changes are asymptomatic. Individual features may fluctuate, microaneurysms and haemorrhages sometimes disappearing, albeit rarely.

completely, on re-examination. However, background retinopathy always raises the possibility of progression to more serious retinopathy.

Action

● *Surveillance.* Careful periodic review is essential; every 6 months or so is usually recommended for all but the most minimal or slowly progressive retinopathy.

● *Explanation.* It is usually appropriate to inform the patient of the discovery of retinopathy; the importance of regular review should be stressed. However, the appearance of retinopathy has alarming implications which are unlikely to be lost on the patient. A considerate and reassuring approach is indicated; the risk of serious visual impairment is greatly reduced with appropriately-timed therapy.

● *Search for other complications.* The discovery of the earliest signs of retinopathy should prompt detailed physical review and a search for evidence of other complications, notably hypertension and nephropathy (see later), which may influence progression of retinopathy.

● *Review of glycaemic control.* The importance of good glycaemic control should be discussed in terms appropriate to the individual. However, the setting of unrealistic glycaemic targets is likely to generate anxiety and frustration.

> **NB** Background retinopathy is asymptomatic: careful ophthalmoscopic review is required.

Pre-proliferative retinopathy (Plate 6)
● Venous loops, beading or reduplication.
● Arterial sheathing.
● Intraretinal microvascular abnormalities (arteriovenous shunts).
● Multiple cotton wool spots (retinal infarcts).
● Multiple, extensive haemorrhages.

These features denote increasing retinal ischaemia. The extent and degree of ischaemia are usually underestimated by the ophthalmological appearances; specialist investigations such as fluorescein angiography may be indicated. Pre-proliferative retinopathy, by definition, carries a relatively high risk of progression to new vessel formation within the subsequent 12 months.

ction

thalmic referral.* In general, specialist opthalmological advice is
ed within a few weeks for pre-proliferative retinopathy.

Proliferative retinopathy

- New vessels (Plate 7).

These arise at the following sites in response to growth factors released by areas of ischaemic retina:

— On the optic disc.
— In the periphery of the retina.

These friable vessels may cause pre-retinal or vitreous haemorrhages. New vessels on the optic disc are the most feared in view of the high risk of haemorrhage. New vessels are asymptomatic in the absence of haemorrhage. If a large haemorrhage occurs, the patient presents with sudden, painless, monocular loss of vision; smaller bleeds may cause the patient to notice 'floaters' in the visual fields. On examination, the new vessels appear frond-like, extending into the subhyaloid space from their origin in the retinal surface. Widespread retinopathy elsewhere is usual. Following a large haemorrhage, there is loss of the normal red reflex on ophthalmoscopic examination. It may be impossible to discern any retinal features on fundoscopy.

Action

- *Urgent referral to an ophthalmologist.* Contact should be made with the ophthalmology service with the minimum of delay; immediate assessment is indicated for acute vitreous haemorrhage.

> **NB** Acute vitreous haemorrhage necessitates immediate referral to an ophthalmologist.

- *Laser photocoagulation.* Timely argon laser therapy can reduce severe visual loss by >50% over 5 years in patients with proliferative retinopathy. It is important that laser therapy is given before visual loss has become too severe and potentially irreversible. Laser therapy is an out-patient procedure. Several sittings may be necessary for extensive laser treatment (panretinal photocoagulation) which may involve thousands of retinal burns. Potential complications include:

- Impaired night vision.
- Visual field constriction.
- Impaired colour vision.
- Progression of macular oedema.

The retina is partially ablated, taking care to preserve the macula and papillomacular bundle. New vessels regress and the stimulus to further new vessel formation is removed by destruction of the ischaemic retina.

Successful photocoagulation may induce permanent quiescence of proliferative retinopathy. However, in most cases, photocoagulation is more appropriately regarded as a palliative procedure which may not completely prevent further haemorrhages. The intraocular haemorrhage must be absorbed before laser treatment can be applied; this may take several weeks.

Advanced diabetic eye disease

- Retinal detachment owing to fibrous traction.
- Rubeosis iridis (new vessels on the iris).

Severe retinal ischaemia may lead to new vessel formation on the iris. Obstruction of the drainage angle by new vessels may cause painful, secondary, rubeotic glaucoma. Retinal detachment – a grey elevation of the retina – may be obscured by vitreous haemorrhage.

Action

- *Urgent referral to ophthalmologist.* In practice, most of these patients will already be under the care of an opthalmologist. Retinal detachment merits immediate expert assessment.

- *Panretinal photocoagulation.* See above.

- *Surgical vitrectomy.* This highly specialized procedure may restore useful vision in selected patients with advanced diabetic eye disease. Microsurgical techniques are employed to remove fibrous plaques, re-attach areas of retina and apply intraocular laser if feasible.

- *Enucleation.* This is a last resort for a painful, blind eye.

Maculopathy

This mainly affects older patients with type 2 diabetes. Three types are recognized:

- *Exudative (Plate 8).* May develop into circinate plaques.

- *Oedematous.* Cystic or diffuse; may be difficult to visualize on direct ophthalmoscopy.

- *Ischaemic.* The least amenable to treatment.

Maculopathy should be suspected if a significant reduction in visual acuity (i.e. by 2 lines on Snellen chart) occurs in the absence of an obvious cause such as cataract formation. Expert slit lamp examination may be required to confirm the diagnosis. Leaking capillaries may be more easily identified by fluorescein angiography.

Action

- *Referral to ophthalmologist.* Hard exudates within two disc diameters of fixation (ask patient to look directly into the light of the ophthalmoscope).

Unexplained deterioration in visual acuity merits referral to an ophthalmologist whether or not retinopathy is visualized.

● *Photocoagulation.* Focal for microaneurysms or grid for diffuse macular oedema.

● *Control of hypertension.* Hypertension should be sought and vigorously treated (see p. 240).

VISUAL HANDICAP

Patients with severe visual impairment should be registered by their ophthalmologist as partially sighted (best corrected acuity 6/60) or blind (3/60, or worse), as appropriate. This triggers compensatory financial benefits and social support.

Low vision aids and adapted everyday appliances are available. Pen injectors and other devices may be useful for patients requiring insulin treatment. With instruction, self-monitoring of capillary glucose is possible; modified glucose meters are available, including devices providing an audible result (see p. 74).

Other potential support includes:

● Braille instruction.
● Large print and audio books.
● Guide dog provision.

Depression is understandably common. Peer support organized through patient organizations can be helpful.

CATARACT

A cataract is an opacity of the crystalline lens of the eye. It is usually asymptomatic in the early stages of development but may progress to cause significant visual impairment or even blindness. The commonest variety of cataract is the so-called senile cataract. Cataracts are features of certain syndromes or therapies which may also be associated with diabetes, for example:

● Myotonic dystrophy (see p. 25).
● Chronic corticosteroid therapy (see p. 22).

Epidemiological studies indicate that diabetes mellitus is a significant risk factor for cataract formation in patients aged up to 70 years. The incidence of cataract is increased several-fold compared with the non-diabetic population; the opacity may also progress more rapidly in diabetic patients. In the UKPDS, improved glycaemic control was associated with a reduction in risk of cataract extraction.

Cataracts are more common in diabetics and appear earlier than in non-diabetics.

Rarely, diabetes is associated with the development of an acute form of rapidly developing lens opacity known as a 'snowflake cataract'. This usually affects young, insulin-dependent patients and typically, though not invariably, follows a period of particularly poor glycaemic control. The cataract may appear and mature within weeks.

TREATMENT

This is indicated if the cataract is:

- Significantly interfering with daily activities.
- Interfering with the assessment of retinopathy.

Surgical extraction with implantation of an intraocular lens is a routine procedure once the cataract has matured. The outcome is usually as satisfactory as for non-diabetics as long as co-existing retinopathy does not impair vision. Cataract extraction can be performed under local anaesthetic and so is feasible even in high-risk patients.

GLAUCOMA

In diabetic patients, glaucoma may be either:

- *Primary*. Chronic open angle glaucoma is more common in diabetic patients; there is a suggestion that its presence may protect against retinopathy to a degree.

- *Secondary*. To advanced diabetic eye disease (rubeosis iridis, see above).

DIABETIC NEUROPATHY

Neuropathy, in its myriad clinical manifestations, is the most common, chronic complication of diabetes and is a cause of considerable morbidity. The diagnosis is essentially clinical; no specialized techniques are usually necessary. Studies have shown that nerve conduction studies are often abnormal at diagnosis of diabetes and tend to improve with control of glycaemia; overactivity of the intraneural polyol pathway (see Section 1) has been implicated but there appears to be a major contribution from microangiopathy of the vasa nervorum. However, only a minority of patients will ultimately develop clinical evidence of chronic neuropathy.

Those that do will have passed through several stages, the earliest of which are usually asymptomatic:

● *Intraneural biochemical abnormalities.* Sorbitol accumulation, myo-inositol depletion (see p. 8).

● *Impairment of electrophysiological measurements.* Decreased nerve conduction velocity; asymptomatic.

● *Clinical neuropathy.* Detectable using clinical methods (see below); may be symptomatic. Histological changes evident.

● *End-stage complications.* Examples are ulceration and Charcot neuroarthropathy. Major derangements of neural structure and function.

CLASSIFICATION

This classification is essentially clinical, reflecting the differing manifestations and natural histories of the various forms (Table 5.2).

TABLE 5.2 Classification of diabetic neuropathies

● Focal neuropathies
— Cranial nerve palsies, carpal tunnel syndrome
● Distal symmetrical polyneuropathy
— Glove and stocking; may be asymptomatic
● Acute painful sensory neuropathy
— Uncommon; may follow initiation of insulin treatment
● Motor neuropathies
— Uncommon; usually resolves
● Autonomic neuropathy
— Erectile dysfunction is the most common manifestation; other forms are rare

---

CLINICAL SYNDROMES

FOCAL NEUROPATHIES

Clinical features
These may affect cranial nerves, e.g. the third, fourth or sixth and certain peripheral nerves, e.g. median, ulnar and common peroneal. Localized vascular lesions are thought to be responsible. Mononeuritis multiplex denotes the involvement of a plurality of peripheral nerves. Distinction from generalized peripheral neuropathy may be difficult; the two often co-exist.

Oculomotor nerve palsies are usually incomplete; diplopia is prominent but the pupil is spared and ptosis uncommon. Transient focal neuropathies can also occur in hyperosmolar states (see p. 185).

Management

Spontaneous recovery of cranial nerve lesions within 3 months is the rule and the patient can usually be reassured without resort to CT imaging or other investigations unless features such as ptosis are present. Recurrence is recognized. Persistent symptoms suggestive of carpal tunnel syndrome merit investigation with nerve conduction studies and consideration of injection therapy or decompression. Foot drop may require an orthopaedic support. Ulnar nerve lesions may cause wasting of the dorsal interossei and hypothenar eminence.

CHRONIC SYMMETRICAL DISTAL POLYNEUROPATHY

Clinical features

This polyneuropathy is common but is often frequently asymptomatic. Symptoms, if present, are usually confined to the legs but advanced neuropathy may also affect the hands leading to difficulties with daily activities, including the administration of insulin. Symptoms may include:

- *Paraesthesiae*. A sensation akin to walking on pebbles is characteristic.

- *Numbness*. Loss of sensation may not be noted by the patient; the complaint may be of subjectively cold feet despite the presence of pedal pulses.

- *Pain*. Unremitting; burning or lancinating in character.

- *Allodynia*. Unpleasant sensations resulting from contact with bedclothes and trousers.

- *Muscular leg cramps* in bed.

- *Impaired position sense*. This may result in unsteadiness of gait; an under-recognized symptom which is sometimes prominent.

Classical signs of diabetic peripheral neuropathy are easily detected on clinical examination:

- *Absent ankle jerks*. An early feature, but age-related loss is common in the elderly.

- *Diminished vibration sense*. A 128 Hz tuning fork is applied to a distal prominence, e.g. the tip of the hallux. If sensation is absent, move proximally to the medial malleolus, upper tibia; avoid testing over soft or oedematous tissue. Vibration sense may also be lost with advanced age. Other more quantitative devices are available, e.g. the Biothesiometer.

- *Reduction in other sensory modalities, position, light touch, pain and temperature*. Can follow loss of vibration sensation. Insensitivity to the application of a 10 g (5.07) Semmes–Weinstein monofilament identifies patients at high risk of neuropathic ulceration (see diabetic foot disease, p. 213). This is a simple and reproducible test in which a nylon filament is applied perpendicularly to a callus-free surface of the sole until it buckles under the gentle pressure. However, sources of error are recognized.

- *Warm dry skin with fissuring caused by local sympathetic denervation.*

- *Dilated superficial veins.* Sometimes bounding pedal pulses as a result of vascular shunting.

- *Clawed toes.* Denervation of intrinsic foot muscles produces 'clawing' of the toes thereby exposing the metatarsal heads and predisposing to ulceration (Plate 9; see diabetic foot disease, p. 213).

Management

- *Education.* Patients may scald insensitive feet by hot bathwater or in front of a fire (Plate 9); injuries by unperceived foreign bodies in footwear may occur; prevention is paramount. Instruction about foot care (Table 5.3, p. 214) is therefore required for patients with evidence of neuropathy. Note that anatomical abnormalities such as hallux valgus predispose to ulceration; their presence should be recorded. Basic elements of foot care are presented in Table 5.3 (p. 214). Repeated discussions with the patient may be required.

- *Exclusion of other causes of neuropathy.* Additional causes, notably chronic excessive alcohol consumption, should be identified. Discontinuation or avoidance of drugs with neurotoxic potential, e.g. nitrofurantoin, phenytoin, is important. Uraemia caused by advanced diabetic neuropathy may exacerbate neuropathy.

- *Glycaemic control.* This should be optimized; the DCCT demonstrated a protective effect of good glycaemic control in young patients with type 1 diabetes (see p. 60). Pancreatic transplantation (see p. 152) has been shown to result in improvements in neuropathy although several years of normoglycaemia are required. The UKPDS found that better glycaemic control preserved neural function as assessed using a Biothesiometer in patients with type 2 diabetes (see p. 65). Finally, it should be acknowledged that the effects of improving glycaemic control have not been substantiated in controlled trials in symptomatic patients. Studies examining the effect of hyperglycaemia on pain thresholds have produced conflicting results.

- *Analgesia.* Therapeutic options are limited for painful syndromes. Analgesia appropriate to the degree of pain must be provided; paracetamol is usually inadequate and opiates may be required. Commence with codeine or dihydrocodeine. Beware the nephrotoxic potential of NSAIDs in patients with renal impairment; in fact, the latter drugs are not very effective for neuropathic symptoms.

- *Antidepressants.* Tricyclic antidepressants – imipramine 25–50 mg before bed or, as a second choice with a higher risk of side effects, amitryptiline – may be useful adjuncts to simple analgesics; rather than working as antidepressants (although this effect may also be useful), these drugs block noradrenaline reuptake thereby reducing pain. Not all patients respond. Their hypnotic effect may also aid sleep although daytime drowsiness may be problematic.

● *Anticonvulsants.* Carbemazepine (starting at 100 mg daily) or phenytoin (100 mg) may sometimes alleviate shooting pains.

● *Other therapies.* Reported benefits of aldose reductase inhibitors have, to date, been unimpressive; these drugs are not licensed in the UK. Capsaicin (0.075% cream) is a recently-introduced, topical alkaloid derived from capsicum peppers. It depletes a peptide neurotransmitter, substance P, in nociceptive C fibre nerve terminals, thereby reducing pains. Clinical experience with the agent to date is limited; transient stinging pain and erythema have been reported. The cream has to be applied three to four times daily.

Alternatively, sheathing painful limbs with surgical adhesives may help alleviate allodynia. A bed-cradle to avoid contact with bedclothes is more practical. Transcutaneous nerve stimulators are occasionally of benefit in patients with intractable pain. Quinine is the traditional therapy for night cramps. Gabapentin is under evaluation for painful neuropathy.

● *Psychological support.* The importance of this should not be underestimated. Support should be underpinned by explanation of the prospect of improvement in acute painful neuropathies.

ACUTE PAINFUL SENSORY NEUROPATHY

Clinical features
This uncommon syndrome presents as acute, severe, distal neuropathy, classically following the institution of insulin therapy (see insulin neuritis, p. 147). Recovery is usual but may be incomplete.

Management
Treatment is symptomatic.

MOTOR NEUROPATHIES

Clinical features
These include classical diabetic amyotrophy of Garland (Plate 10) which may cause constitutional disturbance with weight loss (neuropathic cachexia). The patient is typically a middle-aged male with type 2 diabetes in whom antecedent glycaemic control may have been unremarkable. The presentation is abrupt with:

● Pain in the area of the quadriceps – may be severe.
● Weakness – in one or both quadriceps.
● Muscular wasting – this follows rapidly.

The weakness may be profound, leading to falls and immobility. Painful hypersensitivity of the skin over the anterior aspect of the thigh is characteristic. The symptoms lead to insomnia, anorexia, weight loss and depression. The knee jerk is characteristically absent and it is held that the plantar response may be extensor. The nature of the responsible lesion remains uncertain. Some features point to spinal cord or nerve root damage. An acute vasculopathy of the vasa nervorum is a popular explanation; however, the predilection for the femoral nerve roots is unexplained. Other motor neuropathies are recognized: truncal neuropathies affecting the abdomen are rare. They are usually painful with hyperaesthesia; localized muscular weakness may occur.

Investigation and management
In the classical case of amyotrophy, few, if any, investigations are required. The major differential diagnoses are a nerve root or cauda equina lesion. Plain radiographs of the lumbar spine are usually unrevealing; magnetic resonance imaging (MRI) may sometimes be required. Cerebrospinal fluid protein concentrations may be elevated. Nerve conduction studies may show a localized, femoral neuropathy but evidence of spinal lesions is also recognized. Treatment is symptomatic and supportive with adequate analgesia and physiotherapy. Good glycaemic control is recommended although there is no clear relationship to recovery. Recovery, albeit sometimes incomplete, usually occurs within a few months; however, complete recovery may take more than a year. Ipsilateral recurrence is very uncommon.

AUTONOMIC NEUROPATHY
Clinical features
Diabetes-associated autonomic dysfunction usually remains symptomatic. The most common clinical manifestation is probably erectile dysfunction; this is estimated to affect approximately 30% of men although other factors are often important as well. However, subclinical abnormalities of autonomic function are relatively common amongst diabetic patients, being present in approximately 30% of unselected patients. These may be detected by simple bedside tests of cardiovascular reflex integrity, including:

● *Heart rate variability*. During deep breathing over 1 min – mainly assesses parasympathetic (vagal) function. The mean ratio of the ECG R–R interval in expiration to inspiration is calculated; less than 1.20 is considered abnormal, i.e. heart rate shows reduced variability.

● *Orthostatic BP response*. A test of sympathetic integrity.

Many variations including the heart rate response to standing (the ratio at 30 and 15 seconds) or the Valsalva manoeuvre, for example, have been described. More sophisticated computer-aided systems are also available which provide comprehensive assessments of autonomic function. There are other specialized techniques such as the acetylcholine sweatspot test and measurement of pupillary adaptation to dark. However, these are chiefly used for research purposes. Studies of spectral analysis of heart rate variability and baroreceptor reflex sensitivity may reveal even more subtle abnormalities of autonomic function, the clinical implications of which are uncertain.

Prognosis

Patients with clinically overt autonomic neuropathy have been found to have a relatively high mortality in follow-up studies. Autonomic dysfunction has been implicated in the sudden death of some diabetic patients peri-operatively from cardiorespiratory arrest. The ECG QT interval may be prolonged in diabetic patients; another measure, QTc dispersion, predicted mortality in a recent study of newly-diagnosed patients with type 2 diabetes. There is evidence of imbalance between sympathetic and parasympathetic tone which may dispose to cardiac arrhythmias, particularly during hypoglycaemia. The contribution, if any, of this to the occasional, sudden, nocturnal death of young patients with type 1 diabetes is presently uncertain. However, mounting indirect evidence is persuasive.

Relation to glycaemic control

Improvements in glycaemic control have little beneficial effect on symptomatic autonomic neuropathy since advanced histological changes (axonal loss, demyelination, obliteration of vasa nervorum; see Section 1) within nerves are at best only partially reversible. There is evidence suggesting that long-term restoration of normoglycaemia by pancreatic transplantation (see p. 153) reduces mortality; RCTs are required to confirm this possibility. Patients assigned to intensive glycaemic control in the DCCT had developed fewer abnormal tests of autonomic function tests when assessed after 5 years. However, the prevalence of clinically overt autonomic dysfunction in these young patients was very low. The UKPDS (see p. 65) was unable to demonstrate any benefits of improved glycaemic control on autonomic function.

Erectile dysfunction

This is regarded as the most common manifestation of diabetic autonomic neuropathy. Other major risk factors include:

- Advancing age.
- Type 2 diabetes.
- Antihypertensive drugs – particularly β-blockers and thiazide diuretics.

However, psychological factors are often present and making the distinction between primary organic and psychogenic impotence may prove difficult. Devices enabling detection of nocturnal tumescence may sometimes be helpful but many clinicians adopt a more pragmatic approach. Physical examination concentrates on:

- Genital anatomy – phimosis, Peyronie's disease.
- Evidence of peripheral neuropathy (see p. 206).
- Evidence of peripheral vascular disease (see p. 236).

Hormonal investigations (plasma testosterone, prolactin) are usually not necessary unless there is associated loss of libido or other features suggestive of hypogonadism. Not all patients respond to conventional therapies and personal preferences dictate the acceptability of the various options:

- *Counselling.* By an interested clinician or specialist nurse with demonstration of therapeutic options.

- *Mechanical devices.* Vacuum tumescence devices, occasionally surgical penile implants.

- *Vasoactive drugs.* Prostaglandin E_1 administered intracorporeally or intraurethrally by the patient prior to intercourse; α-blockers (e.g. phenoxybenzamine).

- *Sildenafil.* This recently introduced oral agent is the most popular option. Studies to date suggest that diabetic patients generally require a higher dose than non-diabetics. Sildenafil inhibits the breakdown of cyclic guanosine monophosphate by a specific type 5 phosphodiesterase. The drug is administered in a starting dose of 50 mg approximately 1 hour prior to intercourse. It does not induce an erection; appropriate visual, psychological or physical stimulus is necessary. Sildenafil appears to improve sexual function in 50–60% of diabetic men. The drug is generally well tolerated. No major problems such as priapism (which occasionally complicates injection therapy) have been reported. Other drugs are in development.

However, a major contraindication to sildenafil has emerged: co-administration with nitrate drugs may cause a precipitous fall in BP which has been implicated in some deaths. The drug is contraindicated in approximately 10% of men. In general, care should be exercised by men with cardiovascular disease, particularly severe angina or major impairment of left ventricular function for whom sexual activity may be hazardous.

 Sildenafil is contraindicated in patients taking nitrate drugs.

Small fibre neuropathy
This is an uncommon syndrome characteristically affecting young women with type 1 diabetes in whom severe autonomic dysfunction and Charcot

neuroarthropathy predominate (see p. 218). The selective involvement of unmyelinated nerves preserves light touch and vibration sensation in the feet. However, temperature sensation – which can be quantified using specialized techniques – and pain sensation are markedly impaired. An association with iritis has fuelled speculation about immune-mediated neuropathy.

Orthostatic hypotension
Defined arbitrarily as an otherwise unexplained fall in systolic BP of 30 mmHg or more on standing for 2 min in a volume-replete patient. In fact, BP may continue to fall for up to 15 min. This rare complication may be very disabling and is difficult to manage.

The differential diagnosis includes:

- Addison's disease (more common in patients with autoimmune type 1 diabetes).
- Other causes of autonomic failure, e.g. Shy–Drager syndrome.

Antihypertensive agents and tricyclics may aggravate and should be avoided. Support stockings may help to prevent venous pooling. Careful use of fludrocortisone may be beneficial but risks supine hypertension, oedema and hypokalaemia with higher doses. Other agents include midodrine, an alpha-adrenergic agonist.

Gastroparesis
Recurrent bouts of intractable vomiting may necessitate hospitalization for intravenous fluids and insulin. Barium or radionuclide studies typically reveal delayed gastric emptying but dissociations between the severity of symptoms and abnormalities of tests are recognized; test results may also fluctuate when repeated. Management involves:

- *Pro-kinetic agents.* Regular metoclopramide and erythromycin before meals may be helpful, both acting as pro-kinetic drugs. However, the combination of cisparide and erythromycin is contraindicated because of a risk of serious cardiac arrhythmias; this risk may be especially high in patients with autonomic neuropathy since ECG QT interval may already be prolonged (see p. 210).

- *Good glycaemic control.* This has theoretical benefits on rate of gastric emptying but may be near impossible to attain because of the disruption caused by the vomiting.

- *Gastric surgical procedures.* These have a very limited role; an experienced surgeon and careful selection of patients are crucial.

The pro-motility drugs, cisapride and erythromycin, must not be used in combination.

Diabetic diarrhoea

This unpleasant symptom is classically episodic with nocturnal incontinence; anal sphincter function may be compromised. Short courses of broad-spectrum antibiotics, e.g. tetracycline, sometimes bring rapid benefit; intestinal bacterial overgrowth is postulated but unproven. Other causes of chronic diarrhoea must be excluded:

- Gluten-sensitive enteropathy – more common in patients with autoimmune type 1 diabetes (see p. 11). This may also predispose to hypoglycaemia.
- Pancreatic insufficiency.
- Chronic infective diarrhoea – e.g. giardiasis, amoebic dysentery.
- Inflammatory bowel disease – Crohn's disease, ulcerative colitis.

Intestinal malabsorption is not a feature of neuropathy-associated diarrhoea. Constipation is reportedly a common symptom although rarely causes significant problems.

Bladder paresis

This may rarely produce hesitancy and retention and predispose to urinary infections. Bladder function tests are abnormal. Self-catheterization may be necessary in a few patients.

Gustatory sweating

Rarely, patients may suffer drenching sweats of the head and upper torso while eating, unrelated to hypoglycaemia. Anticholinergic drugs have been tried but often have intolerable side effects.

Peripheral oedema

Rare; ephedrine may help. Avoid exacerbation of lower limb oedema by drugs such as nifedepine and amlodipine.

DIABETIC FOOT DISEASE

Diabetic patients have a 10–20-fold increased risk of non-traumatic, lower-limb amputation compared with the non-diabetic population. Thus, foot disease is an important cause of morbidity in diabetic patients and is theoretically preventable in many cases. Rehabilitation is often impossible in the older patient. In the elderly, there is also a significant mortality rate associated with major amputation, probably largely reflecting serious comorbidity in this group.

In the UK, foot complications remain the most common reason for hospitalization amongst diabetic patients. All districts should establish a specialist foot clinic to which patients can be referred, or self-refer, for urgent assessment of serious lesions. Combined foot clinics with input from a podiatrist, vascular surgeon and diabetologist can reduce amputation rates.

> **NB** Diabetic patients with foot disease are at greatly increased risk of requiring surgical amputation.

The syndrome of diabetic foot disease includes elements of:

● *Peripheral neuropathy.* The major factor acting through insensitivity, motor imbalance with abnormal pressure distribution and the consequences of local sympathetic denervation.

● *Peripheral vascular disease.* Leading to impaired tissue, perfusion is present in approximately half of all cases; the combination comprises the neuro-ischaemic foot.

● *Tissue infection.* Secondary to trauma or neuropathic ulceration.

THE NEUROPATHIC FOOT

As discussed above, the neuropathic foot is insensitive (owing to sensory neuropathy), dry (owing to sympathetic denervation) and warm (well-perfused in the absence of co-existing peripheral vascular disease, see p. 236). Areas of high pressure develop during weight-bearing because of alterations in foot anatomy consequent upon denervation of intrinsic foot muscles. This exposes the metatarsal heads to abnormally high local pressures during normal gait. Callus develops over these areas. Neuropathic toes may be compressed painlessly by ill-fitting shoes. Patients should receive instruction about foot care verbally and, where appropriate, as a written leaflet (Table 5.3); advice should be reinforced by regular contact with a podiatrist.

TABLE 5.3 Basic rules for care of the neuropathic foot

- Inspect feet daily (or have someone else inspect them)
- Check footwear for foreign objects before wearing
- Have feet measured carefully when purchasing shoes
- Buy lace-up shoes with plenty of toe room
- Attend for regular podiatry
- Keep feet aways from heaters, fires and hot water bottles
- Check temperature of bathwater before bathing
- Avoid walking barefoot especially outdoors
- Avoid unaccustomed lengthy walks when on holiday

Callus formation indicates chronic local high foot pressures.

TISSUE DAMAGE

Shearing forces during walking cause disruption of underlying tissues which may lead to haemorrhage under the callus (a danger sign; Plate 11), subsequently to ulceration, secondary infection and ultimately gangrene (Plate 12). Major risk factors are presented in Table 5.4. Previous ulceration is particularly important; recurrence is common. Elderly, socially isolated patients who perhaps cannot inspect or even physically reach their feet are also at high risk. Oedema, from congestive cardiac failure, nephropathy, immobility or calcium antagonists renders feet vulnerable as does the chronic deformity associated with Charcot neuroarthropathy (see p. 218).

 Visible haemorrhage within a plantar callus is a danger sign of impending ulceration.

TABLE 5.4 Indicators of feet at increased risk of ulceration

- Neuropathy – especially with callus, blisters or fissures
- Ischaemia
- Previous ulceration
- Previous amputation
- Impaired mobility owing age or comorbidity
- Social isolation or low socio-economic status

TREATMENT

Patients should be referred to the podiatry service if they have any of the indications presented in Table 5.5. Amateur chiropody by the patient directed against lesions such as corns or deformed toenails should be discouraged. Regular debridement of callus is required to reduce the risk of ulceration. For established ulcers, particularly indolent or recurrent ulcers, innovative but expensive therapies have recently become available. The role of these treatments has not been clearly defined:

TABLE 5.5 Indications for referral to a podiatrist

- Patients with peripheral neuropathy
- Patients with significant ischaemia
- Patients with other foot lesions, e.g. callus, corns, ingrowing toenails
- Patients requiring detailed foot assessments for other indications

● *Cultured dermis.* This is a preparation reminiscent of a skin graft constructed from neonatal fibroblasts embedded in a synthetic matrix. Studies to date suggest that the proportion of ulcers that are healed is increased by its use. Infection must be controlled prior to application.

● *Platelet-derived growth factor.* In conjunction with good wound care, becaplermin (0.01% gel) has also been shown to improve ulcer healing in chronic, uninfected ulcers compared with placebo. Further studies are required.

● *Hyaluronic acid.* Under evaluation.

Health care professionals such as district nurses, general practice nurses and community podiatrists should be able to refer urgently to the local hospital specialist foot clinic. Patients should also be able to self-refer, if necessary; this requires appropriate education. Referral criteria are presented in Table 5.6.

TABLE 5.6 Criteria for referral to a specialist diabetes foot clinic

● Patients with neuropathic ulceration which has not responded to treatment within 4 weeks
● Patients with a foot infection not responding to antibiotics
● Acute or chronic Charcot neuroarthropathy
● Patients requiring special shoes or insoles
● Patients requiring weight-relieving casts

Infection with spreading cellulitis and/or deep infection represents a threat to the foot, and sometimes to the patient's life. Unless there is a prompt and convincing response to initial, out-patient treatment, the following action is required:

● *Hospital admission.* Bedrest facilitates ulcer healing. An ulcer will not heal if the patient continues to walk – pressure relief is essential; its failure is usually responsible for recurrences. If infection is controlled, the application of a removable or lightweight plaster cast can allow healing; a window is left in the plaster to enable inspection. Great care must be taken to avoid consequences of immobility, notably neuro-ischaemic heel ulcers in debilitated patients. These can be difficult to heal. Action should be directed towards relevant comorbidity such as peripheral oedema.

 Care must be taken to avoid neuro-ischaemic heel ulcers in debilitated patients.

● *Assessment.* Assessment of the extent of infection – by plain radiographs to exclude osteomyelitis in deep infections – and of the peripheral vasculature (see p. 237) is essential. Neuropathy in the absence of bone infection may produce translucency of the metatarsal heads. Arterial calcification is asymptomatic but may be visible on plain radiographs of the feet of patients with extensive diabetic neuropathy.

It is important to document its presence in patients with diabetic foot disease since the results of Doppler studies of the peripheral vasculature may be misleading (see p. 237). Chronic, deep-seated infection has a general debilitating effect; hypoalbuminaemia and a normochromic normocytic anaemia are commonly found.

> **NB** Plain radiographs of the feet with deep or chronic infection should be taken to exclude osteomyelitis.

- *Antibiotics.* A mixed growth is usual, the most common organisms being:

- *Streptococcus pyogenes.*
- *Staphylococcus aureus.*
- Anaerobic species.

Anaerobic organisms such as bacteroides are common; this is often apparent from the odour. Occasionally, gas formation may result – check radiographs. Gram-negative bacilli may contribute to deep infections. Deep wound swabs will guide the choice of antibiotics but action against all the above organisms is required for serious infections. Intravenous antibiotic therapy may be required initially. Oral treatment may need to be continued for several weeks for deep tissue infection or osteomyelitis. Examples of antibiotic regimens are presented in Table 5.7.

TABLE 5.7 Examples of antibiotic regimens for diabetic foot infections

Superficial infections
- Oral ampicillin–flucloxacillin
- Oral amoxycillin–clavulanate
- Azithromycin (if penicillin allergy)

Deep tissue infections
- Intravenous ampicillin + flucloxacillin + metronidazole
- Intravenous amoxycillin–clavulanate
- Intravenous ciprofloxacin + clindamycin

- *Surgery.* Judicious debridement, amputation of digits, drainage of deep abscesses (beware the patient with neuropathy who complains of increasing discomfort in the foot – classical signs of infection are not always present) can be performed by a trained podiatrist or surgeon, as appropriate. The aim is always to preserve the limb but the point must be recognized when life-threatening infection demands more major surgery such as mid-foot or, as a last resort, below-knee amputation.

> **NB** Increasing discomfort in an infected neuropathic foot raises the possibility of abscess formation

- *Rehabilitation.* Following amputation, if feasible (see below).

- *Prevention of recurrence.* Education of the patient and relevant carers, provision of special footwear, home help and careful follow-up in the foot clinic aim to prevent recurrence. For patients with severe deformities, assessment by an orthotist is essential. Ready-to-wear boots may be helpful in the short term but are unaesthetic. Shoes made to order may be required to accommodate insoles. Devices are available which identify high-pressure sites thereby aiding insole design. Trainers are worn by some patients; these represent a relatively inexpensive and acceptable alternative.

Amputation
Minor, or less commonly, major amputation may be required for:

- Non-healing lesions.
- Gangrene.
- Osteomyelitis.
- Recurrent lesions at a single site.

Removal of digits may suffice; however, an inadequate peripheral blood supply may result in a non- or slow-healing amputation site. A ray amputation of the second, third or fourth toes, taking the associated metatarsal head, may result in a very satisfactory outcome although healing will take some weeks. Fore-foot and mid-foot amputations are generally avoided, if possible. Below- rather than through- or above-knee is the best option if major amputation is required.

Rehabilitation
Major amputation is usually a devastating event. The prospects for successful rehabilitation are often remote. Walking using a below-knee prosthesis increases energy expenditure by 50%, an impossible target in elderly or debilitated patients. The risk of ulceration in the contralateral foot may be increased owing to altered weight-bearing. Confinement to a wheelchair may be the unfortunate consequence.

CHARCOT NEUROARTHROPATHY

Increased blood flow through the foot, secondary to local autonomic denervation, together with abnormal pressure loading may lead to unsuspected fractures with minimal normal daily trauma (Plate 13); the presence of callus may indicate previous metatarsal fractures. The patient may present acutely with a foot which is warm, tender and oedematous; pedal pulses are characteristically present. These features strongly suggest an acute

Charcot neuroarthropathy; however, an erroneous diagnosis of infection or inflammatory arthritis is not uncommon. Contrary to common belief, some discomfort is usual; the foot is rarely completely painless.

NB Radiographs must be taken if a patient with neuropathy presents with an acutely swollen hot foot.

Radiographs will usually confirm the diagnosis. Initially, fractures may be apparent which progress rapidly to extensive subluxation and disorganization with remodelling (Plate 13). Isotope bone scans are unhelpful in distinguishing acute neuroarthropathy from infection, being positive in both circumstances. MRI and CT are more helpful in delineating the nature and extent of the process. Plasma levels of bone alkaline phosphatase are often elevated. When remodelling has been completed, the patient is left with a deformed neuroarthropathic foot which is at high risk of ulceration (Plate 14); a 'rocker bottom' deformity is characteristic. Bilateral changes are usually apparent if radiographs are obtained.

Management
Treatment during the acute stages is controversial; no RCTs have been performed to guide clinicians.

● *Immobilization*. A walking plaster or removable cast is usually favoured, taking care to avoid trauma and ulceration from the cast itself.

● *Intravenous bisphosphonates*. These drugs inhibit osteoblast activity and are used with the aim of suppressing bone remodelling. Custom-made footware subsequently helps to prevent ulceration (if worn, ask the patient, inspect the shoes). Monitor plasma alkaline phospatase during therapy.

● *Reconstructive orthopaedic techniques*. Realignment techniques have been described recently which may help patients who develop a deformed and unstable hind foot. Such surgery should only be contemplated by experienced surgeons.

NB Charcot neuroarthropathy is a major complication of diabetes associated with high risk of recurrent foot ulceration.

DIABETIC NEPHROPATHY

INCIDENCE

It is estimated that approximately 25–30% of patients with type 1 diabetes will develop nephropathy. The incidence amongst patients with type 2 diabetes is similar. However, certain ethnic groups, e.g. Blacks, South Asians, native Americans, appear to be at higher risk than Caucasians. Reports, not entirely consistent between studies, have suggested that the incidence of nephropathy in patients with type 1 diabetes has fallen during recent decades. This may reflect generally better glycaemic control and greater attention to control of hypertension. However, the rapidly increasing global incidence of type 2 diabetes seems set to ensure that diabetic nephropathy continues to be a major consumer of health care resources. Indeed, diabetic nephropathy is already the single largest cause of end-stage renal failure in Westernized countries.

> **NB** Diabetes is now the single largest cause of end-stage renal failure in Westernized countries.

Diabetic nephropathy not only results in progressive renal failure; morbidity and mortality from CHD, cerebrovascular disease and peripheral vascular disease are also very high, particularly amongst patients with type 2 diabetes, most of whom will die from atherosclerotic disease rather than renal failure. Thus, diabetic nephropathy, in common with other causes of chronic renal failure, may be regarded as a state of accelerated atherosclerosis.

> **NB** Diabetic nephropathy is associated with a greatly increased incidence of atherosclerosis.

NATURAL HISTORY

As for other chronic microvascular complications of diabetes, several distinct phases are recognized in the natural history of nephropathy. The earliest stages are asymptomatic. The important prognostic implications of nephropathy necessitate regular testing of urine for albumin.

> **NB** Proteinuria is the clinical hallmark of diabetic nephropathy.

In recent years, much emphasis has been placed on early pharmacological intervention, particularly with angiotensin-converting enzyme (ACE) inhibitors, even in the absence of overt hypertension. However, both the selection of methodology used for screening and the timing and choice of pharmacotherapy remain areas of controversy. This debate reflects the absence of long-term follow-up data demonstrating that very early intervention ultimately reduces the incidence of end-stage renal failure.

Outcome studies of diabetic nephropathy are hampered by the long natural history of this complication. For this reason, most interventional studies to date have been relatively small and short term. Moreover, they have tended to rely on surrogate endpoints such as transition from microalbuminuria to clinical nephropathy. To complicate the situation, microalbuminuria (see p. 222) is much less specific a predictor of nephropathy in type 2 diabetes. Microalbuminuria in patients with type 2 diabetes is a marker of cardiovascular risk (see p. 228); this also applies to the non-diabetic population. Thus, transitions, defined as crossing arbitrary thresholds of progression, provide limited information, and extrapolation to the longer term is fraught with difficulties. These caveats notwithstanding, evidence has been amassed suggesting that delaying the progression of diabetic nephropathy may now be a therapeutic possibility.

NB Annual testing for proteinuria is required to detect the development of diabetic nephropathy.

DEVELOPMENTAL CONTINUUM

Although the natural history outlined below suggests distinct stages the development of nephropathy is, in fact, a continuum:

● *Stage 1.* Functional changes include increased renal plasma flow and renal hypertrophy at diagnosis; these subclinical changes are very common but reversible with control of glycaemia.

● *Stage 2.* Renal lesions; early structural changes may be present after 2–3 years; subclinical.

● *Stage 3.* Microalbuminuria (see below). BP starts to rise, although remains within the normotensive range; asymptomatic.

● *Stage 4.* Overt clinical nephropathy. Standard dipstick tests for protein become positive, initially intermittently then persistently. Nephrotic syndrome may develop. Plasma creatinine starts to rise as creatinine clearance declines. Hypertension is now usually established.

● *Stage 5.* Progression to end-stage renal failure. Plasma creatinine rises above 500 μmol/L, usually at a relatively constant rate for the individual over 7–10 years from the onset of clinical nephropathy. The point at which dialysis will be required may be predicted using sequential plots of the reciprocal of the plasma creatinine concentration once this exceeds 200 μmol/L.

BP is usually difficult to control by this time. Fluid retention may result in pulmonary or peripheral oedema. In addition, the incidence of macrovascular events – MI, stroke, severe peripheral vascular disease (Plate 15) – is greatly increased.

DIAGNOSIS

MICROALBUMINURIA

In the earliest clinically-detectable stage, urinary albumin excretion is increased to between 30–300 mg/day (the so-called 'microalbuminuria' range); sensitive radioimmunoassays are required to quantitate proteinuria accurately, best performed on a timed overnight collection. An albumin concentration <20 mg/L is considered normal. A urinary albumin/creatinine ratio, measured in the first-voided sample of the morning, is a more practical alternative to timed collections. The following levels are diagnostic of microalbuminuria, assuming exclusion of alternative possibilities:

- Adult men – 2.5 mg/mmol.
- Adult women – 3.5 mg/mmol.

CLINICAL PROTEINURIA

When albumin excretion exceeds 300 mg/day, the Albustix dipstick test becomes positive. This marks the development of clinical nephropathy. Nephrotic syndrome may sometimes develop with:

- Urinary protein excretion >5 g daily.
- Hypoalbuminaemia.
- Peripheral oedema.

However, lesser degrees of urinary protein excretion may be influenced by several factors:

- *Hyperglycaemia.* Tests at diagnosis and during periods of poor glycaemic control may be misleading.

- *Intercurrent illness.* Urinary tract infection is most common, may be asymptomatic and therefore must be excluded.

- *Posture.* Upright posture increases protein excretion. Testing the first-voided sample of the day avoids this effect.

- *Exercise.* This increases urinary protein excretion.

- *Congestive cardiac failure.*

- *Other renal pathology.* Examples are glomerulonephritis, drug-induced renal disease (e.g. penicillamine, gold).

Thus, care must be exercised before concluding that proteinuria is attributable to diabetic nephropathy. The finding of microalbuminuria or a positive Albustix test should prompt exclusion of the other possibilities. The albuminuria must be confirmed on at least one additional sample, especially if treatment is being considered; this is especially so for levels within the microalbuminuria range. Dipstick tests for lesser degrees of albuminuria require confirmation with a laboratory test. The following screening strategy has been suggested by expert groups:

- Once the diabetes has been stabilized, albumin/creatinine ratios may be checked annually in patients aged 12–70 years.
- Positive results should prompt re-testing and exclusion of alternative possibilities.
- Timed overnight urine samples are regarded as the best test; failing this, repeat early morning albumin/creatinine ratios are an acceptable alternative.
- Persistently positive tests should lead to careful assessment of glycaemic control, BP, plasma lipids, plasma creatinine and other micro- and macrovascular complications. However, with the exception of creatinine and lipids, these should be checked for annually in most patients.

Patients with type 1 diabetes who have persistent microalbuminuria are at relatively high risk of progression to clinical nephropathy. However, patients with diabetes of long duration may sometimes have stable microalbuminuria. Other patients may regress to normal albumin excretion rates in the absence of therapeutic intervention.

Further investigations
Renal biopsy is usually necessary when there are atypical features, particularly:

- A very rapid deterioration in renal function.
- Absence of significant retinopathy.
- Sudden development of nephrotic syndrome.
- Features suggesting alternative pathology, e.g. haematuria, evidence of relevant autoimmune disease.

Note that when diabetic nephropathy is well advanced, microscopic haematuria is often detectable on dipstick testing. However, IgA nephropathy, which presents with haematuria, should be excluded by measurement of plasma immunoglobulins.

Comorbidity
By the time dialysis is required, most patients will have significant, additional complications of diabetes. In particular, retinopathy will have resulted in visual impairment or blindness in some patients. Indeed, the association between severe retinopathy and nephropathy is so close that the absence of the former should prompt consideration of alternative reasons for renal failure. However, exceptions occur to this general rule. Patients are also likely to have neuropathy, not infrequently with features of autonomic dysfunction (see p. 209). Problems such as postural hypotension may pose management difficulties, particularly in relation to

haemodialysis (see p. 227). The incidence of peripheral gangrene is greatly increased with chronic renal failure. Other macrovascular complications are also common.

MANAGEMENT

● *Glycaemic control*. The DCCT (see p. 60) demonstrated that good glycaemic control reduces the incidence of microalbuminuria. There has been a suggestion from other retrospective data that a threshold effect for microalbuminuria may operate, the risk increasing sharply at levels of HbA_{1c} consistently greater than 8%. However, no precise threshold could be identified in the DCCT. Tightening glycaemic control has no proven benefit in the later stages of nephropathy. In patients with type 2 diabetes, observational studies suggest a synergistic deleterious effect of proteinuria and elevated HbA_{1c} levels on survival.

The UKPDS showed a 30% reduction in the risk of microalbuminuria at 15 years' follow-up with intensive therapy (see p. 65). A multifactorial approach may be beneficial (see Evidence-based Medicine 5.1).

● *Control of hypertension*. BP gradually rises as urinary albumin excretion increases. However, in the initial stages, it may remain within the accepted normotensive range; nonetheless, BP is elevated for the individual patient concerned. Glomerular filtration declines with progression to end-stage renal failure over 7–10 years (although with considerable inter-individual variation). Control of hypertension is essential.

ACE inhibitors may also have a renoprotective effect even at lower BPs; in the UK, lisinopril is licensed for normotensive patients with type 1 diabetes and microalbuminuria. Care must be taken in women of childbearing age in view of the teratogenic potential of these drugs. A report suggesting that lisinopril may also retard the progression of retinopathy in such patients requires confirmation.

There is some evidence that non-dihydropyridine calcium antagonists (e.g. diltiazem) have greater antiproteinuric effects than dihydropyridines (e.g. nifedipine). When plasma creatinine concentrations are elevated, there is clear RCT evidence that captopril reduces the rate of decline of renal function, largely independently of its effects on systemic BP; the higher the BP, the greater the renoprotective effect of captopril. Care is required to avoid the development of hyperkalaemia in patients with overt nephropathy; sometimes this necessitates withdrawal of ACE inhibitor therapy.

 Hyperkalaemia is a hazard with potassium-retaining drugs in patients with nephropathy.

Polymorphisms of the ACE gene may have prognostic and therapeutic implications for patients with diabetic nephropathy. Patients with the DD genotype are homozygous for deletion of a 287 base pair repeat sequence within intron 16 of the gene. Patients with type 2 diabetes who also have the DD genotype have higher circulating levels of ACE. Such patients have been shown to have a more rapid loss of renal function and may require higher doses of ACE inhibitors. The D allele has also been linked with an increased risk of nephropathy in patients with type 1 diabetes.

> **NB** Genetic factors have been identified which may increase susceptibility to nephropathy in diabetic patients.

The potential dangers posed by bilateral renal artery stenosis in patients with type 2 diabetes are discussed below. A combination of antihypertensive drugs is often required, particularly in patients with type 2 diabetes and clinical nephropathy. Use of loop diuretics, β-blockers, long-acting calcium antagonists and centrally-acting drugs may all be necessary. In particular, the early addition of a loop diuretic such as frusemide is helpful; as plasma creatinine concentrations rise, large doses may be required.

> **NB** Combinations of antihypertensive agents are usually required for patients with clinical nephropathy.

- *Treatment of dyslipidaemia.* The high toll from accelerated macrovascular disease warrants the use of statins. Note that the risk of myositis is increased when statins are co-prescribed with cyclosporin following renal transplantation. Unfavourable alterations in lipid profiles – increased LDL-cholesterol, increased triglycerides, reduced HDL-cholesterol – can be detected before creatinine levels rise; increases in plasma levels of atherogenic lipoprotein(a) may also contribute. Fibrates (see p. 256) should be used with caution in renal impairment.

- *Cigarette smoking.* This should be completely avoided.

- *Protein restriction.* Modest restriction to 0.6–0.7 g/kg daily is usually recommended for clinical nephropathy. Vegetable protein may be less nephrotoxic than animal-derived protein, but the benefit is unproven.

EVIDENCE-BASED MEDICINE 5.1

STENO TYPE 2 STUDY

(Lancet 1999; 353: 617–622.)

STUDY DESIGN

Randomized, unblinded trial comparing intensive, multifactorial therapy (low-fat diet and exercise, smoking cessation, ACE inhibitors, vitamins C and E, aspirin and stepwise therapy directed against hyperglycaemia, dyslipidaemia and hypertension) in a specialized hospital diabetes centre (n=80) with standard treatment by GPs (n=80). Mean age of patients 55 years; mean follow-up 3.8 years.

RESULTS

Compared with patients in the standard treatment group, those in the intensive group had reduced risks for clinical nephropathy (56% relative risk reduction; P=0.01), progression of retinopathy (40%; P=0.04), blindness in one eye (85%; P=0.03), progression of autonomic neuropathy (62%; P=0.01) and the combined endpoint of death and macrovascular events (37%; P=0.03).

INTERPRETATION

Multifactorial intervention reduced the development of nephropathy and other complications. However, the relative contribution of each intervention to outcomes is uncertain.

● *Dialysis.* Survival rates have improved for patients with diabetes on dialysis. If the patient is considered not suitable for transplantation, dialysis is used as sole long-term therapy. Although advanced retinopathy is common, visual impairment is not a contraindication to renal replacement therapy. Because of their tendency to fluid retention, dialysis may have to be introduced at an earlier stage in diabetic patients. Thus, when plasma creatinine has reached 500 μmol/L, dialysis should be under active consideration. CAPD is the favoured form of therapy.

NB Dialysis should be considered when the plasma creatinine concentration has reached 500 μmol/L.

CAPD is relatively inexpensive, avoids rapid fluctuations in vascular volume and so is regarded as well suited to patients with cardiovascular disease or autonomic neuropathy. Moreover, no vascular access is required. Insulin may be delivered into the peritoneal cavity by injection into the dialysate; the pharmacokinetics are altered by factors including the volume of dialysate and the tonicity (i.e. isotonic vs hypertonic); approximately 50% of the injected dose is systemically absorbed. Reported survival rates are somewhat less favourable for diabetic patients compared with non-diabetics. However, survival of diabetic patients on peritoneal dialysis is similar to haemodialysis. Peritonitis is the principal complication.

Haemodialysis requires the construction of vascular access either as an arteriovenous fistula or artificial graft; these tend to fail more rapidly in diabetic patients and distal necrosis of digits may occur. Autonomic neuropathy-related hypotension may make removal of excess fluid problematic and glycaemic control may be difficult to stabilize. Survival is generally less good in elderly patients but may exceed 10 years in some cases.

• *Renal transplantation.* Renal transplantation – usually cadaveric but sometimes from a living, related donor (particularly in the USA) – is the treatment of choice for patients with end-stage diabetic nephropathy. Patient and graft survival rates remain inferior to those for non-diabetic recipients. Rehabilitation is usually good, c.f. haemodialysis. Several key selection criteria must be fulfilled (Table 5.8):

TABLE 5.8 Criteria for renal transplantation in diabetic patients

- Age <65 years
- Absence of severe cardiovascular or cerebrovascular disease
- Absence of significant sepsis
- Absence of life-limiting comorbidity
- Availability of a suitable donor organ

Assessment of the coronary vasculature is routine; coronary angiography is required in most centres. The diabetogenic effects of immunosuppressive agents (corticosteroids, cyclosporin and tacrolimus) may necessitate increased insulin doses post-transplantation. Dyslipidaemia may also be exacerbated by immunosuppression. The main causes of death post-transplantation are atheromatous cardiovascular disease and sepsis; autonomic neuropathy may also be a factor (see p. 209). There is an increase in the risk of neoplastic disease with long-term, immunosuppressive therapy.

• *Combined pancreas and renal transplantation.* Patients with type 1 diabetes who require a renal transplant must receive lifelong, immunosuppressive therapy to prevent rejection. In these circumstances, a pancreatic graft, whole organ or segmental either simultaneously or sequentially, is an additional consideration (see pp. 152–153).

MACROVASCULAR DISEASE

CORONARY HEART DISEASE

MORTALITY

CHD is the commonest cause of mortality among diabetic patients; it is the major cause of death in patients >40 years and in patients with disease duration exceeding 30 years.

 CHD is the principal cause of premature mortality in patients with diabetes.

Patients with proteinuria (see microalbuminuria or greater) are at significantly greater risk of atheromatous cardiovascular disease for reasons which remain only partially understood. It has been hypothesized that (micro)albuminuria reflects generalized endothelial dysfunction which may predispose to atheroma. Nonetheless, diabetes per se is a major risk factor for CHD. This is amply demonstrated by the observation that the normal protection from CHD afforded to pre-menopausal women is negated by diabetes.

 The normal protection from CHD afforded to pre-menopausal women is negated by diabetes.

RISK FACTORS FOR ATHEROSCLEROSIS

In longitudinal and interventional studies, glycaemic control has emerged as an independent risk factor for atherosclerotic cardiovascular disease. Current evidence suggests that there is a linear association between glycated haemoglobin levels and cardiovascular risk in patients with type 2 diabetes. However, the main modifiable risk factors for atherosclerosis in diabetic patients are identical to those operative in non-diabetics:

- Hypertension.
- Dyslipidaemia.
- Cigarette smoking.

Importantly, however, the adverse effects of hypertension and dyslipidaemia are amplified by the presence of diabetes. This also pertains for levels of lipids and BP which might be regarded as normal in non-diabetics. Moreover, when a multiplicity of risk factors is present, the risk of macrovascular disease is greatly enhanced (Fig. 5.1).

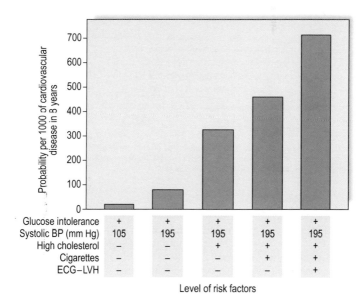

Glucose intolerance	+	+	+	+	+
Systolic BP (mm Hg)	105	195	195	195	195
High cholesterol	–	–	+	+	+
Cigarettes	–	–	–	+	+
ECG–LVH	–	–	–	–	+

Level of risk factors

Fig. 5.1 Multiple risk factors for CHD. (Reproduced with permission from Kannel WB, McGee DL. Diabetes Care 1979; 2: 120–126.)

> **NB** The coronary risk associated with dyslipidaemia, hypertension or cigarette smoking is amplified by the presence of diabetes.

The higher risk of CHD in patients with diabetes was forcefully demonstrated in a recent population-based study from Finland in which patients with type 2 diabetes who had no overt CHD were found to be at as high a risk of death as non-diabetics who had already sustained an MI (Fig. 5.2). Thus, patients with type 2 diabetes have a high absolute risk as high as non-diabetics in whom secondary preventative measures, notably the use of statins, are now well established. The patient with type 2 diabetes may therefore be regarded as a candidate for therapeutic measures hitherto reserved for patients with established CHD.

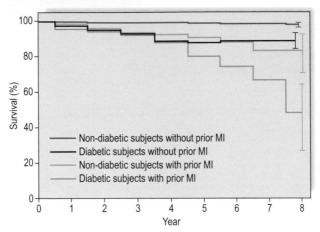

Fig. 5.2 Kaplan–Meier estimates of the probability of death from CHD in 1059 subjects with type 2 diabetes and 1378 non-diabetics without prior MI. (Reproduced with permission from Haffner SM, et al. N Engl J Med 1998; 339: 229–234.)

ACUTE MYOCARDIAL INFARCTION

Even in the thrombolytic era, the mortality rate of patients with diabetes following MI remains approximately 2-fold higher than non-diabetic subjects. Both immediate and late mortality rates are increased. Left ventricular failure and cardiogenic shock are the principal causes of death. However, there is no conclusive evidence that infarct size is larger in diabetics. The histology of CHD in diabetic patients does not differ appreciably from that in the non-diabetic population. However, coronary artery disease may progress more rapidly in diabetics. Moreover, a specific diabetic cardiomyopathy has been postulated which may contribute to the development of cardiac failure in some patients.

> **NB** Immediate and later mortality rates following MI are higher in diabetic patients.

The symptoms of MI may be modified by diabetes. Clinically 'silent' infarcts are more common in patients with diabetes; neuropathy affecting the autonomic fibres which also transmit pain sensation from the myocardium is held to be responsible. Angina pectoris may also be less prominent. Acute coronary ischaemia may therefore present atypically with symptoms such as:

• Dyspnoea.

- Syncope.
- Acute confusion in the elderly.

An ECG should be considered if a patient presents with such symptoms. Ischaemic ECGs are more commonly found in asymptomatic diabetic patients than non-diabetics. Abnormalities of the QT interval may also have prognostic implications in patients with type 2 diabetes (see p. 210).

> **NB** Acute MI may present with minimal or atypical symptoms in diabetic patients.

Management of acute myocardial infarction in diabetics
There is no evidence for diminished efficacy of interventions in patients with diabetes. The effect of aspirin is similar in diabetics and non-diabetics. Because of their higher absolute risk, diabetic patients may derive even greater benefit from interventions such as thrombolysis and beta-blockers than non-diabetics. There is evidence that these drugs are under-used.

> **NB** The benefits of thrombolysis and beta-blockers are greater in diabetic patients reflecting their higher absolute risk.

Thus, in addition to analgesia, this should include the following measures, as appropriate:

- *Aspirin.* Chewed at presentation and in the long term if no contraindications exist (300 mg daily enteric-coated).

- *Thrombolysis.* As for non-diabetics. The small risk of vitreous haemorrhage in patients with advanced retinopathy should not deter the use of thrombolysis.

- *ACE inhibitors.* For cardiac failure or impaired left ventricular function on echocardiogram.

- *Beta-blockers.* Particularly beneficial in diabetic patients.

> **NB** The small risk of intraocular haemorrhage from retinopathy should not deter use of thrombolytic agents.

In addition, control of the metabolic disturbances associated with acute MI may help reduce mortality. The hormonal stress response associated with MI has several potentially adverse metabolic consequences:

- Acute exacerbation of insulin resistance (see p. 28).

- Acute hyperglycaemia.
- Increased lipolysis (see p. 6; fatty acids may increase infarct size and may be pro-arrhythmic).
- Suppression of endogenous insulin secretion.

A proportion of non-diabetic patients with acute MI develop transient hyperglycaemia as a consequence of this hormonal stress response; the HbA_{1c} level will be normal reflecting satisfactory glucose levels prior to the infarct. Glycated proteins are relatively insensitive for diagnostic purposes, particularly minor degrees of glucose intolerance. If there is any continuing doubt, a 75 g oral glucose tolerance test (see Section 2) 6 weeks after the infarct is the definitive test.

Glucose–insulin infusions

Even in the absence of diabetes, intravenous infusions of glucose–insulin–potassium reduce infarct size in experimental animal models. Clear evidence for benefit in hyperglycaemic patients came with the publication of a multi-centre RCT from Sweden – the Diabetes Mellitus Insulin Glucose Infusion in Acute Myocardial Infarction (DIGAMI) study; Evidence-Based Medicine 5.2.

EVIDENCE-BASED MEDICINE 5.2

THE DIABETES MELLITUS INSULIN GLUCOSE INFUSION IN ACUTE MYOCARDIAL INFARCTION (DIGAMI) STUDY

(Br Med J 1997; 314: 1512–1515.)

STUDY DESIGN

620 subjects, more than 80% of whom were considered to have type 2 diabetes, were randomly assigned (a) to intensive treatment with an intravenous insulin–glucose infusion on the coronary care unit followed by multiple daily insulin injections (*n*=306), or (b) to a control group who received insulin only if clinically indicated (*n*=314).

Approximately 13% were previously undiagnosed. Thrombolysis, aspirin, ACE inhibitor and beta-blocker use was similar between the groups.

→

At discharge, 87% of the intensive treatment group were taking insulin compared with 43% in the control group. Although 15% of the intensive treatment group experienced hypoglycaemia, this was not associated with any adverse events.

RESULTS

HbA_{1c} decreased significantly in both groups during follow-up, the reduction being greater in the intensively treated group at the 3- and 12-month follow-up.

- A relative reduction in mortality of 30% was observed in the intensively treated group during the first year of follow-up.
- A significant reduction ($P<0.05$) in mortality of 11% was still evident after nearly 3.5 years (Fig. 5.3).

The reduction in mortality was most pronounced in a pre-defined subgroup of patients who had:

- Not previously received insulin treatment.

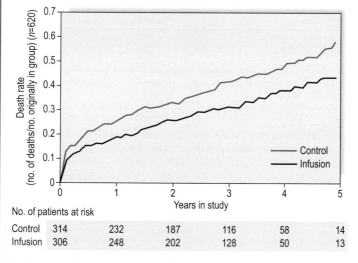

No. of patients at risk

Control	314	232	187	116	58	14
Infusion	306	248	202	128	50	13

Fig. 5.3 Actuarial mortality curves during long-term follow-up in patients receiving insulin-glucose infusion followed by subcutaneous insulin and the control group among the total DIGAMI cohort. (Reproduced with permission from Malmberg K, et al. Br Med J 1997; 314: 1512–1515.)

- A lower predicted cardiovascular risk as a consequence of being younger (<70 years) with no prior history of MI or congestive cardiac failure.

The protocol used on coronary care units for the DIGAMI study is presented in Table 5.9.

TABLE 5.9 Protocol used on coronary care units for the DIGAMI study

Infusion
500 mL 5% glucose with 80 units of soluble insulin, i.e. ~1 unit insulin per 6 mL infusate
Commence with 30 mL/h. Check blood glucose after 1 h. Adjust infusion rate aiming for a level of 7–10 mmol/L. Check glucose every 2 h, but 1 h after change of infusion rate. If initial decrease in glucose is >30%, the infusion rate should be left unchanged if blood glucose is >11 mmol/L but reduced by 6 mL/h if glucose is 7–10.9 mmol/L. If blood glucose is stable at <11 mmol/L after 10 pm, reduce infusion rate 50% during the night.

Blood glucose (mmol/L)	Action
>15	Give 8 units insulin as i.v. bolus and increase infusion rate by 6 mL/h
11–14.9	Increase infusion rate by 3 mL/h
7–10.9	Leave infusion rate unchanged
4–6.9	Decrease infusion rate by 6 mL/h
<4	Stop infusion for 15 min. Test glucose every 15 min until blood glucose >7 mmol/L. If symptoms of hypoglycaemia are present, administer 20 mL of 30% glucose intravenously. Restart infusion with an infusion decreased by 6 mL/h when blood glucose is >7 mmol/L.

NB Careful monitoring by trained staff is required for safe implementation of the DIGAMI protocol.

As a secondary prevention measure, the glucose–insulin protocol used in this study compares favourably in terms of cost-effectiveness with established interventions such as thrombolysis; for the cohort as a whole, 11 patients had to be treated to save one life at 3.5 years. The precise explanation for the improvement in survival remains uncertain. Insulin-mediated suppression of plasma fatty acid levels may be relevant. Another intriguing, but largely theoretical, possibility is that the reduced mortality in the intensively treated patients might, at least in part, have resulted from withdrawal of sulphonylureas. However, the impressive results of the subgroup analysis may reflect the higher, intrinsic, cardiovascular risk of patients previously treated with oral antidiabetic agents.

Concerns about the cardiovascular safety of sulphonylureas were initially raised by the findings of the University Group Diabetes Program in the 1970s. This controversial study reported an increased risk of cardiovascular mortality in patients randomized to tolbutamide. However, the UKPDS (see p. 65) did not demonstrate any difference in risk of CHD between patients treated with sulphonylureas or exogenous insulin. This issue is discussed in more detail in Section 3.

> **NB** Intravenous infusion of insulin + glucose followed by subcutaneous insulin reduces mortality in diabetic patients following MI.

The intravenous infusion is continued for 24 hours. At this point, the patient is transferred to small doses of subcutaneous insulin. Whether twice-daily insulin is as effective as multiple daily injections is presently undetermined; it is more acceptable to most patients. Long-term insulin therapy may not be feasible for some patients and clinical judgement is therefore required. Insulin should probably be continued as long as possible. However, recurrent hypoglycaemia with small doses may necessitate withdrawal of insulin. Metformin should be withdrawn in patients with acute ischaemic heart disease because of the potential for lactic acidosis in the setting of tissue hypoxia; insulin–glucose infusion is the treatment of choice.

To summarize:

- Discontinue oral antidiabetic agents on admission.
- Check blood glucose; if >11 mmol/L commence insulin–glucose infusion.
- Previously undiagnosed patients should also be treated.
- Continue the insulin–glucose infusion for 24 hours.
- Transfer to subcutaneous insulin and continue after discharge wherever possible.

> **NB** In the DIGAMI study, patients with type 2 diabetes considered to be at relatively low risk of death showed the greatest benefit from insulin therapy.

Revascularization procedures

Although symptomatic relief is similar to that obtained in non-diabetics, in general, revascularization procedures (angioplasty, coronary artery bypass grafting) appear to be less effective in diabetics; reported patient and graft survival rates are lower. Re-stenosis following angioplasty may be more common in diabetics. Therapeutic developments, e.g. increasing use of intracoronary stents, new agents directed against platelet aggregation, are being evaluated. Recent data suggest that plalelet glycoprotein IIb/IIIa receptor inhibitors are beneficial.

Cardiac failure

Studies in diabetic animals and humans provide support for a specific defect in myocardial function independently of atheroma of the coronary vasculature. Echocardiographic abnormalities of left ventricular function have been reported; these may remain subclinical. Microangiopathy and fibrosis of the myocardium are reported histological features to which systemic hypertension may contribute. It is hypothesized that these abnormalities may help to explain the well-documented excess incidence of cardiac failure observed in diabetic patients which is increased up to 5-fold that for non-diabetics.

 NB Diabetes is associated with an increased risk of cardiac failure.

The Hypertension in Diabetes Study (see p. 243) documented a significant reduction in the incidence of cardiac failure with intensive control of BP. The role of insulin resistance – a metabolic feature of cardiac failure – is being examined with respect to possible novel therapeutic strategies.

PERIPHERAL VASCULAR DISEASE

Together with neuropathy and infection, peripheral vascular disease contributes to foot disease in patients with diabetes (see p. 213). The incidence of peripheral vascular disease is increased approximately two-fold in diabetic patients. Abnormalities of circulating lipids, hypertension and smoking are recognized risk factors for peripheral vascular disease.

 NB Peripheral vascular disease is increased approximately two-fold in diabetic patients.

CLINICAL FEATURES

Atherosclerosis has a predilection for the distal vessels, i.e. below the popliteal fossa. Thus, the typical picture is palpable femoral pulses with absent pulses below this level. Patients are asymptomatic until significant arterial stenoses develop. Symptoms, which will depend on the site and degree of the stenosis, may then include:

- *Intermittent claudication.* Classical calf claudication.

- *Rest pain.* Denotes critical ischaemia; usually distal sites.

- *Leriche syndrome.* Buttock and leg claudication, erectile impotence as a result of major stenosis of the aortofemoral vessels.

- *Ischaemic foot lesions.* Ischaemia in isolation accounts for less than 10% of diabetic foot ulcers. However, ischaemia is the co-pathology in neuro-ischaemic lesions which comprise approximately 50% of all ulcers (see p. 215).

Co-existing vascular disease may impede healing of ulcers that are predominantly of neuropathic origin, particularly when there is superadded infection in soft tissues or bone. Finally, atherosclerotic disease may result in renal artery stenosis which is of relevance to the pathogenesis and treatment of hypertension (see p. 240).

 NB In diabetic patients, atherosclerosis has a predilection for vessels below the popliteal fossa.

ASSESSMENT OF PERIPHERAL VASCULATURE

• *Clinical evaluation.* The history should include enquiry about: claudication, rest pain, features of Leriche syndrome (see p. 236), foot ulceration – past or present, smoking habits, family history of atherosclerotic disease, other manifestations of atherosclerosis – history of MI, transient ischaemic attacks, stroke (see earlier), and lipid status.

• *Physical examination.* This includes palpation of peripheral pulses and auscultation for bruits. Trophic changes in the skin are sought and limb temperature is assessed. The limb is pale and cold in the presence of significant ischaemia but may appear red with critical impairment of blood flow ('sunset foot'). Buerger's sign may be positive: the limb blanches on being raised from the horizontal, then assumes a dusky-red colour on being hung over the edge of the bed. Evidence of additional risk factors for atherosclerosis should be sought, including corneal arcus, xanthelasma and hypertension. Aggravating disorders (e.g. anaemia) should also be sought.

• *Doppler studies.* These are readily performed at the bedside using a hand-held probe; however, interpretation requires experience and training since information is potentially open to misinterpretation in patients with diabetes. The ratio of the Doppler-measured ankle pressure to the brachial artery pressure is normally 1.0. Values less than 0.5 indicate severe disease. However, the ratio may be falsely elevated by arterial calcification in diabetes. This renders the vessel highly resistant to compression by the ankle pressure cuff. The clue comes in the quality of the Doppler signal. Normally three components may be discerned (i.e. the signal is triphasic). With arterial calcification, there is a reduction to a bi- or mono-phasic signal. Further assessment is then indicated.

• *Duplex scanning.* This is a useful, non-invasive technique combining ultrasound imaging with Doppler assessment of blood flow to provide information about the haemodynamic effects of lesions. Once again, however, calcification may limit the quality of the information obtained.

Duplex scanning is usually a prelude to angiography if surgery is contemplated.

● *Oxygen tension*. This can be measured transcutaneously on the dorsum of the foot using a laser Doppler probe allowing confirmation of critical ischaemia.

● *Angiography*. This remains the investigation to delineate the site and extent of the lesions which often affect the distal arterial tree. Digital subtraction of bone improves the quality of the imaging of below-knee vessels. There is also the major advantage of being able to perform angioplasty or thrombolytic agents during the procedure. However, care should be taken to ensure adequate hydration in patients with renal impairment undergoing angiography.

MANAGEMENT

● *Aspirin*. This reduces mortality from cardiovascular disease and should be given where there are no contraindications.

● *Foot care*. This is of great importance and patients should receive appropriate instruction (see p. 214). Timely podiatry may avert more serious lesions.

● *Vasodilators*. Oral agents are usually ineffective. Intravenous praxilene and low-molecular weight dextran may sometimes be helpful in selected patients with severe ischaemia.

● *Surgical sympathectomy*. Lumbar sympathectomy is ineffective for intermittent claudication. In any case, patients with severe co-existing neuropathy will often have clinical features suggestive of sympathetic denervation.

● *Reconstructive surgery or angioplasty*. These may preserve limbs although major amputation is still sometimes the only option. Two major patterns are seen, which carry different prospects for successful intervention:

1. Proximal disease. Patients with weak femoral pulses, and absent pulses more distally, may be suitable for angioplasty or arterial bypass grafting (aortofemoral and femoropopliteal). Localized short stenoses are most suitable for angioplasty.
2. Distal disease. More commonly encountered in diabetes; normal femoral and popliteal pulses with absent foot pulses. This is much more difficult to treat by angioplasty or bypass grafting, particularly when there is diffuse disease below-knee.

● *Amputation*. If required for major arterial occlusion, this may have to be radical.

● *Rehabilitation*. See p. 218.

CEREBROVASCULAR DISEASE

The incidence of cerebrovascular disease is increased by a factor of 1.5–2 in diabetic patients. Histologically, atheroma of the cerebral circulation is indistinguishable from that observed in non-diabetics. An important role for the central nervous system in the regulation of glucose metabolism has long been recognized; Claude Bernard described piqûre diabetes in animals – glycosuria following puncture of the floor of the fourth ventricle – in the 19th century. In a manner analogous to the situation in acute MI, hyperglycaemia after an acute stroke has been postulated to be a response to the stress response in some patients not previously recognized as diabetic. However, there is some evidence that hyperglycaemia at presentation with acute stroke is an independent marker of adverse clinical outcome, principally mortality within the first month.

TRANSIENT DEFECTS ASSOCIATED WITH ACUTE METABOLIC DERANGEMENTS

• *Hemiplegia.* In addition to atheromatous cerebrovascular disease, transient hemiplegia has a recognized but rare association with hypoglycaemia, particularly nocturnal episodes (see p. 162). It has long been postulated that a subcritical stenosis becomes clinically manifest when neural dysfunction owing to hypoglycaemia is superimposed; however, supportive evidence is scant.

• *Other focal neurologies.* Reversible focal neurology is also recognized in patients presenting with DKA, and in particular, non-ketotic hyperosmolar pre-coma or coma (see p. 185).

• *Convulsions.* Epilepsy may be triggered in susceptible patients by hyperglycaemia particularly with hyperosmolarity (see Section 4).

COGNITIVE DYSFUNCTION

Atherosclerotic dementia may contribute to impaired psychomotor performance, learning and memory in older diabetic patients. In addition, correlations between psychological dysfunction and degree of chronic hyperglycaemia have been reported in the elderly. Hypertension (see p. 240) and other factors are also implicated. There is some evidence suggesting that better glycaemic control may improve cognition. On the other hand, chronic severe neuroglycopenia may rarely cause a dementia-like syndrome.

ATRIAL FIBRILLATION

Diabetes is regarded as an additional risk factor for stroke when considering anticoagulation for atrial fibrillation. In the UKPDS (see p. 65), atrial fibrillation was identified as a major risk factor for stroke.

> **NB** Atrial fibrillation is a major risk factor for stroke in patients with type 2 diabetes.

HYPERTENSION

Hypertension is now recognized as an important and modifiable risk factor for both macro- and microvascular complications of diabetes. In type 1 diabetes, hypertension is principally encountered in patients with nephropathy. For type 2 diabetes, by contrast, the prevalence of hypertension is much higher; in this group, hypertension is closely associated with insulin resistance (see p. 28). There is considerable evidence that hypertension in these high-risk patients is both under-diagnosed and inadequately treated. Regular monitoring of BP is an important and undervalued aspect of diabetes care.

> **NB** In type 1 diabetes, hypertension is largely confined to patients with nephropathy.

Another important distinction is that in type 2 diabetes, hypertension may go undetected for many years prior to diagnosis. Thus, risk factors for cardiovascular disease – hypertension, hyperglycaemia (and associated dyslipidaemia) – are present and operative during the pre-diabetic period. Atheromatous disease may be well established by the time that diabetes is diagnosed; this has been likened to a 'ticking clock' for CHD which starts many years before the patient's diabetes becomes clinically apparent.

> **NB** Cardiovascular risk factors are frequently present in combination for many years prior to the diagnosis of diabetes.

HAEMODYNAMIC ABNORMALITIES IN DIABETES

Subtle alterations in diabetic patients may increase the risk of tissue damage attributable to hypertension. The suggestion is that for any specified level of systemic BP, patients with diabetes are more susceptible. Postulated mechanisms include:

● *Failure of autoregulation.* Impaired autoregulation in vulnerable vascular beds such as the retinal and renal glomerular systems caused by hyperglycaemia results in the direct transmission of systemic BP to the microvasculature; the implication is that any elevation of systemic BP will cause greater tissue damage when hyperglycaemia is present.

● *Decreased vascular compliance.* Decreased compliance of major vessels (e.g. the aorta), perhaps resulting from non-enzymatic glycation (see Section 1), may result in transmission of higher pressures to vascular beds.

● *Increased BP variability.* Increased variability of BP in diabetic patients has been reported during 24-hour recordings.

● *Decreased nocturnal BP decline.* Failure of the physiological decline ('dipping') in BP during sleep is a reported early feature of microalbuminuria. Thus, the mean BP over a 24-hour period is increased.

ASSESSMENT OF THE DIABETIC PATIENT WITH HYPERTENSION

● *Exclusion of secondary hypertension.* The history and physical examination will usually reveal any endocrine cause of hypertension and diabetes (Table 5.10) or other forms of secondary hypertension. However, most of the former, which with the exception of thyrotoxicosis are uncommon, are associated with relatively minor glucose intolerance. The association with primary hyperparathyroidism is controversial. However, insulin resistance is a reported feature of this common disturbance of calcium metabolism.

● *Signs of target organ damage.* Including left ventricular hypertrophy, arterial bruits, absent pedal pulses (increased risk of renal artery stenosis, see p. 249), hypertensive retinal changes should be sought.

● *Assessment of other cardiovascular risk factors.* See page 228.

TABLE 5.10 Endocrine causes of diabetes and hypertension

● Thyrotoxicosis
● Acromegaly
● Cushing's syndrome
● Conn's syndrome
● Phaeochromocytoma

INVESTIGATIONS

For most patients these should include:

● *Urinalysis.* For microalbuminuria or clinical grade proteinuria.

● *Renal function and electrolytes.* For renal impairment, hypokalaemia (Conn's syndrome, but usually caused by diuretics), hyperkalaemia (renal impairment, hyporeninaemic hypoaldosteronism in patients with type 2 diabetes).

• *ECG.* For evidence of left ventricular hypertrophy (indicates adverse prognosis, echocardiography is more sensitive), ischaemia (may be subclinical), atrial fibrillation (relatively common – increased risk of stroke).

• *Plasma lipids.* See page 246.

• *Ambulatory BP recording.* The role of ambulatory BP recording and home measurements by patients in diagnosis and management has not been clearly delineated. Ambulatory measurements may be useful if there is unusual variability in clinical pressures, hypertension apparently resistant to three or more drugs, symptoms suggesting hypotension or a suspicion of 'white-coat hypertension'. The 1999 British Hypertension Society guidelines suggest an optimal mean daytime ambulatory pressure or home measurement of <130/75 for diabetics.

Other investigations (e.g. treadmill exercise testing, isotope imaging studies to exclude renal artery stenosis) may be indicated in individual patients.

TYPE 1 DIABETES

Hypertension is particularly associated with diabetic nephropathy and plays an important role in determining the rate of decline of renal function (see p. 219). Degrees of hypertension below currently accepted diagnostic criteria may be clinically important, hence recent recommendations for a target BP of 130/80 in the presence of nephropathy. Impairment of the physiological fall in BP that occurs during the night may also be important in patients with microalbuminuria (see p. 228). Nephropathy is more prevalent among patients who have hypertensive parents suggesting that hypertension may be an inherited factor which increases the risk of renal disease. A high rate of sodium/lithium countertransport in erythrocytes appears to have negative prognostic implications for patients with nephropathy.

TYPE 2 DIABETES

The prevalence of hypertension is especially high in type 2 diabetes. Amongst a subgroup of participants in the UKPDS (see p. 65), the prevalence (defined rather loosely as a BP >160/90 or receiving antihypertensive medication) was approximately 40% at age 45; this rises to more than 60% in the over-75s. Factors, which are closely related to type 2 diabetes, will also influence BP levels, notably:

• Increasing age.
• Increasing body weight.

The effect attributable to sex is less clear; some studies have suggested that women are at higher risk. While hypertension is more common in patients with type 2 diabetes, the prevalence reflects the general background of the population studied. Black patients, for example, are at particular risk, reflecting the predilection for hypertension and its sequelae in this group as a whole. By contrast, amongst patients with diabetes, South Asians in the UK have a prevalence somewhat lower than the indigenous white population. In type 2 diabetes, hypertension is associated with insulin resistance and it has been hypothesized that the two conditions may be causally related (see Section 1). However, there is continuing uncertainty about the strength and nature of the association.

> **NB** Hypertension in type 2 diabetes is regarded as a component of the insulin resistance syndrome in some ethnic groups.

HYPERTENSION IN DIABETES STUDY

In 1987, this randomized study of BP control was embedded within the main UKPDS in a factorial design. The study provided important confirmation of the adverse effect of hypertension in patients with type 2 diabetes. Evidence-Based Medicine 5.3 provides a summary of the key points of the study. Whether any particular class of antihypertensive drugs is associated with advantages or disadvantages for diabetic patients remains uncertain. The results suggested that the most important consideration is the level of BP attained rather than the agents used; similar efficacy was demonstrated for atenolol and captopril. The results of other studies in non-diabetic patients have not revealed any major consistent differences between older and newer agents.

> **NB** The attained BP level appears to be more important than the drugs used in patients with type 2 diabetes.

EVIDENCE-BASED MEDICINE 5.3

THE HYPERTENSION IN DIABETES STUDY. UKPDS 38 AND 39.

(UKPDS 38. Br Med J 1998; 317: 703–713.)
The study compared (a) tight control of BP (target <150/85, n=758) either with the ACE inhibitor, captopril (25–50 mg twice daily, n=400) or atenolol (50–100 mg daily, n=358) plus additional agents as necessary (suggested sequence: frusemide, slow-release nifedepine, methyldopa and prazocin) with (b) less tight (<180/105, n=390) control.

RESULTS

- Mean BP was reduced to 144/82 vs 154/87 mmHg (a difference of 10/5 mmHg) for the tight and less tight control groups, respectively ($P<0.0001$).
- Multiple drug therapy (three or more agents) was required more often in the tight control group (29% vs 11%, respectively). However, at 9 years, only 56% of patients in the tight control group had attained the target BP of <150/85.
- Tight control reduced diabetes-related endpoints (fatal or non-fatal) by 24% ($P=0.0046$; Fig. 5.4), diabetes-related deaths by 32% ($P=0.019$), stroke by 44% ($P=0.013$) and microvascular disease by 37% ($P=0.0092$).

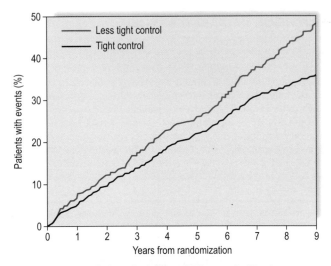

Fig. 5.4 Hypertension in Diabetes Study. Effect of tight control of blood pressure on diabetes-related endpoints (fatal or non-fatal). (Reproduced with permission from UK Prospective Diabetes Study Group. Br Med J 1998; 317: 703–713.)

- The reduction in microvascular complications was predominantly attributable to a reduced risk of photocoagulation for retinopathy; there were associated reductions in the progression of retinopathy (34%, $P=0.0004$). In addition, a measure of visual loss (equivalent of a reduction from 6/6 to 6/12 or 6/9 to 6/18 on the Snellen chart) was reduced suggesting prevention of maculopathy, the main cause of visual impairment in type 2 diabetes (47%, $P=0.004$).

→

- A transient reduction in microalbuminuria (P=0.009) at 6 years in the tight control group was not sustained at 9 years; there was no difference in clinical grade proteinuria or serum creatinine between the groups by the end of the study.
- All-cause mortality was not significantly reduced (18%, P=0.17) by tight BP control. However, there was a 34% reduction in combined macrovascular endpoints (i.e. MI, sudden death, stroke and peripheral vascular disease, P=0.019).
- Although the reduction in MI (21%) was not statistically significant ECG Q-wave abnormalities were reduced by 48% (P=0.007). In addition, the risk of cardiac failure was reduced by 56% (P=0.0043).

UKPDS 39 BR MED J 1998; 317: 713–720

- Captopril and atenolol were equally effective in reducing the incidence of diabetic complications.
- The mean gain in weight was, however, higher in the atenolol group (3.4 vs 1.6 kg) while glycated HbA_{1c} concentrations were slightly higher over the first 4 years. No difference in the rate of hypoglycaemia was observed between the drugs.
- Captopril was better tolerated than atenolol with 78% vs 65% of patients still taking their allocated drug at their last clinic visit (P<0.0001).

METABOLIC EFFECTS OF ANTIHYPERTENSIVE DRUGS

Much debate has surrounded the effects of antihypertensive agents on risk factors for cardiovascular disease. While the clinical significance of these effects remains uncertain, treatment of hypertension has not produced the expected reduction in mortality from CHD in trials using beta-blockers and thiazides. It has been suggested that adverse metabolic effects might have offset some of the beneficial effects of these drugs:

- *Insulin action.* Beta-blockers (particularly non-selective agents) and high-dose thiazide diuretics aggravate insulin resistance (whereas ACE inhibitors and alpha-blockers can improve insulin action, see p. 246). Interestingly, in the Hypertension in Diabetes Study (Table 5.12), the HbA_{1c} in the atenolol-treated group was significantly higher than that for the captopril-treated group during the first few years of the study; more antihyperglycaemic therapy was required in the atenolol-treated patients. Both beta-blockers and thiazides, particularly in combination, have been implicated in the pathogenesis of type 2 diabetes in patients with essential hypertension during longitudinal studies.

- *Lipids*. The adverse effect of these antihypertensive agents on plasma lipids (increased very-low density lipoproteins (VLDL) and hypercholesterolaemia, respectively) has also received attention. Associated haemostatic abnormalities (increased fibrinogen and factor VII, reduced activity of plasminogen activator inhibitor-1) may contribute to atherogenesis.

- *Hypokalaemia*. There have been reports of increased risk of sudden death in diabetic and non-diabetic patients with ECG abnormalities treated with thiazides. However, these reports have not been confirmed in RCTs.

The metabolic effects of thiazides can be minimized by the use of low doses, e.g. bendrofluazide 2.5 mg daily, or less. Higher doses have limited additional antihypertensive effect and greatly increase the risk of adverse effects. Dihydropyridine calcium antagonists with a short duration of action, e.g. nifedipine, may also impair insulin action. However, longer-acting drugs (e.g. amlodipine) and modified-release preparations, together with non-dihydropyridine drugs (e.g. diltiazem, verapamil) appear to have neutral effects. By contrast, several classes of more recently introduced antihypertensive agents may have beneficial effects of insulin sensitivity:

- *ACE inhibitors*. These agents are either neutral or may improve insulin sensitivity in non-diabetic and diabetic patients. ACE gene polymorphisms may have implications for insulin action (see p. 4) in addition to therapeutic responses to ACE inhibitors. In the HOPE study (Evidence-based Medicine 5.4) the risk of developing diabetes was reduced by rampiril.

- *Angiotensin II receptor antagonists*. There are reports of improved insulin action with these agents.

- *Alpha$_1$ blockers*. Doxazocin can improve insulin sensitivity and lipids but there are doubts about its cardioprotective effects.

- *Selective imidazoline receptor agonists*. Moxonidine improves insulin action in animal models and in obese hypertensive patients. Rilmenidine, another agent in this class, has also been shown to improve metabolic defects in animals; effects on glucose and lipid metabolism in humans with diabetes appear to be neutral to date.

In addition to the Hypertension in Diabetes Study, data from several other RCTs in recent years (Evidence-Based Medicine 5.4) have demonstrated substantial benefits from treating hypertension in patients with type 2 diabetes; these trials used regimens based on thiazides and long-acting calcium antagonists. In these studies, the therapeutic benefit in the diabetic subgroups was greater than that observed in non-diabetics, reflecting the higher absolute risk associated with diabetes. However, there has been controversy about reports of higher cardiovascular event rates in patients treated with calcium antagonists compared with other agents such as ACE inhibitors. Resolution of this uncertainty may come with the publication of additional large comparative studies. Studies in non-diabetics have not suggested any significant differences between the major classes of antihypertensive agents to date.

Concerns about another long-running controversy – the 'J-shaped curve' (i.e. very low BP being associated with adverse outcomes) – have now effectively been allayed; thus, the lower the attained BP, the greater the clinical benefit. The 1999 WHO–International Society for Hypertension guidelines state that any of the main classes of antihypertensive drugs may be considered suitable as first-line therapy.

┌─ EVIDENCE-BASED MEDICINE 5.4 ┐

Other RCTs of antihypertensive therapy involving patients with type 2 diabetes.

1. SHEP (SYSTOLIC HYPERTENSION IN THE ELDERLY PROGRAM)

(JAMA 1996; 276: 1886–1892.)
• Total $n=4736$; diabetic $n=583$.
• Chlorthalidone ± atenolol or reserpine vs placebo.

FINDINGS

Reduction in major cardiovascular events (cerebral and cardiac) with active treatment vs placebo. Greater benefit in diabetic subgroup reflecting higher absolute risk.

2. HOT (HYPERTENSION OPTIMAL TREATMENT TRIAL)

(Lancet 1998; 351: 1755–1762.)
• Total $n=18790$; diabetic $n=1501$.
• Felodipine + other agents as required to attain BP targets.
• Aspirin vs. placebo.

FINDINGS

Reduction (by 50%) in major cardiovascular events with target diastolic of 80 mmHg vs 90 mmHg in diabetic patients.

→

3. SYST-EUR

(Lancet 1997; 350: 757–764 and N Engl J Med 1999; 340: 677–684.)
- Total n=4695; diabetic n=492.
- Nitrendipine + enalapril or thiazide vs placebo.

RESULTS

Excess risk of diabetes almost completely eliminated by antihypertensive therapy with major reductions (approx 70%) in cardiovascular mortality and all cardiovascular endpoints.
Beneficial effect of aspirin.

4. HOPE (HEART OUTCOME PREVENTION EVALUATION)

(N Engl J Med 2000; 342: 145–153 and Lancet 2000; 355: 253–259.)
- Total n=9927 with pre-existing CHD, stroke or peripheral vascular disease; 38% with diabetes.
- Ramipril vs. placebo.

RESULTS

Overall, 25% reduction in risk of cardiovascular death, 20% for MI and 32% for stroke with ramipril vs placebo. For diabetic subgroup, 17% risk reduction in diabetic complications.

CAUTIONS AND CONTRAINDICATIONS

Diabetic patients are at risk of developing long-term tissue complications which may render certain antihypertensive drugs unsuitable (Table 5.11). The most appropriate drug should be selected initially (Table 5.12). Treatment of hypertension in patients with diabetes is also complicated by other considerations:

- *Risk of hypoglycaemia.* Problems of impaired recognition of warning symptoms and recovery from hypoglycaemia (see p. 156) with beta-blockers are uncommon with cardioselective drugs, e.g. atenolol. Insulin treatment should not be regarded as a contraindication to the use of such drugs, which are of proven benefit in diabetic patients. Reports of an increased risk of hypoglycaemia in insulin-treated patients have not been substantiated. In the

TABLE 5.11 Cautions and contraindications to antihypertensive therapy in diabetic patients

Caution or contraindication	Drugs
Dyslipidaemia	Beta-blockers Thiazides (high doses)
Erectile dysfunction	Beta-blockers Thiazides
Gout	Thiazides
Peripheral vascular disease	Beta-blockers
Renal artery stenosis	ACE inhibitors All receptor antagonists

TABLE 5.12 Indications for particular antihypertensive drugs in diabetic patients

Indication	Drugs of choice
Nephropathy	ACE inhibitors (+ loop diuretics) Non-dihydropyridine calcium antagonists
Ischaemic heart disease	Beta-blockers Long-acting calcium antagonists
Cardiac failure	ACE inhibitors Loop diuretics Beta-blockers (in selected patients)

(ACE inhibitor, angiotensin converting enzyme inhibitor.

UKPDS (see p. 65), there was no difference in the risk of severe hypoglycaemia between the atenolol and captopril treatment groups. Hypoglycaemia attributable to ACE inhibitors appears to be uncommon in clinical practice (see p. 156).

● *Renal artery stenosis.* A minority of patients with type 2 diabetes who have absent pedal pulses because of peripheral vascular disease also have clinically significant renal artery stenosis. Certain drugs – ACE inhibitors and angiotensin II antagonists – should be used with caution in view of the risk of precipitating an acute deterioration in renal function. Where there are functional stenoses of both renal arteries, glomerular filtration is maintained by the vasoconstrictor effect of angiotensin II on efferent glomerular arterioles. Removal of this effect by these drugs may cause a major decrease in glomerular filtration. Under certain circumstances (patients with congestive cardiac failure with generalized atherosclerosis), deterioration in renal function may be encountered with unilateral renal artery stenosis. This risk may have been overstated in the past but it is prudent to check plasma creatinine and electrolytes within a week of commencing ACE inhibitor therapy in at-risk patients.

ETHNICITY AND CHOICE OF TREATMENT

Black patients, who tend to have low plasma renin levels, respond better to beta-blockers and calcium antagonists than to ACE inhibitors. In South Asian patients with multiple components of the insulin resistance syndrome, metabolically neutral or advantageous drugs are logical, first-line choices.

STRATEGIES FOR THE MANAGEMENT OF HYPERTENSION IN DIABETES

● *Non-pharmacological.* Attainment of ideal body weight, reduced salt intake (see p. 86), regular aerobic physical exercise (see p. 100).

● *Drug therapy.* When BP targets are not achieved, commence with the most appropriate drug for the particular patient. Add or substitute drugs in logical combinations (e.g. ACE inhibitor and diuretic or calcium antagonist). Use low doses to minimize unwanted effects. Diuretics are often useful since hypertension in diabetics is associated with an expanded plasma volume. Multiple drug regimens are often required. Loop diuretics are often necessary for patients with significant renal impairment in whom hypertension may be particularly difficult to control. Patients with diabetes will often require a multiplicity of other drugs such as oral antidiabetic agents, lipid-lowering agents and aspirin. Since hypertension is largely asymptomatic, once-daily dosing and use of well-tolerated drugs are likely to improve compliance.

DIABETIC DYSLIPIDAEMIA

Quantitative and qualitative alterations in plasma lipids in diabetic patients increase the risk of atheroma. Furthermore, the impact of dyslipidaemia is magnified by diabetes. Nephropathy is associated with additional disturbances of plasma lipids which further increase risk. Common genetic dyslipidaemias, e.g. familial combined hyperlipidaemia, are just as common in diabetics as non-diabetics. The rare syndromes of lipodystrophy may be associated with marked hyperlipidaemia.

TYPE 1 DIABETES

Patients with good glycaemic control usually have relatively normal plasma lipid profiles. Acute metabolic decompensation, particularly DKA, may be associated with marked hyperlipidaemia, sometimes with clinical manifestations such as eruptive xanthomata and lipaemia retinalis. The success of insulin therapy in such circumstances reflects the actions of the hormone on several aspects of lipid metabolism:

- The stimulatory effect of insulin on the endothelial enzyme lipoprotein lipase which hydrolyzes circulating triglycerides in VLDLs and chylomicrons. This leads to a secondary reduction in LDL-cholesterol levels.
- The suppression of adipocyte lipolysis (via hormone-sensitive lipase) which in turn reduces the delivery of non-esterified fatty acids to the liver (see p. 6).
- The suppression of hepatic VLDL secretion by insulin.

Nephropathy has a major impact on lipids. The development of diabetic nephropathy leads to dyslipidaemia with elevated levels of total cholesterol, LDL-cholesterol and triglycerides in concert with reduced levels of cardioprotective HDL-cholesterol. In addition, the plasma concentration of lipoprotein(a), an independent risk factor for CHD, increases.

TYPE 2 DIABETES

The most common abnormalities of plasma lipids in patients with type 2 diabetes are:

- Hypertriglyceridaemia.
- Reduced HDL-cholesterol levels.

Elevations of total and LDL-cholesterol concentrations are not as prevalent, the total cholesterol level in general is similar to that in non-diabetics. Hypertriglyceridaemia is associated with insulin resistance and impaired insulin action as outlined above. Decreased breakdown of VLDL increases the circulating concentration of atherogenic, triglyceride-rich, remnant, lipoprotein particles. Low HDL-cholesterol levels are closely associated with hypertriglyceridaemia, arising from increased transfer of cholesteryl ester from HDL to VLDL and chylomicrons by the action of cholesteryl ester transfer protein. LDL-cholesterol particle size is reduced by increased activity of hepatic lipase. This produces smaller, more dense, apoprotein-rich LDL particles (so-called pattern B on electrophoresis) which are regarded as having enhanced atherogenicity. The prevalence of these abnormalities appears to be approximately twice as high in patients with type 2 diabetes as in non-diabetics. However, any specified level of cholesterol has a greater impact on coronary risk in the presence of diabetes. The risk of coronary event is particularly high when the following triad is present:

- Low HDL-cholesterol.
- High ratio (>5.0) of total cholesterol/HDL-cholesterol.
- Hypertriglyceridaemia.

It is suggested that the atherogenicity of disordered lipid metabolism in diabetes may be further increased by additional factors:

● *Glycation of lipoproteins.* Apoprotein B, the major protein component of LDL, is susceptible to non-enzymatic glycation (see Section 1). This reduces the affinity for tissue LDL receptor thereby reducing clearance from the plasma.

● *Oxidative modification.* The uptake of LDL by scavenger pathways which lead to atherosclerosis may be increased by oxidation. This, in turn, may be increased by glycation.

Management

The greatly increased risk of atherosclerotic disease in patients with diabetes, in concert with recent results from clinical trials of lipid-modifying drugs, has led to an increased awareness of the importance of detecting (see Section 2) and treating dyslipidaemia. Although measurement of lipids in the fasting state is usually performed (in order to include triglycerides and HDL-cholesterol), there are practical difficulties involved in patients treated with insulin. Increasing research attention is being focused on post-prandial lipid status. In patients with type 2 diabetes, post-prandial clearance of lipoproteins from the circulation is impaired; it is hypothesized that this post-prandial hyperlipidaemia contributes to the development of atheroma.

Although many subtle alterations in plasma lipids have been described, therapeutic decisions rest on measurement of some or all of the following:

● Total cholesterol.
● Triglycerides.
● LDL-cholesterol (calculated with reasonable accuracy using the Friedewald formula when fasting triglycerides are <4.5 mmol/L).
● HDL-cholesterol (which also allows calculation of ratio of total cholesterol/HDL-cholesterol).

Therapeutic decisions, particularly when to introduce lipid-modifying drugs, must take into consideration the impact of other key cardiovascular risk factors (see p. 228).

THERAPEUTIC TARGETS IN DIABETIC DYSLIPIDAEMIA

Although observational studies suggest that low HDL-cholesterol and hypertriglyceridaemia may be more predictive than elevated LDL-cholesterol levels, the results of interventional RCTs using statins strongly favour LDL-cholesterol lowering as the primary aim of therapy (Evidence-Based Medicine 5.5).

NB Reduction of LDL-cholesterol concentrations is currently regarded as the primary therapeutic aim of lipid-lowering therapy.

┌─ **EVIDENCE-BASED MEDICINE 5.5** ─────────────────────────

Placebo-controlled trials that have demonstrated benefits of lowering
LDL-cholesterol concentrations in patients with diabetes.

THE SCANDINAVIAN SIMVASTATIN SURVIVAL STUDY (4S)

(Diabetes Care 1997; 20: 614–620.)
- Significant (55%) reduction in incidence of major coronary events in
  diabetic men with high LDL-cholesterol levels (5.5–8.0 mmol/L) and
  prior CHD.

THE CHOLESTEROL AND RECURRENT EVENTS (CARE) STUDY

(Circulation 1998; 98: 2513–2519.)
- Pravastatin significantly reduced the incidence of CHD events in
  diabetic patients with average LDL-cholesterol levels and prior CHD.

  Note. Results are derived from analyses of diabetic subgroups in each
  trial.

To date, no studies have been published exclusively in diabetic patients;
both the 4S and CARE studies contained relatively small diabetic subgroups.
Clinical guidelines produced by expert committees are being regularly
updated as evidence from trials accumulates. For diabetic patients with
established cardiovascular disease, current guidelines for secondary
prevention with lipid-modifying drugs should be followed. The situation
pertaining to primary prevention is less clear at present. Differences in
recommendations between some expert groups have generated confusion
for clinicians faced with therapeutic decisions. Examples of two recent
guidelines, those of the Joint British Societies (1998) and those of the ADA
(2000) are presented in Table 5.13.

The magnitude of benefit derived from drugs such as the hydroxymethyl
glutaryl coenzyme A (HMG-CoA) reductase inhibitors (or statins) depends
on the absolute cardiovascular risk. The available data strongly suggest that
diabetic patients should be regarded at high risk of cardiovascular events. In
the CARE study, for instance, in high-risk patients with diabetes and

established CHD 22 new coronary events were prevented in every 100 patients treated with simvastatin for 5 years. By contrast, in a primary prevention study in non-diabetic men in the West of Scotland with no risk factors other than LDL-cholesterol levels of 4.5–6.0 mmol/L, similar treatment with pravastatin prevented only one event. Calculation of absolute cardiovascular risk is widely regarded as a logical approach, the aim being to target drug therapy to those at highest risk of cardiovascular events. However, risk cut-off levels are ultimately arbitrary and once again there are inconsistencies between available published guidelines. The 1998 Joint British guidelines (Table 5.13) attempt to identify those at highest coronary risk (i.e. >30% over next 10 years) as a priority but they also set targets for lipids and BP (including the use of pharmacological agents as necessary) in patients whose risk is >15% over 10 years.

TABLE 5.13 Suggested targets for plasma lipids and other coronary risk factors in diabetic patients

1. Joint British Societies recommendations on prevention of CHD in clinical practice

Targets for (a) patients (diabetic or non-diabetic) with CHD or other major atherosclerotic disease or (b) high-risk groups (coronary risk >15% over next 10 years) such as diabetics with no clinical evidence of atherosclerosis (particularly when risk factors are present in combination).

Risk factor	Target
Total cholesterol	<5.0 mmol/L
LDL-cholesterol	<3.0 mmol/L
BP	<130/85 mmHg

Also recommended: good glycaemic control (with use of insulin during and immediately after MI), aspirin and other cardioprotective drugs as indicated (e.g. beta-blockers, ACE inhibitors).

Reference: Heart 1998; 80 (suppl 2): S1–S29.

2. American Diabetes Association, 2000

LDL thresholds for initiation and targets of drug therapy in diabetes

| | Macrovascular disease | |
	No evidence	Present
Initiation level	<3.4	<2.6
LDL goal	<2.6	<2.6

All levels in mmol/L. To convert to mg/dL divide by 0.02586. Macrovacular disease includes clinically evident CHD, cerebrovascular and peripheral vascular disease.
Note. Initiation levels may be lower for patients with no evidence of macrovascular disease but who have multiple risk factors (low HDL-cholesterol, hypertension, family history of cardiovascular disease, microalbuminuria or clinical grade proteinuria). Diabetic men and women are considered to be at equal risk.

Reference: Diabetes Care 2000; 23 (suppl 1): S57–S60.

NON-PHARMACOLOGICAL TREATMENT

This includes:

● *Dietary measures*. Attainment of ideal body weight, reduction in saturated fat consumption to around 30% of total calories, increasing intake of mono-unsaturates. Excessive alcohol consumption may exacerbate hypertriglyceridaemia.

● *Aerobic physical exercise*. This may improve hypertriglyceridaemia and raise HDL-cholesterol levels.

● *Optimization of metabolic control*. Hepatic LDL receptors, the major regulators of plasma LDL levels, are dependent on insulin; total and LDL-cholesterol levels may therefore decline with improved glycaemia. Elevated triglyceride levels may respond even more to measures such as use of insulin to attain good glycaemic control.

● *Avoidance of drugs which exacerbate dyslipidaemia*. This includes beta-blockers as well as higher doses of thiazide diuretics. However, the Hypertension in Diabetes Study (see p. 243) found no consistent trends in lipid levels between the atenolol and captopril groups. Other drugs such as corticosteroids exacerbate dyslipidaemia as well as hyperglycaemia. Oestrogens in contraceptive preparations may exacerbate dyslipidaemia (see p. 270). However, post-menopausal low-dose oestrogen replacement therapy tends to improve plasma lipid profiles.

● *Exclusion of other factors*. Hepatic dysfunction, renal impairment (of any cause) and hypothyroidism may cause or exacerbate dyslipidaemias and should be excluded.

If these measures prove inadequate, specific lipid-lowering drugs will be indicated for many patients.

● *Statins*. The HMG-CoA reductase inhibitors reduce intracellular cholesterol synthesis thereby upregulating the expression of LDL receptors; this leads to increased clearance of LDL-cholesterol from the circulation. They are generally very well-tolerated drugs with an excellent safety record. Clinical trials have clearly demonstrated the beneficial effects of lowering LDL-cholesterol levels using statins. Statins, particularly at higher doses, may also reduce elevated plasma triglycerides; improvements in low HDL-cholesterol concentrations are less marked. Current clinical trial evidence favours statins as the drugs of choice for patients with established CHD with total cholesterol concentrations >5.0 mmol/L. The incidence of stroke may also be reduced by certain statin therapy in these circumstances.

NB Statins are currently regarded as the lipid-modifying drugs of choice for patients with established CHD.

• *Fibric acid derivatives.* The fibrates represent a logical alternative choice, particularly for mixed dyslipidaemias. However, the evidence from clinical trials (see below) is less convincing than the results for the statins. Triglyceride levels are reduced and HDL-cholesterol levels may rise to a lesser extent. Although glycaemic control may be slightly improved by lowering plasma fatty acid levels and reducing the activity of the glucose–fatty acid (Randle) cycle, this is rarely clinically apparent. Some fibrates also decrease plasma fibrinogen levels, another risk factor for atheroma. Several trials have reported reductions in coronary events in non-diabetic and diabetic patients using fibrates (Evidence-Based Medicine 5.6).

EVIDENCE-BASED MEDICINE 5.6

Placebo-controlled randomized trials of effects of fibrates on coronary events.

I. HELSINKI HEART STUDY

(N Engl J Med 1987; 317: 1237–1245 and Diabetes Care 1992; 15: 820–825.)
• Total n=4081 men; diabetics n=135.
• Non-signficant reduction in CHD in diabetics with gemfibrozil.

2. BEZAFIBRATE INFARCTION PREVENTION STUDY (BIP)

(Kaplinsky E. Data presented at European Society of Cardiology meeting, 1998.)
• Total n=2855 men, n=367 women (mean age 60 years).
• Patients with diabetes largely excluded.
• No significant reduction in events for the total cohort.
• Benefits for subgroup with hypertriglyceridaemia, i.e. 40% reduction in combined coronary endpoints (P=0.03).

3. VETERANS ADMINISTRATION HDL INTERVENTION TRIAL (VA-HIT)

(N Engl J Med 1999; 341: 410–418.)
• Total n=2531 men with CHD; diabetics comprising 25%.

→

- Mean HDL-cholesterol at entry 0.8 mmol/L.
- Reduction in combined non-fatal and fatal coronary events (22%, $P=0.006$) and stroke (27%, $P=0.05$) with gemfibrozil.

The optimal choice between statins and fibrates is the focus of several comparative clinical trials. Further information on efficacy and safety will emerge in the next few years. Combination therapy using statins and fibrates together is not generally recommended since the risk of myositis may be increased (although clinically evident myositis is uncommon). Other options include:

- *Resins.* Unpalatable; may increase triglyceride levels.

- *Nicotinic acid.* Reduces triglycerides but is contraindicated in diabetes – hyperglycaemia may be exacerbated.

- *Acipimox.* The nicotinic acid analogue acipimox reduces triglycerides; there is no evidence that clinical events are reduced. Insulin resistance may be reduced.

- *Fish-oil supplements.* Reduce triglycerides and mortality in survivors of MI. However, deterioration in glycaemic control has been reported.

- *Plant sterols.* Lower plasma cholesterol; no pharmacological preparations but now included in some products, e.g. margarine; minor effects.

Specialist advice should be sought in the management of major or resistant dyslipidaemias.

DERMATOLOGICAL FEATURES OF DIABETES

The skin of diabetic patients may be affected by:

- Lesions that are virtually specific to diabetes.
- Lesions associated with aspects of the diabetic syndrome (e.g. insulin resistance).
- Lesions associated with diabetic complications.
- Skin disorders that also occur in non-diabetics but which occur more frequently in diabetics.
- Reactions to therapy with oral agents or insulin preparations.

- *Necrobiosis lipoidica diabeticorum.* This uncommon lesion (Plate 16) is closely associated with diabetes (particularly type 1 diabetes) although it reportedly sometimes antedates the development of glucose intolerance. The lesions typically affect the pre-tibial skin but may be multiple and develop at sites of trauma. The lesion does not appear to be closely related to glycaemic control but conversely may be found in the presence of chronic microvascular complications. Treatment with topical steroids, skin grafts or cryotherapy is often unsatisfactory. The lesion heals leaving white scars.

● *Diabetic dermopathy.* This appears as red/brown papules on the shins which progress to shiny hyperpigmented or depressed scaly scars. Minor trauma – perhaps unrecognized or underestimated in the presence of neuropathy are speculative factors in its pathogenesis.

● *Vitiligo.* This is a cutaneous marker of autoimmunity.

● *Bullae.* Rarely, bullae may occur in patients with neuropathy, probably reflecting unrecognized trauma.

● *Granuloma annulare.* This occurs in non-diabetics and it is uncertain whether there is more than just a chance association with diabetes.

● *Acanthosis nigricans.* This is a marker of marked insulin resistance (see p. 28).

● *Hyperandrogenism.* Features include hirsutism, acne and male-pattern alopecia in females; these are features encountered in the polycystic ovary syndrome (see p. 33), or less commonly, Cushing's syndrome (see p. 24).

● *Pigmentation.* This is a feature of haemochromatosis ('bronze diabetes', see p. 21).

● *Allergic reactions.* Allergies to sulphonylureas or insulin preparations are uncommon.

● *Glucagonoma syndrome.* This very rare syndrome (see p. 24) is associated with a characteristic rash (necrolytic migratory erythema).

● *Eruptive xanthomata.* Very high plasma triglycerides during periods of major, acute, metabolic derangements, e.g. DKA (see p. 168) may cause transient cutaneous eruptions; these resolve with restitution of metabolic control.

MUSCULOSKELETAL AND CONNECTIVE TISSUE DISEASE

● *Osteopenia and fractures.* Patients with type 1 diabetes of long duration may have reduced bone mineral densities compared with the non-diabetic population. The clinical significance of this is uncertain since fractures, other than of the metatarsal bones in neuropathic patients (see p. 204), are uncommon.

• *Localized osteopenia*. This appears to be of importance in the pathogenesis of Charcot neuroarthropathy (see p. 218). Increased blood flow through the neuropathic foot may be an important contributory factor.

• *Limited joint mobility*. Diabetes of long duration may result in thickening of the subcutaneous tissues producing limited mobility and stiffness around joints. The 'prayer' sign may be elicited, i.e. the patient may not be able to closely oppose some or all fingers when palms are placed together. In addition, the skin of affected patients may have a waxy appearance reminiscent of scleroderma.

• *Capsulitis*. Adhesive capsulitis of the shoulder (and sometimes hips) appears to be associated with diabetes and may differ histologically from the idiopathic forms of these conditions.

• *Gout*. An increased serum uric acid concentration is a marker for CHD and is associated with glucose intolerance (see Sections 1 and 2). Hyperuricaemia is also more prevalent amongst individuals with obesity, hyperlipidaemia, and hypertension and so has been considered by some investigators to be part of the insulin resistance syndrome (see p. 31). In non-diabetic individuals, plasma uric acid concentrations are inversely related to rates of insulin-mediated glucose disposal as determined using the glucose clamp technique.

• *Spontaneous muscle infarction*. This rare condition presents acutely with severe pain and swelling in the thigh or calf; MRI demonstrates intramuscular oedema and inflammation. Treatment of uncomplicated cases is symptomatic with bedrest and analgesia. An acute compartmental syndrome may complicate the condition; this requires urgent surgical decompression (fasciotomy).

• *Rhabdomyolysis*. This complication of acute metabolic decompensation is discussed on page 184.

INFECTION AND DIABETES

PREVALANCE OF INFECTION AND DIABETES

Although fungal and bacterial infections may be encountered more frequently in diabetic patients, particularly at times when metabolic control is poor, it remains uncertain whether the overall incidence of infection is increased. Diabetes has long been considered a risk factor for pulmonary tuberculosis. Recurrent cutaneous or urogenital infections, e.g. vulvovaginal candidiasis or balanitis, may be the presenting feature of diabetes and their occurrence should prompt appropriate investigations (see p. 44).

> **NB** Recurrent cutaneous or urogenital infections may be the presenting feature of diabetes.

Predisposing factors

● *Physical factors.* Severe invasive infections may develop because of particular predisposing factors which arise from the diabetic state. For example, chronic complications such as foot ulcers provide a portal of entry of microorganisms to soft tissues and bone. Polymicrobial infections are usual in this situation. Autonomic neuropathy (see p. 209) predisposes to urinary stasis and ascending infections. Pyelonephritis is occasionally complicated by necrosis and sloughing of renal papillae demonstrable on retrograde pyelography. Necrotizing otitis externa may be encountered, particularly in elderly diabetic patients.

● *Metabolic factors.* The ability of neutrophil leukocytes to migrate, ingest and kill organisms may be compromised by hyperglycaemia; overactivity of the polyol pathway is implicated (see p. 8). Through stimulation of counter-regulatory hormone secretion (see p. 3) and cytokine release (tumour necrosis factor-α and interleukins induce insulin resistance), infections may lead to a deterioration in metabolic control; infections are the commonest identifiable precipitating cause of DKA (see p. 168).

> **NB** Acute infections may lead to a deterioration in metabolic control.

Attainment of good metabolic control is therefore important in the management of infections in diabetic patients; this may necessitate temporary insulin therapy in diet- or tablet-treated patients with type 2 diabetes. The association between the rare and serious complication of invasive infection with the saprophytic mucor species (rhinocerebral mucormycosis) with DKA (see p. 168) is noteworthy; this condition is encountered in some other states associated with severe metabolic acidosis.

Viral infections

As discussed in Section 1, some viruses (rubella, mumps, coxsackie B4) have been implicated in the aetiology of type 1 diabetes. Intrauterine rubella infection leads to autoimmune type 1 diabetes in 20–40% of children. Recent concerns that immunization against common childhood infections might lead to an increased risk of type 1 diabetes have not been substantiated.

SPECIAL TOPICS

CHILDHOOD AND ADOLESCENCE

Diabetes is one of the most common, chronic diseases in childhood; the prevalence, aetiology and pathophysiology of type 1 diabetes are considered in more detail in Section 1. The principal aims of treatment of diabetes in childhood are:

- Achievement of good metabolic control.
- Attainment of normal growth and development.
- Avoidance of serious hypoglycaemia.
- Prevention of long-term complications of diabetes.

The difficulties posed by insulin treatment in children mean that these ideals are rarely achieved. Emphasis should, however, be placed on the favourable prospects for the child with diabetes; diabetes should be a bar to few recreational activities or occupations.

PRESENTATION

With rare exceptions, many of these being genetic syndromes, diabetes developing in childhood is autoimmune type 1 diabetes (see p. 11). The incidence of childhood diabetes has been increasing in the UK and some other countries during recent decades. Presentation is usually with a short history (days to weeks) of typical symptoms (see p. 38); enuresis is well recognized. DKA is the presentation in approximately 25% of children in the UK (see p. 168). Non-specific complaints may include weight loss, growth failure and general malaise. A caveat is the fact that glycosuria is common in children (see p. 44); the diagnosis of diabetes must be confirmed by appropriate blood tests (see p. 45). Moreover, ketonuria may develop rapidly during acute illness in children; however, the absence of glycosuria with a normal blood glucose concentration will confirm that this is an appropriate physiological response to decreased carbohydrate intake. In the USA, attention has been drawn to the range of diabetes presenting in the second decade of life:

- *Type 1 diabetes.* In all races.

- *Type 2 diabetes.* Increasingly encountered in the USA amongst obese youths from ethnic minorities, e.g. Native Americans.

- *Atypical diabetes.* In Black Americans; presenting in DKA but subsequently following a course more characteristic of type 2 diabetes.

- *MODY.* Caucasians (see p. 26).

DIAGNOSIS

Diagnosis will usually be straightforward if typical symptoms are present; a fingerprick glucose concentration will be unequivocally elevated with glycosuria and ketonuria on urinalysis (see Section 2). The provisional diagnosis of diabetes in childhood should always prompt emergency admission to a children's ward; DKA may develop rapidly and confirmation of the diagnosis on a laboratory-analyzed blood specimen should not delay admission. The occasional absence of ketonuria should not deter the admission of a child with typical symptoms and an elevated blood glucose concentration.

 Diabetes may progress rapidly to DKA in children; prompt hospital admission is indicated at diagnosis.

Transient hyperglycaemia in childhood in the setting of an acute illness or following trauma should always be followed up; although many cases appear to settle spontaneously this presentation may occasionally be attributable to one of the less common forms of diabetes, e.g. MODY (see p. 26). A family history of an autosomal dominant inheritance of diabetes appearing under the age of 25 years is highly suggestive and it is not uncommon for young people with MODY to be diagnosed when they present with an intercurrent illness. In the occasional child in whom an oral glucose tolerance test (see p. 48) is deemed necessary to confirm or exclude the diagnosis:

- 1.75 g per kg body weight glucose is administered, up to a maximum of 75 g (see p. 48).

TREATMENT AND PROGNOSIS

- *Initiation of therapy.* A short period of hospitalization on a paediatric ward may be all that is required to initiate insulin and provide basic instruction to the parents and child concerned; follow-up at home is usually provided by a specialist diabetes nurse with back-up from other members of the multidisciplinary, paediatric diabetes care team. Some units avoid hospitalization and initiate therapy at home wherever possible; clearly this requires adequate support from nurses in the community. Anxieties and feelings of guilt are common in parents and require considerate and informed handling.

The long-term prognosis is an obvious cause for concern. An optimistic response is appropriate since the great majority of children should be able to live relatively long and healthy lives; improvements in care will hopefully result in still better outcomes in the future. Questions concerning the risks to existing or future siblings are frequently raised (see p. 13). Guidelines are required on the principles of diet and insulin therapy (see Section 3), recognition and management of hypoglycaemia (see p. 156) and intercurrent illness (sick day rules, see p. 283). Initial education is reinforced and expanded by continuing contact with the paediatric diabetes care team.

● *DKA*. The principles of therapy for this medical emergency are similar to those for adults (see p. 171). Soluble insulin is infused intravenously at a rate of 0.1 units/kg/h. Particular care should be exercised with intravenous fluid replacement in view of the particular risk to children of the uncommon but potentially fatal complication of cerebral oedema during treatment (see p. 184). Characteristically, the patient has initially responded well to treatment prior to the development of neurological deterioration and deepening coma. Immediate treatment with intravenous mannitol (0.5–2.0 g/kg body weight, repeated as necessary) is regarded as the treatment of choice.

Subclinical elevations in cerebrospinal pressure are common during the treatment of DKA owing to alterations in cerebral osmolarity; cerebral swelling has been demonstrated in children using CT. Experiments in animal models have suggested that rapid reductions of plasma glucose concentration below approximately 15 mmol/L may be important in the pathogenesis of cerebral oedema; however, there is relatively little support for this view in case reports. The use of hypotonic fluids during treatment has also been implicated although the evidence is inconclusive.

 Children are at particular risk of developing cerebral oedema during treatment of DKA.

Electrolyte replacement also requires due care with frequent monitoring of plasma potassium concentration.

● *Nutrition*. Diet and insulin doses are tailored with the aim of achieving normal physiological development. Nutritional advice is similar in essence to that given to adults with type 1 diabetes (see p. 86). Appropriate calories and nutrient balance are required to allow normal rates of growth; individual prescriptions are necessary. Progress should be monitored using appropriate growth charts. Dietary indiscretions are common; the child may also use non-cooperation with meals as a powerful weapon against parents only too aware of the risks of hypoglycaemia.

● *Insulin therapy*. For initial stabilization, a dose of approximately 0.5 units/kg daily is typical, albeit with inter-individual variability. In general, twice-daily insulin is recommended for children from the age of 5 years or so. Biphasic, premixed insulins are useful (see p. 138); convenient pen injector devices may encourage compliance and have become the standard means of insulin delivery. Self-injection is the ultimate aim for all children although the age at which this is accomplished varies. A pronounced 'honeymoon' period may be observed shortly after initiation of insulin therapy during which glycaemic control is temporarily excellent with minimal doses of insulin. This may last for several months (occasionally years) but ultimately the need for increased insulin doses becomes apparent from rising blood glucose concentrations. Many physicians would aim to continue insulin at the lowest dose in recognition of the inevitability of the need for lifelong insulin treatment.

• *Monitoring of control.* Self-testing of blood glucose (see p. 73) is favoured as soon as the child is able. Glycated haemoglobin measurements (see p. 71) provide an additional measure of control. Good glycaemic control is often difficult to attain in children with pre-breakfast hyperglycaemia posing a particular challenge. Fear of the consequences of nocturnal hypoglycaemia (which may impose limits on evening insulin doses) must be recognized (see p. 162).

• *Schooling.* Diabetes in childhood is entirely compatible with normal schooling and activities; educational attainment should not be impaired. The main metabolic complication is hypoglycaemia (see p. 156). The school should be made aware of the diagnosis and teachers given basic advice on treatment and the likelihood of hypoglycaemia and its management. Less frequent is DKA (see above and p. 168). Summer camps for children with diabetes are popular and combine socialization, sporting activities and informal diabetes education.

• *Hypoglycaemia.* Severe hypoglycaemia is common in insulin-treated children; approximately 25% of children will experience one or more episodes of severe hypoglycaemia during the first few years following diagnosis.

> **NB** Children with diabetes are at high risk of recurrent severe hypoglycaemia.

In very young children, symptoms and signs of developing hypoglycaemia may be difficult to recognize; generalized convulsions may complicate neuroglycopenia. The developing brain of younger children (particularly under the age of 7 years) is susceptible to damage from recurrent severe hypoglycaemia (see p. 156). Impairment of memory, visuospatial and verbal performance have been reported in cross-sectional studies. The implications of such studies remain uncertain but it is well recognized that severe hypoglycaemia may result in permanent neuronal damage. Reassuringly, the DCCT (see p. 60) found no evidence of impaired neuropsychological performance in the intensively-treated patients who experienced higher rates of severe hypoglycaemia; however, children were not included in this trial. Nocturnal hypoglycaemia, often prolonged and unrecognized, is also common in children (see p. 162). The longer period between evening meal and breakfast may result in depletion of limited hepatic glycogen stores in children.

 Recurrent severe hypoglycaemia in young children is associated with impaired cognitive performance.

Hypoglycaemia is understandably a major fear for parents who find themselves responsible for recognition and prompt corrective therapy. For the child who is cooperative, 15–20 g oral, rapidly-absorbed, simple carbohydrate is required. Viscous glucose gels which can be applied to the oral mucous membranes in the uncooperative or unresponsive child and intramuscular glucagon (see Section 3) are also helpful. Appropriate instruction in the use of these therapies, which can be administered by parents or carers, is required. Intravenous glucose injection may sometimes be necessary but must be administered by a trained professional (see Section 3).

● *Idiopathic brittle diabetes.* This is also considered in Sections 3 (p. 147) and 4 (p. 165). It is now generally acknowledged that most cases of brittle diabetes are attributable to deliberate interference or non-compliance with insulin regimens. Such behaviour may be exceedingly disruptive but is relatively uncommon. Temporary escape from difficult home circumstances or relationships may be the underlying motive for repeated hospitalization with hyper- or hypoglycaemia. The emotional tensions of adolescence may contribute. Resolution of the behaviour may follow improvement in life circumstances, e.g. the development of a supportive, long-term, personal relationship. Limited studies suggest that the long-term prognosis for patients with so-called brittle diabetes is worse than for patients with type 1 diabetes in general. Premature death (e.g. from DKA, see p. 168) and an excessive burden of chronic tissue complications such as nephropathy (see p. 219) are recognized consequences of long-duration brittle diabetes. Management often proves difficult; general emotional and personal counselling and support may be required. There appears to be little role for conventional psychotherapy in the absence of an obvious disturbance such as depression.

NB Chronic brittle diabetes behaviour is associated with an increased risk of long-term complications.

● *Psychological disorders.* Closely related are the syndromes of disordered eating patterns – anorexia nervosa and bulimia nervosa. Omission or dramatic reduction of insulin doses by adolescent girls may be used as a means of controlling body weight; this appears to be a common and underestimated problem.

> **NB** Non-compliance with insulin regimens is a common cause of poor metabolic control in adolescence.

When the daily rigours of, and anxieties associated with, type 1 diabetes and its management are considered, it is not surprising that psychological problems such as eating disorders are relatively common, if frequently underdiagnosed. By contrast, major depression and intentional overdoses with insulin are infrequent. The emotional turmoils associated with adolescence provide an ample source of anxiety which may be accentuated by the additional burden of diabetes and may lead to difficulties with control. Alcohol and recreational drugs may also be factors in some individuals. The patient's agenda should always be considered.

● *Sports and exercise.* Regular physical exercise and participation in most sports are to be encouraged (see p. 100). Insulin-treated diabetes is by no means necessarily a bar to high levels of achievement in sporting pursuits. Hypoglycaemia during or following exercise is an obvious risk (see above and p. 156). Exercise in patients with type 1 diabetes is considered in greater detail in Section 3 (p. 100).

● *Growth and development.* The arrival of puberty, which is not usually delayed in diabetic children, may be associated with increasing insulin requirements; this is held to reflect the effects of growth hormone secretion on insulin sensitivity and so may be regarded as a physiological cause of insulin resistance (see p. 28).

> **NB** Puberty is associated with increased insulin requirements in type 1 diabetes.

Insulin doses may rise to 1.0–2.0 units/kg/day; the development of obesity with continuing unsatisfactory control and escalating insulin doses may be a problem, particularly for girls. Menstruation may be associated with cyclical disturbances of metabolic control. Normal adult height is ultimately attained by most children with diabetes. Temporary impairment of growth rates during periods of very inadequate glycaemic control may be correctable subsequently if satisfactory control is achieved. Mauriac syndrome describes a syndrome of growth retardation, obesity and hepatomegaly; it is rarely encountered with modern insulin regimens.

● *Diabetic complications.* Clinically overt diabetic complications are uncommon in childhood. There has been much debate about the contribution, if any, of pre-pubertal years to the subsequent risk of chronic tissue complications (see Section 5). Although the general principle is attainment of metabolic control which is as close to normal as possible, intensive insulin therapy is contraindicated in children (see pp. 131–152).

● *Organization and integration of care.* The hospital-based, multidisciplinary, paediatric diabetes care team will have primary responsibility for care (see p. 78). This comprises paediatrician, specialist nurse and dietician with ready access to social workers and psychologists as necessary. Close support for families is essential and 24-hour telephone advice should be available for emergencies. Children's clinics should be welcoming and appropriately stocked with toys, games and videos.

At an appropriate juncture, the older teenager is referred to a clinic for young persons which may be run jointly by a paediatrician and an adult-oriented diabetologist. Such clinics, ideally held in the late afternoon or early evening, are preferable to immersing the young patient in an unselected adult diabetes clinic. Monitoring for early evidence of complications is an important aspect of care at this stage. Continuing contact with the clinic is important and efforts should be directed towards encouraging regular attendance; defaulters should always be welcomed back. A sympathetic and non-judgemental approach from the diabetes care team is required.

> **NB** Regular contact with the hospital clinic should always be encouraged.

DIABETES IN THE ELDERLY

Diabetes, mainly type 2 diabetes, is particularly common in the elderly; more than 50% of patients in the UK (the majority having type 2 diabetes) are over the age of 60 years (see Section 1). In many Western countries 10–20% of those aged 65 or above have diabetes. Although glucose tolerance declines with advancing age, there is continuing controversy about whether progressive insulin resistance is primarily responsible. Symptoms of diabetes may be non-specific, vague or absent (see p. 38).

● *Aims of treatment.* The aims of treatment may be modified by considerations of life expectancy and concomitant medical conditions (see p. 58). In the UKPDS (see p. 65), which did not enter any patients over 65 years at diagnosis, the benefits of glycaemic control were not apparent until nearly a decade after randomization. Thus, a limited life expectancy might discourage an intensive approach to antidiabetic therapy. In such circumstances, the emphasis might be more appropriately focused on avoidance of symptoms with the minimum of unwanted effects from treatment rather than delaying the development of microvascular disease. However, the role of insulin should not be neglected; many patients derive a feeling of well-being from better control of their diabetes. A trial of insulin therapy may therefore be warranted.

 NB Non-specific malaise caused by chronic hyperglycaemia can be relieved by appropriate insulin therapy.

• *Comorbidity*. Co-existing cardiovascular and cerebrovascular disease are especially common; polypharmacy is often necessary and carries risks of adverse effects and drug interactions. Degrees of renal impairment, arising for a multiplicity of reasons, e.g. diuretic therapy, prostatic obstruction, are relatively common in the elderly population; care must be exercised with renally-excreted drugs. In addition, impaired hepatic function, e.g. hepatic congestion secondary to cardiac failure, may render certain antidiabetic medications inappropriate (see p. 106).

NB Impairment of major organ function in the elderly increases the risk of adverse events with antidiabetic medication.

The prevalence of hypertension rises with age (see p. 240) together with the risk of cardiovascular events. Attention should be directed towards modifiable cardiovascular risk factors, notably hypertension, as appropriate for the individual. Cardiovascular events may present with atypical symptoms in the elderly, e.g. acute confusion.

• *Oral antidiabetic agents*. Care should be exercised with sulphonylureas since severe hypoglycaemia, although uncommon, carries a relatively high mortality rate (see p. 115). Agents with a short duration of action are preferred (see Section 3, pp. 106–131). Metformin should in general be avoided in the elderly.

• *Insulin treatment*. Although the majority of elderly patients have type 2 diabetes, insulin therapy becomes necessary in a significant proportion as oral agents lose their capacity to provide adequate glycaemic control (see p. 131). Other patients will require insulin because of contraindications to oral agents arising from comorbidity (see above). The relationship between glycaemic control and cognitive function merits further scrutiny in the elderly. Physical and psychological disabilities allied to social isolation may act as limitations to successful insulin therapy; compromise may be necessary. Avoidance of insulin-induced hypoglycaemia is often paramount for the very elderly and those living alone (see p. 163). Conversely, consideration should also be given to discontinuation of insulin therapy in selected patients (see p. 151). Insulin may be appropriately commenced during an intercurrent illness and continued thereafter when oral agents may suffice.

● *Institutional care of the elderly diabetic.* This is an expanding area and has tended to be overlooked; the standards of care in many residential and nursing homes, which may not have trained nursing staff, need to be improved. Common medical problems make management of diabetes more complex in institutionalized patients (Table 6.1). Patients may not receive regular detailed physical reviews; complications may develop unnoticed. Community support from appropriately-trained nursing staff who are able to liaise with other members of the district diabetes care team (see p. 78) is necessary. Educational and training programmes for the staff of residential and nursing homes should be established.

Table 6.1 Problems complicating the management of diabetes in institutionalized patients

- Confusion and anorexia – may render dietary intake erratic
- Recurrent chest or urinary tract infections leading to poor metabolic control
- Disordered swallowing – commonly the result of stroke
- Pressure ulcers – cause debilitation, poor control; neuropathy and peripheral vascular disease may exacerbate the problem
- Impaired communication – dysphasia, major sensory impairment
- Physical disability may serve to discourage regular surveillance for diabetic complications

---

PREGNANCY, CONTRACEPTION AND THE MENOPAUSE

PREGNANCY

PRE-GESTATIONAL DIABETES

This is defined as diabetes pre-dating conception; it is usually type 1 diabetes (see p. 11). However, type 2 diabetes may already be established, particularly in older, more obese women especially if belonging to populations with a high prevalence of diabetes (see p. 15). Pregnancy in women with diabetes is associated with risks to both mother and child for the reasons listed in Table 6.2. In the leading industrialized nations, improved care has dramatically improved the outcome for mother and child; this is not, however, the case in many developing nations. This improvement is due to several factors, central being the appreciation that abnormal fetal development is linked to maternal hyperglycaemia:

- The introduction of insulin therapy in the 1920s and subsequent refinements in insulin regimens which allow the attainment of excellent glycaemic control (see p. 70).
- The routine use of self-monitoring of blood glucose.
- Use of retrospective methods for assessment of glycaemic control, i.e. glycated haemoglobin and fructosamine (see pp. 71 and 73).
- Improvements in general obstetric and neonatal care.

TABLE 6.2 Maternal and fetal risks associated with diabetic pregnancy

Maternal
- Metabolic control deteriorates in the 2nd and 3rd trimesters
- Pre-existing complications such as retinopathy and nephropathy may progress
- Risk of pre-eclamptic toxaemia is increased 2-fold
- Subclinical CHD may be unmasked
- Increased risk of urinary tract infection
- Increased rates of caesarean section

Fetal
- Risk of congenital malformations is increased
- Rates of stillbirth are increased
- Perinatal mortality is increased
- Higher incidence of neonatal complications (e.g. hypoglycaemia, birth trauma)
- Increased lifetime risk of diabetes in offspring

Fertility is not usually affected in women with well-controlled type 1 diabetes in the absence of complications; this contrasts with the dismal prognosis for women of reproductive age in the pre-insulin era for whom successful pregnancy was a rare event. However, the development of major complications, particularly renal failure owing to nephropathy (see p. 219) may result in anovulation. Autoimmune premature ovarian failure may be more common in women with type 1 diabetes, particularly when other features of autoimmunity are present (see Section 1). Young women with polycystic ovary syndrome may have an increased lifetime risk of type 2 diabetes associated with insulin resistance, hyperandrogenism and anovulation.

In women with pre-existing diabetes, pregnancy is associated with alterations in the regulation of glucose metabolism owing to the actions of human placental lactogen and progesterone; these hormones antagonize the actions of insulin leading to a state of relative insulin resistance as pregnancy progresses. Lipolysis is also accelerated, despite hyperinsulinaemia.

> **NB** Pregnancy is a physiological state of insulin resistance.

In women with no impairment of B-cell function, the insulin resistance associated with pregnancy remains subclinical since increased insulin secretion compensates. However, the additional insulin resistance means that women with pre-existing type 1 diabetes need higher doses of insulin as pregnancy progresses. Women with type 2 diabetes treated with diet or tablets often require insulin during pregnancy. Finally, glucose intolerance or diabetes may be precipitated in predisposed women who previously had normal glucose tolerance (gestational diabetes, see p. 278).

● *First trimester.* During the first trimester, fasting glucose concentrations decline modestly in non-diabetic women reaching a nadir at approximately 12 weeks. The renal clearance of glucose (see Section 2) is increased, reflecting an increase in glomerular filtration rate (in the absence of any change in maximal reabsorption via the renal tubules). Post-prandial glucose levels, by contrast, tend to rise whereas plasma insulin concentrations are unchanged. Effects on insulin requirements may also be influenced by pregnancy-associated nausea and vomiting. Note that hyperemesis gravidarum may rarely be a presenting feature of autoimmune thyrotoxicosis; the latter condition is more common in patients with type 1 diabetes.

● *Second and third trimesters.* The regulatory effects of insulin on carbohydrate and fat metabolism become impaired, i.e. a state of relative insulin resistance develops (see p. 28). It is hypothesized that these metabolic changes facilitate transfer of maternal nutrients to the fetus. In insulin-treated women, insulin requirements may increase markedly between weeks 28 and 32 of gestation. Insulin requirements tend to fall to some extent after 35 weeks although this does not have any adverse prognostic implications for fetal well-being.

● *Parturition.* With delivery of the placenta, insulin requirements very rapidly fall to pre-pregnancy levels. If the higher insulin doses of later pregnancy are continued post-partum, severe hypoglycaemia may result.

 Insulin requirements rapidly return to pre-pregnancy levels post-partum.

Effect of pregnancy on diabetic complications
Pregnancy has important implications for women with diabetes of long duration with pre-existing retinopathy and nephropathy; these complications may progress rapidly during pregnancy. Acceleration of

retinopathy carries risks of visual loss whereas nephropathy and hypertension may threaten both mother and fetus. Such complications should be carefully assessed; wherever possible this should be done in a pre-conception clinic in order that appropriate action can be taken (see p. 277).

● *Diabetic nephropathy.* As mentioned above, diabetic nephropathy may impair fertility. Advanced nephropathy (i.e. plasma creatinine concentrations >250 μmol/L) is also associated with high rates of fetal loss (Table 6.3). During pregnancy, hypertension and proteinuria may progress requiring pre-term delivery; pre-eclampsia, which is more common in diabetic pregnancy, may cause diagnostic difficulties. ACE inhibitors (see Section 5) are contraindicated in pregnancy. These agents should be avoided in women of childbearing age because of their teratogenic potential. Drugs with a proven safety record, e.g. methyl dopa, should be used instead. Severe hypertension is regarded as a contraindication to pregnancy (Table 6.3).

TABLE 6.3 Contraindications to pregnancy in diabetic women

● Advanced nephropathy
 — Plasma creatinine >250 μmol/L
 — Nephrotic syndrome
 — Severe hypertension
● Severe CHD
 — MI
 — Congestive cardiac failure
● Clincial autonomic neuropathy
 — Especially gastroparesis

ACE inhibitors are contraindicated in pregnancy.

Nonetheless, successful pregnancies have been reported in diabetic women receiving CAPD (see p. 226) and even following renal transplantation (see p. 227).

● *Retinopathy.* Advanced retinopathy (i.e. pre-proliferative or proliferative) is likely to progress during pregnancy. Retinopathy may also appear for the first time. Ideally, retinopathy should be stabilized with laser photocoagulation as necessary prior to conception; pregnancy should be deferred under these circumstances.

NB Proliferative retinopathy should be stabilized by photocoagulation prior to pregnancy wherever possible.

Progression, which may result in irreversible visual impairment, may be accelerated by co-existing hypertension. Stable photocoagulated retinopathy does not usually progress. Reduced retinal perfusion, which may result from any acute improvement in glycaemic control, has been implicated as a factor in the progression of retinopathy during diabetic pregnancy. Careful assessment of retinopathy is therefore required during each trimester of pregnancy with prompt referral if significant progression is detected.

● *Macrovascular disease.* Although this is rarely encountered in pre-menopausal women, the risk of complications such as MI or cardiac failure is higher in older diabetic women (see p. 228). MI during pregnancy is associated with a high risk of fetal mortality; severe ischaemic heart disease is regarded as a contraindication to pregnancy; termination may be indicated (Table 6.3). Pregnancy may result in severe cardiac decompensation.

Outcome of diabetic pregnancy
Perinatal mortality for diabetic pregnancies has improved considerably although remains higher than for non-diabetic pregnancies. In part, this may reflect the fact that only a minority of women receive appropriate pre-pregnancy counselling.

The causes of excess perinatal mortality include:

● Stillbirth.
● Major congenital malformations.

The overall risk of congenital malformations is increased by maternal diabetes; the rate rises to 10-fold or higher in women with poor control. This reflects putative teratogenic effects of hyperglycaemia during embryogenesis. Rates of stillbirth are also significantly increased in comparison to non-diabetics.

> **NB** The overall risk of congenital malformations is increased 3-fold by maternal diabetes.

Prevailing maternal glycaemia during fetal organogenesis (early in the first trimester) is inversely related to the risk of malformations. Pre-pregnancy counselling with attainment of excellent glycaemic control before conception is the ideal since anomalies may have been initiated before the patient even realizes that she is pregnant.

> **NB** The risk of congenital anomalies is inversely associated with the degree of glycaemic control at conception.

● *Hypoglycaemia*. There is no evidence that episodes of maternal hypoglycaemia (which are common in insulin-treated patients) are harmful to fetal development. Thus, the emphasis is on the attainment of excellent glycaemic control during pregnancy. Pre-prandial plasma glucose targets are typically set at <5.5 mmol/L with post-prandial levels <7–8 mmol/L; however, pre-bed glucose levels should be >6 mmol/L in order to avoid nocturnal hypoglycaemia. Attaining these targets necessitates frequent (q.d.s.) self-monitoring of blood glucose with adjustment of insulin doses.

The aim is to maintain glycated haemoglobin or fructosamine levels (see pp. 71 and 73), measured monthly, within the non-diabetic range. It is well recognized that pregnancy is a unique state in which, for either psychological or physiological reasons, excellent control is usually achievable.

● *Maternal DKA*. This has much more serious implications, often resulting in miscarriage. Although DKA (see p. 168) is much less common than hypoglycaemia, pregnancy is associated with an acceleration in lipolysis which predisposes to ketosis; this may result in DKA in the absence of marked hyperglycaemia.

> **NB** DKA during pregnancy is associated with a high risk of fetal loss.

Effects of maternal diabetes on the fetus

In addition to an increased risk of late intrauterine death (which in some cases appears to be related to polyhydramnios), the neonate is at risk of the following complications:

● *Macrosomia*. This is held to be a consequence of increased placental transfer of glucose and aminoacids resulting in fetal B-cell hyperplasia and hyperinsulinaemia causing accelerated growth of insulin-sensitive tissues, but possibly acting via cellular receptors for insulin-like growth factors.

Macrosomia increases the risk of shoulder dystocia and is an indication for elective caesarean section. A birth weight in excess of 4.5 kg is the conventional, if arbitrary, definition of macrosomia. Birthweight is also related to maternal height and weight but the incidence of large-for-dates infants (>90th centile) is increased approximately 2-fold by diabetes. The rates for caesarean section vary considerably between centres for reasons which are not always readily apparent; diabetes per se is not an indication for caesarean section. Generally accepted indications for caesarean section are listed in Table 6.4.

> **NB** Rates of caesarean section are increased in diabetic pregnancy.

TABLE 6.4 Indications for caesarean section

- Malpresentation
- Suspected disproportion
- Intrauterine growth retardation
- Fetal compromise
- Pre-eclampsia

Asphyxia and birth trauma are other consequences of macrosomia; the Apgar score is often low and the routine presence of a paediatrician at delivery is recommended.

- *Neonatal hypoglycaemia.* Although this is difficult to define (5% of normal neonates having glucose levels <1.7 mmol/L), infants of diabetic mothers are at increased risk. This is thought to reflect hyperinsulinaemia in macrosomic babies; early institution of oral feeds is usually sufficient.

- *Polycythaemia.* This rarely produces clinical problems; enhanced fetal haemopoiesis is thought to be a consequence of hyperinsulinaemia and fetal hypoxia.

- *Respiratory distress syndrome.* This has become much less common reflecting the trend in recent years towards later delivery (see p. 278) and improvements in obstetric care. It is mainly a risk when delivery before 36 weeks is indicated.

- *Neonatal jaundice.* This occurs in over 50% of babies, being more common in those with macrosomia; phototherapy may be required. Impaired availability of glucuronic acid for conjugation in concert with increased bilirubin production caused by polycythemia and haemolysis are suggested mechanisms.

- *Hypocalcaemia and hypomagnesaemia.* These may occur occasionally for reasons which are uncertain; transient functional hypoparathyroidism has been invoked. Intravenous treatment is rarely required.

- *Cardiomyopathy.* Uncommon and usually temporary with no long-term sequelae; supportive care is required.

- *Increased lifetime risk of diabetes.* The risk of diabetes developing in the offspring will depend on the type of diabetes affecting the mother (see Section 1).

- *Congenital malformations.* The main categories of major congenital malformations, together with some specific examples, are presented in Table 6.5.

TABLE 6.5 Classification of major congenital anomalies

- Cardiovascular
  — Septal defects; transposition of the great vessels
- Skeletal
  — Sacral agenesis; pes equinovarus
- Genitourinary
  — Renal agenesis; duplex ureter
- Neural tube defects
  — Anencephaly; spina bifida
- Gastrointestinal
  — Anorectal atresia; tracheo-oesophageal fistula

Management of diabetic pregnancy

All diabetic women should be seen early in the first trimester in a joint clinic with an experienced obstetrician, diabetologist, specialist nurse and dietician. Ideally, this visit would follow pre-pregnancy counselling and planning of the time of conception. Follow-up is usually every 2 weeks, then weekly after 24 weeks.

- *Pre-pregnancy.* Optimize glycaemic control – consider change to b.d. free mixing of soluble and isophane or q.d.s. regimen (see Section 3, p. 131); caution with insulin analogues – although apparently safe, experience in pregnancy is currently limited; a change to human or animal insulin should be considered and discussed with the patient (see p. 135); institute daily self-monitoring of blood glucose; check glycated haemoglobin; if treated with oral agents, an early change to insulin is usually indicated since control is likely to deteriorate in the second and third trimesters; assess and stabilize retinopathy with photocoagulation as necessary; check for nephropathy and hypertension; discourage tobacco and alcohol (see Section 3); check rubella immunity; start oral folate supplements; review diet – no major changes are usually necessary (see p. 86); provide education re: aims and risks of pregnancy; genetic counselling if requested (see p. 25). Test for proteinuria – check plasma creatinine and exclude urinary tract infection if present.

- *First trimester.* As above, plus ultrasound scan for anomalies, gestational age, multiple pregnancy.

- *Second trimester.* Increase insulin dose as appropriate; ultrasound scan; check for obstetric complications (e.g. pre-eclampsia).

- *Third trimester.* Insulin dose may continue to increase up to 35 weeks; ultrasound for macrosomia and polyhydramnios; monitor for pre-eclampsia; risk of preterm labour; cardiotocograph monitoring during labour.

- *Post-partum.* Early discussion of contraception (see p. 281); arrange follow-up for patients with gestational diabetes (see p. 278).

Timing of delivery will depend on indicators of maternal and fetal well-being. Most patients will go to term although many clinicians recommend induction at 38 weeks because of the unpredictable risk of late intrauterine death with either vaginal delivery or caesarean section, as appropriate. However, induction as early as 36 weeks has fallen out of favour. Pre-term labour may present particular problems for the diabetic mother: intravenous infusions of β-adrenergic agonists (ritodrine or salbutamol) are usually combined with high-dose dexamethasone, the latter to encourage fetal lung maturation. The combination of drugs induces marked insulin resistance and accelerated lipolysis (see Section 1); hyperglycaemia and even DKA may ensue without carefully judged, and sometimes high, infusion rates of intravenous insulin. Hypokalaemia is another risk; plasma potassium should be monitored.

 Management of pre-term labour with β-agonists and dexamethasone may cause major metabolic decompensation in diabetics.

Management of diabetes during delivery

At the onset of labour, short-acting insulin (see p. 136) is infused using a syringe-driver at a rate of 1–2 units/h in conjunction with a constant infusion of 5% dextrose at a rate of 100 mL/h. The aim is to avoid hypo- and hyperglycaemia by adjusting the insulin infusion rate according to bedside measurements of capillary glucose using a test-strip/meter system (see p. 73). As mentioned above, the use of β-agonists and dexamethasone can lead to a substantial increase in insulin requirements. Following delivery of the placenta, insulin requirements fall immediately to pre-pregnancy levels; the insulin infusion rate should be halved and the patient's usual pre-pregnancy regimen of subcutaneous insulin should be administered when she is ready to eat again.

GESTATIONAL DIABETES

In the 1997 re-classification of diabetes (see p. 9), gestational diabetes was recognized as a special category which now includes former categories of impaired glucose tolerance.

Diabetes which is first diagnosed during pregnancy is known as gestational diabetes (see p. 10). Thus, both pre-existing (but undiagnosed) diabetes and diabetes which has been precipitated by pregnancy are included in this category. In the majority of the latter group, glucose tolerance returns to normal post-partum although the long-term risk of permanent type 2 diabetes is substantially increased; the magnitude of this risk reflects the frequency of type 2 diabetes in the population concerned. The incidence of gestational diabetes varies from low rates of 1–2% in White Europeans to 4–5% in South Asians. As mentioned above, impaired glucose tolerance (see Sections 1 and 2) in pregnancy is now included in the category of gestational diabetes. Women with MODY (see p. 26) are not infrequently first diagnosed during pregnancy.

> **NB** Impaired glucose tolerance in pregnancy is classified as gestational diabetes mellitus.

Diagnosis

There is no consensus on the diagnostic criteria for gestational diabetes mellitus. In the absence of an unequivocal elevation of blood glucose, the diagnosis rests on the results of 75 g oral glucose tolerance tests (see Section 2).

A higher risk of gestational diabetes is conferred by the clinical factors presented in Table 6.6.

TABLE 6.6 Groups at increased risk of diabetes in pregnancy

- Older women
- Those with a previous history of glucose intolerance
- Those with a history of large-for-gestational age babies (birthweight >4.5 kg or >90th centile for gestational age)
- Women from certain, high-risk, ethnic groups
- Women with glycosuria on two occasions in pregnancy
- Women with obesity
- Pregnancy with polyhydramnios
- Women with a family history of diabetes in a first-degree relative

---

Since glycosuria is common during pregnancy, in the absence of any other risk factors a random blood glucose measurement or two may be sufficient to allay concerns about diabetes. In other circumstances, the 75 g oral glucose tolerance test (see p. 48) remains the definitive test. In high-risk populations, a case can be made for screening early in pregnancy for pre-existing diabetes. The physiological changes in fasting glucose levels (see p. 47) during the first trimester invalidate the use of this measurement as a screening test. A complex and confusing literature has built up around the concept of gestational diabetes and views about the importance of its detection and clinical implications have become polarized. Concerns have been voiced that the diagnosis of gestational diabetes may lead to a higher rate of caesarean section in the absence of clear indications. However, there is an opposing view that some form of screening for glucose intolerance in pregnancy is appropriate. This usually takes the form of a blood test between 24 and 28 weeks' gestation to detect new-onset diabetes. Glycated proteins (see p. 71) are not sufficiently sensitive and cannot be used for this purpose. The O'Sullivan test is the one most widely used in the USA:

● *The O'Sullivan screening test.* This has a cut-off value of ≥7.8 mmol/L 60 min after an oral 50 g glucose challenge, having a high sensitivity and specificity (>80% for each) for glucose intolerance at 20–28 weeks. The test may also be applied to high-risk populations in the first trimester.

The sensitivity of clinical risk factors listed above is generally lower (<70%). It should be borne in mind that the O'Sullivan screening test was designed to determine the risk of diabetes in the mother, rather than to predict the outcome of the index pregnancy.

Management

The detection of gestational diabetes raises important questions about the aims of therapeutic interventions. It has been argued that there is insufficient data to justify universal screening for gestational diabetes since there is no reliable evidence that therapeutic intervention is effective, except perhaps in reducing the proportion of babies with macrosomia. However, macrosomia is confounded by maternal obesity. Dietary measures may suffice to maintain blood glucose levels within the aforementioned target range.

● *Calorie restriction.* For obese women, a 30% calorie reduction in daily calorie consumption will reduce hyperglycaemia. The US National Academy of Science recommends that total weight gain during pregnancy for women with obesity should be limited to <6 kg, if possible:

Body mass index (kg/m^2)	Recommended weight gain (kg)
20–26	11.5–16.0
26–29	7.0–11.5
>29	<6.0

● *Oral antidiabetic agents.* These are usually avoided (see p. 106), although fears about teratogenicity have not been substantiated.

● *Insulin.* Insulin is required in approximately 30% of women with gestational diabetes. The merits of judging control by measurement of pre-prandial vs post-prandial blood glucose levels have been debated; no clear answer has emerged with respect to prevention of fetal macrosomia. Insulin lispro has been used successfully in gestational diabetes, albeit in a relatively small number of women. There is a suggestion from a randomized study that the frequency of hypoglycaemia may be lower than with conventional soluble insulin; further studies are required to establish the safety of insulin analogues during embryogenesis. However, lispro is not detectable in cord blood. The risk of producing underweight babies by the institution of very strict maternal glycaemic control raises theoretical concerns about programming a higher risk of diabetes in the offspring according to the Barker–Hales hypothesis (see p. 17).

Follow-up

Follow-up and counselling of mothers with gestational diabetes with advice about (a) avoidance of obesity and (b) the protective effect of regular exercise (see p. 100) are offered with the aim of preventing or delaying the onset of permanent type 2 diabetes. Follow-up studies suggest that maintenance of desirable body weight can reduce the risk of conversion to type 2 diabetes by approximately 50%.

 NB Maintenance of ideal body weight reduces the risk of developing type 2 diabetes following gestational diabetes.

After delivery, another 75 g oral glucose tolerance test should be performed. Most patients (>90%) will revert to normal glucose tolerance post-partum. The rate of progression to type 2 diabetes depends both on the degree of glucose intolerance during pregnancy and the ethnicity of the patient. Additional factors include:

- Body weight during pregnancy.
- Subsequent weight gain (see p. 280).
- Parity.
- Family history of diabetes.

Follow-up is often incomplete; an annual fasting blood glucose and instructions to present for testing symptoms of diabetes should be regarded as minimal requirements (see p. 78). In high-risk populations, e.g. Hispanic American women, approximately 40% of gestational diabetes which resolves immediately after the index pregnancy will become established as permanent diabetes within 6 years. In European populations, the rate of progression is much lower, making follow-up more problematic. In addition, a small proportion of women with gestational diabetes subsequently develop type 1 diabetes; it is suggested that these patients have slow-onset, autoimmune, B-cell destruction which is unmasked by the insulin resistance of pregnancy (see p. 28); positivity for anti-GAD antibodies (see Section 1) has been shown to be predictive but this test is presently confined to research studies.

CONTRACEPTION

Selection of appropriate contraception should not present difficulties for the majority of women with diabetes. The importance of planned pregnancy in women with diabetes is discussed above; contraception is obviously an important component. The main options are as follows; standard contraindications should be observed:

● *Oral combined contraceptive.* With modern, low-dose oestrogen preparations, deleterious metabolic effects are usually minimal. There is a reluctance to use the oral combined pill in women with vascular complications of diabetes because of adverse changes in plasma lipid profiles; hypertriglyceridaemia, in particular, may be aggravated and the progesterone-only pill or other methods are preferred. Induction of a prothrombotic state is well recognized; certain progestogens (desogestrel, gestodene) are associated with somewhat higher risks.

● *Progesterone-only pill.* No appreciable metabolic effects. Reports of reduced efficacy may reflect non-compliance. These preparations may be used during breast-feeding.

● *Long-acting depot progestogens.* May be particularly useful if compliance is a problem. Potential for menstrual irregularities and adverse effects on lipids.

● *Intrauterine contraceptive devices.* Effective; no metabolic effects; there are no specific contraindications in diabetic women.

● *Mechanical barrier methods.* Effective; as for non-diabetics.

Sterilization or vasectomy may be preferred by some couples. In the few situations in which pregnancy is contraindicated, e.g. severe maternal CHD, sterilization offers definitive, long-term protection.

THE MENOPAUSE

The risk of cardiovascular disease (see p. 228) increases after the menopause (although for diabetic women it is well established that the normal protection afforded by the pre-menopausal state is negated). The transition to the post-menopausal state represents an opportunity for therapeutic intervention with oestrogen replacement therapy which, it has been suggested, may be of particular long-term benefit in women with diabetes. Observational studies suggest that the risk of cardiovascular disease may be significantly reduced; since diabetic women are at increased risk, the effects of oestrogen replacement on plasma lipids, insulin sensitivity and vascular reactivity may theoretically be even more advantageous than for non-diabetic women. However, such cardiovascular protection has not yet been demonstrated in RCTs in either population.

In a recent large RCT, no net effect of recurrence of CHD was observed over 4 years of follow-up. Moreover, risk was increased during the first 4 months in the hormone replacement group. However, a trend towards protection was observed with longer duration treatment. The role of oestrogen replacement therapy in primary prevention of CHD remains uncertain. Other potential benefits (relief of menopausal symptoms, skeletal protection) should be judged on their merits and on the patient's preferences. Standard contraindications should be observed. Care should be taken in women with hypertriglyceridaemia in whom severe hypertriglyceridaemia with risk of pancreatitis may be precipitated; transdermal preparations are less likely to cause exacerbations.

Oral oestrogen preparations may occasionally cause marked exacerbation of hypertriglyceridaemia.

INTERCURRENT ILLNESS

Intercurrent illness may cause derangements of hitherto stable metabolic control; major metabolic disturbance (i.e. DKA or hyperosmolar non-ketosis) may ensue without an appropriate compensatory response to acute severe illness. It is therefore vital that patients or their carers understand the principles of managing diabetes during intercurrent acute illness. In daily life, occasional episodes of self-limiting hyperglycaemia are frequently encountered in insulin-treated patients. These episodes are often a limited high reading or two, and arise for a number of potential reasons; it is usually difficult to discern the precise reason. Examples of common causes are presented in Table 6.7.

TABLE 6.7 Common causes of temporary deterioration in metabolic control

- Insufficient insulin (e.g. error, omission)
- Dietary indiscretion (without a sufficient increase in insulin dose)
- Emotional disturbances (mechanisms uncertain; may be multifactorial)
- Menstruation (in some women – mechanisms uncertain)
- Infection
- Surgery or trauma
- MI
- Drug therapy (e.g. corticosteroids)

SICK DAY RULES

A major problem is overcoming the understandable fear of severe hypoglycaemia if the patient is unable to take food or liquids; this misconception continues to be difficult to root out even amongst health care professionals. The basic rules are outlined in Table 6.8. It should be recognized that (a) the blood glucose levels at which action is required are somewhat arbitrary and (b) severe ketosis may occasionally develop in the absence of marked hyperglycaemia (see Section 4).

TABLE 6.8 Sick day advice for diabetic patients

Your blood glucose may rise even if you are unable to eat your normal food or drink any liquids. It is very important that you DO NOT STOP TAKING YOUR INSULIN OR TABLETS in these circumstances.

Blood glucose testing
- Test your blood glucose every 2–4 hours and adjust insulin according to the advice of your doctor or diabetes specialist nurse. You may feel confident adjusting your own insulin.
- If your glucose is less than 11 mmol/L, continue with your usual insulin dose. Extra doses of short-acting (clear) insulin may be required.
- If your blood glucose is between 11 and 15 mmol/L, take an extra 4 units of clear insulin (or cloudy if this is the only insulin you take) with each injection, even if you are unable to eat.
- If your blood glucose is more than 15 mmol/L, take an extra 6 units of clear insulin (or cloudy if this is the only insulin you take) with each injection, even if you are unable to eat.
- If you are not sure, CONTACT YOUR DOCTOR OR DIABETES NURSE IMMEDIATELY FOR ADVICE.

Ketones and ketoacidosis
- If your blood glucose is staying at levels of 15 mmol/L or higher or if you are vomiting TEST URINE FOR KETONES. Ketones are acids produced when your body does not have enough insulin and starts to burn fats.

  KETOACIDOSIS is a dangerous condition which requires prompt hospital treatment – ketones in your urine in these circumstances usually means that hospital admission is required WITHOUT DELAY – call an ambulance if you are unable to contact your doctor.

Dietary advice
- Try to drink 4–6 pints of sugar-free liquids throughout the day (e.g. water, tea, low-calorie soft drinks).
- If you don't feel like eating, replace the carbohydrate in your food with alternatives (such as milk, ice cream, fruit juice, honey or jam).

Consult your doctor – as an emergency – if:
— **You are vomiting**
— **You are not improving quickly**
— **Your blood glucose levels remain high**
— **Your blood glucose levels are too low**
— **You are concerned about the situation**

Diet- or tablet-treated patients
Vomiting may mean that oral antidiabetic therapy is not absorbed; this alone may result in rising blood glucose levels. However, intercurrent

illness, particularly conditions such as severe sepsis, major trauma or MI can cause rapid metabolic decompensation. Insulin, subcutaneously or by intravenous infusion if vomiting (together with intravenous dextrose), may be required temporarily (see Table 6.9, p. 287). The management of diabetes following acute MI is considered in detail in Section 5. Finally, metformin should be avoided in the presence of severe sepsis or tissue hypoxia because of the small risk of lactic acidosis (see p. 188); again, insulin is the treatment of choice.

> **NB** Insulin is the treatment of choice in patients with type 2 diabetes during severe intercurrent illness.

SURGERY AND OTHER INVASIVE PROCEDURES

Patients with diabetes are more likely to require surgical treatment than non-diabetics, e.g. for foot complications (see p. 213). Furthermore, they are also more likely to have concurrent conditions (e.g. CHD, autonomic neuropathy, renal impairment) which may adversely affect the outcome of surgery. Invasive procedures such as upper GI endoscopy, arteriography (peripheral or coronary) or percutaneous angioplasty, for example, require that patients fast for several hours before and afterwards.

> **NB** Patients with diabetes are at increased risk of requiring surgery and invasive diagnostic or therapeutic procedures.

For patients treated with oral agents or subcutaneous insulin, measures are required:

a. To avoid hypoglycaemia.
b. To maintain good metabolic control.

The hormonal stress response induced by surgical trauma may cause metabolic decompensation (see Sections 1 and 4), the resulting catabolic state compromising tissue repair and recovery. Even laparascopic surgery may be associated with adverse metabolic effects. Fluid and electrolyte disturbances may also be compounded by uncontrolled diabetes. For all patients:

• Liaison with the anaesthetist is recommended.

- Metabolic control should be optimized in good time if possible (this may require initiation of temporary insulin treatment for some tablet-treated patients).
- On the day of operation, the patient should be placed near the start of a morning list, if possible.
- If emergency surgery is necessary, the aim should be to correct any major metabolic disturbance as far as possible. The effect of previously administered antidiabetic therapy, e.g. oral agents already taken that day, necessitates frequent monitoring and use of dextrose and insulin as indicated.
- Electrolyte disturbances should be corrected prior to surgery, wherever possible.

Diet- or tablet-treated diabetes

In well-controlled patients, omission of short-acting sulphonylureas (see p. 110) on the morning of elective surgery and avoidance of glucose- and lactate-containing intravenous fluids may be sufficient for minor procedures.

- Blood glucose levels should be monitored every 1–2 h pre- and postoperatively.
- Long-acting sulphonylureas (e.g. chlorpropamide, glibenclamide) should be discontinued several days prior to surgery since they may cause serious and prolonged postoperative hypoglycaemia; insulin or short-acting agents (e.g. tolbutamide) should be substituted as a temporary measure.
- Metformin should also be avoided peri-operatively and at the time of radiological contrast investigations because of the risk of lactic acidosis (see pp. 120 and 188).
- For major surgery, management should be as for insulin-treated patients.

Insulin-treated patients

- *Intravenous dextrose and insulin.* For all but the most trivial procedures, patients should be stabilized peri-operatively using intravenous infusions of dextrose and insulin as outlined in Table 6.9. These regimens may also be used for patients who are vomiting or anorexic.

- *Plasma electrolytes.* These should be checked frequently and the amount of potassium adjusted accordingly. When prolonged dextrose infusions are required (e.g. for postoperative ileus), an appropriate infusion of sodium chloride should also be administered since hyponatraemia may develop if dextrose alone is infused. For the patient who is not taking carbohydrate by mouth, the dextrose should not be interrupted as this is likely to result in hypoglycaemia. Saline, as required, should be co-infused with dextrose-insulin via a Y-connector.

- *Transfer to subcutaneous insulin.* Subcutaneous insulin is restarted with a meal as appropriate. When subcutaneous insulin is reinstated, the initial injection should include a short-acting insulin and the intravenous infusion should be terminated 30–60 min after the injection to minimize the risk of transient insulinopenia.

● *Other special situations.* The management of diabetes during labour is discussed above; acute MI is considered on page 230. Open heart surgery with cardiopulmonary bypass requires considerably more insulin to compensate for the glucose-containing fluids used in the procedure.

TABLE 6.9 Dextrose and insulin infusions for control of diabetes peri-operatively

---

Combined infusion regimen
● Short-acting insulin (15 units) is added to 500 mL 10% dextrose (usually with 10 mmol potassium chloride – caution if renal impairment)
● Infusion is commenced at 100 mL/h, i.e. delivering 10 g glucose and 3 units insulin hourly.
● Blood glucose is monitored hourly at the bedside using a meter system (appropriate quality control is essential)
● If blood glucose rises >10 mmol/L or falls <5 mmol/L the ratio of glucose to insulin can be altered, e.g. reduce insulin to 10 units or increase to 20 units as necessary

Advantages:
1. Simple fixed-ratio of glucose to insulin
2. Electromechanical infusion pump not required

Disadvantages:
1. Changing rate necessitates complete change of infusate
2. Care must be taken to ensure insulin and potassium injections clear the injection bung of the dextrose bag; mix well

---

Dextrose + insulin via separate lines
● Glucose is administered via a drip-counter at a rate of 100 mL per hour of 10% dextrose (containing appropriate potassium)
● Short-acting (soluble) insulin (50 units) is added to 50 mL saline (0.9%) in a 50 mL syringe and delivered via a variable rate electromechanical pump (with built-in battery supply)
● The insulin (approximately 1 unit per mL) is co-infused via a Y-connector at a variable rate aiming to maintain blood glucose concentrations between approximately 5–10 mmol/L
● Commence with 2 units per hour, increasing or reducing the insulin infusion rate according to hourly blood glucose measurements

Advantages:
1. Ajustable ratio of insulin to glucose
2. No need to change dextrose infusion

Disadvantage:
1. Risk of hypo- or hyperglycaemia if insulin infusion rate incorrect or delivery interrupted

---

 Symptoms and signs of hypoglycaemia are masked by anaesthesia – frequent monitoring of blood glucose is necessary during surgery.

SOCIAL AND LEGAL ASPECTS OF DIABETES MELLITUS

EMPLOYMENT

Iatrogenic hypoglycaemia is the principal concern which limits employment prospects in some professions where this might result in injury to the patient or to others.

Diet- or tablet-treated patients

Patients should encounter few barriers to employment. Employers are encouraged to view potential employees according to their suitability and to be sympathetic to diabetic patients who in general have good attendance and performance records.

Insulin-treated patients

Insulin-treated patients are barred from entry into the armed forces, police or fire service in the UK. They are also excluded from driving most passenger-carrying vehicles or large goods vehicles, each of which requires a special licence (see below). However, the situation pertaining to taxi licences depends on the local regulatory authority and is more variable. A private pilot's licence is not permissible nor is employment as an air-traffic controller or as a member of the aircrew. Certain occupations (e.g. steeplejack, railway track worker) present obvious risks for any patient at risk of hypoglycaemia. Shift work, especially when periods of working days alternate with nights, can be disruptive.

VEHICLE DRIVING

Ordinary driving licences

For the average car driver, diabetes should not interfere materially with usual social or business driving. However, patients should be discouraged from employment which entails regular long-distance driving. The basic rules of driving safely with insulin-treated diabetes are outlined in Table 6.10. All patients to whom these apply should be provided with this information, both verbally and in writing; periodic checks of knowledge and application are advised (many patients do not observe these simple rules). Diabetic patients should be strongly advised not to drink alcohol before driving (see Sections 3 and 4).

Diabetes poses special potential risks related to driving:

- Danger of hypoglycaemia with sulphonylureas or insulin.
- Development of chronic visual or neuropathic complications.

In the UK, diabetic patients treated with oral agents or insulin are legally required to inform the national licensing authority, the Driver and Vehicle Licensing Agency (DVLA), at diagnosis and thereafter if clinically significant

---

TABLE 6.10 Standard advice for diabetic drivers

- If driver taking insulin, readily accessible glucose tablets (or a suitable alternative) must be carried in the car
- Plan each journey
- Make provisions for unexpected delays
- Check blood glucose before and periodically during long journeys
- Take regular breaks on long journeys
- Avoid fatigue
- Have regular meals and snacks at the designated time
- If hypoglycaemia develops, stop the car at the earliest safe opportunity, switch off the engine and remove the ignition key, vacate the driver's seat (be careful on busy roads)
- Carry an identity card or bracelet confirming the diagnosis
- **Never** drink alcohol before driving

---

complications develop, e.g. retinopathy with visual impairment, neuropathy with loss of proprioception, or if there are important changes in treatment (e.g. starting insulin). Although the risk of severe hypoglycaemia with sulphonylureas is relatively low (see p. 110), patients should be informed of the possibility when treatment is commenced. Monotherapy with metformin, however, carries no danger of hypoglycaemia (see p. 120).

In fact, despite the theoretical dangers there is little evidence that diabetic patients are more likely to be involved in road traffic accidents. However, this generalization has to be tempered by the not uncommonly encountered problems relating to diminished symptomatic awareness of hypoglycaemia.

Regulations for drivers
Many countries require diabetic drivers to declare their condition; failure to do so may invalidate insurance policies (see p. 291). National licensing authorities should be consulted in cases of doubt. In the UK, patients treated with antidiabetic agents or insulin are legally obliged to inform the DVLA. Although the responsibility rests with the patient, it is incumbent on the professional providing diabetes care (be this the hospital physician or GP) to ensure that the patient is made aware of this requirement. Regulations vary considerably between different countries, particularly in relation to vocational licensing (see p. 291).

NB In the UK, any patient treated with oral antidiabetic agents or insulin must inform the DVLA.

In the UK, a 3-year licence will usually be issued by the DVLA which is renewed subject to satisfactory reports. If the questionnaire completed by the patient at the time of renewal gives any cause for concern, a supplementary report (or occasionally medical examination) will be requested from the patient's physician by the DVLA's medical advisors. The DVLA also routinely requests brief medical reports in a proportion of cases. If the medical advisor is concerned that the patient's state poses an unacceptable risk, the licence may be suspended pending a further report. If an irreversible disability has arisen, e.g major visual impairment from retinopathy, then the suspension will be permanent. For patients with reduced or absent warning symptoms of hypoglycaemia (see p. 159), the licence may be reissued subsequent to a satisfactory follow-up report.

Although the patient's doctor does not make decisions about the licence, he or she does have a responsibility to warn patients not to drive if circumstances suggest there is an undue risk; making such a judgement can be difficult if accurate quantification of the defect is not possible, e.g. neuropathy-associated impaired proprioception. However, there are specific situations in which the patient should be advised not to drive (Table 6.11). If there is major concern on the part of the physician, it is prudent to reinforce the advice in writing. For some of the more common cautions and contraindications to driving, there are no guidelines and sensible advice has to be given according to individual circumstances.

TABLE 6.11 Situations in which a driver with diabetes should cease driving

- Newly diagnosed patients at risk of hypoglycaemia – this includes all insulin-treated patients and some sulphonylurea-treated patients. Driving should be avoided until glycaemic control is stabilized
- Acute deterioration in glycaemic control, especially if leading to refractive visual disturbances
- Recurrent hypoglycaemia, particularly if severe
- Impaired warning symptoms or recognition of hypoglycaemia
- Best corrected visual acuity worse than 6/12 (Snellen chart – monocular vision is acceptable if acuity satisfactory)
- Distal sensory neuropathy, particularly with loss of proprioception

---

- *Awareness of hypoglycaemia.* Symptomatic unawareness of hypoglycaemia is a particular risk. Hypoglycaemia impairs driving ability thereby increasing the risk of an accident. Importantly, patients may be unable to recognize that their driving ability is impaired. Even more serious, automatism (unconscious but complex and sometimes irrational motor behaviour) may occur leading the patient (and others) into potentially dangerous situations.

- *Visual impairment.* Retinopathy, particularly maculopathy, may impair visual acuity. In addition, patients who have received extensive laser therapy may have impaired night vision and restricted visual fields. Perimetry testing may be required by the licensing authority. Cataracts may also present problems with the glare from car headlights when driving at night.

Following the instillation of mydriatic eye drops for fundoscopy (see p. 197), visual acuity may be transiently reduced to levels below the legal requirement in the UK (which approximates to 6/10 on the Snellen chart). Dazzle from headlights or reflected light is another potential hazard and it is sensible to avoid pharmacological mydriasis if the patient is driving home after the consultation. Attempts at reversal using constricting pilocarpine drops are not recommended since the pupil tends to become fixed at mid-point.

 Mydriatic eye drops may cause a temporary reduction in visual acuity to below the legal requirement.

Vocational driving licences
In the UK, insulin-treated patients are barred from applying for licences for vehicles in excess of 3.5 tonnes (including large goods vehicles or passenger carrying vehicles which contain more than 16 seats). However, insulin-treated patients who held vocational licences prior to 1991 may continue to have their licence renewed subject to careful, regular, medical evaluation. Recent European Union legislation has placed restrictions on insulin-treated patients driving any vehicles over 3.5 tonnes; the DVLA is considering the circumstances of each patient in the light of a medical report from the patient's supervising physician. Harmonization of regulations between member states has yet to be achieved. In the UK, taxi and ambulance drivers are subject to local authority regulations which show wide variations in their requirements.

Driving insurance
Many insurance companies unfairly charge higher premiums for diabetic patients; this practice is not justified by the statistics (see p. 289). However, failure to declare diabetes may invalidate insurance (as well as exposing the patient to the possibility of legal action).

Life insurance
As diabetes carries risks of long-term microvascular and neurological complications, severe metabolic derangements (mainly a risk to younger patients) and macrovascular disease (the main cause of excess mortality, see Sections 4 and 5), life insurance premiums are usually (although not invariably) higher than for the general population. However, there is considerable variation in this weighting between individual companies which often appears unjustified. Moreover, the weighting is based on historical actuarial data, which are, by definition, a reflection of diabetes management in previous decades and may therefore overestimate the risks

pertaining to patients managed with modern approaches. The patient may be forced to shop around for the best deal. National patient organizations may be able to recommend companies with whom they have negotiated more favourable terms. It is important that the risks posed by adverse prognostic indicators are assessed by an experienced physician who is able to make a realistic judgement about the effects on life expectancy of, for example, clinical nephropathy in a patient with long-duration type 1 diabetes; the presence of CHD or a history of poor compliance is likely to be regarded unfavourably by insurers. Some companies will simply not accept diabetic patients, regardless of the presence or absence of long-term complications.

Long-distance travel

Diabetes should rarely prove to be a bar to recreational or occupational long-distance travel. Altered meal times and time zone changes may pose problems for insulin-treated patients but these can usually be overcome without too much difficulty; advance planning is required to minimize the chances of a mishap. Avoidance of destinations which are hostile or desolate, unless accompanied, is an obvious precaution. National patient self-help associations may be able to offer assistance with advice about certain destinations, reciprocal health agreements and availability of insulins. The International Diabetes Federation can provide contact numbers for diabetes member associations in various countries. Prior discussion with the diabetes nurse specialist is also recommended, particularly with regard to air-travel across several time zones; these flights require careful assessment according to the circumstances:

- Airlines should be informed of the diagnosis at the time of booking.
- The main risk is hypoglycaemia; unexpected delays can be particularly difficult – reliance on small doses of short-acting insulin to cover meals every 4–6 hours may be necessary. For long-haul flights, an additional meal (and small dose of short-acting insulin) interposed between usual main meals may be required for east-to-west (e.g. transatlantic) flights; conversely, omission of a medium-acting injection may be indicated for long-distance travel in the opposite direction.
  Other points which may require discussion include:
- Travel insurance – comprehensive cover is required for countries that do not offer free or reduced-cost medical treatment, e.g. European Union member states (E111 form required).
- Immunization.
- Anti-malarial prophylaxis.
- Foodstuffs and drink (including safety of local water supplies).
- Precautions for travel with and storage of insulin and delivery devices (see p. 136), e.g. avoiding exposure to extremes of temperature (do not pack insulin in checked luggage as it will freeze in the baggage hold), avoid direct sunlight at destination.

- Pack sufficient (and extra) insulin, syringes, test strips, lancets. A travelling companion should carry half of the supplies.
- Identity cards or bracelets (useful for custom officers if carrying syringes). Carriage of a card detailing diagnosis and treatment in the local language is recommended.
- Carry dextrose tablets and carbohydrate snacks in case of delayed meals.
- Use prophylactic antiemetics (if prone to travel sickness).
- Consider the hazards of excess sun exposure.
- GI disturbances – pack antidiarrhoeals; broad-spectrum antibiotics from doctor may be advisable.
- Take care to avoid injury, e.g. moped rental.
- Patients with neuropathy should be cautious with new footwear; unaccustomed prolonged walking or climbing may cause serious trauma. Abrasions from rocks are another potential hazard; appropriate footwear should always be worn.

SECTION I

REFERENCES AND BIBLIOGRAPHY

Alberti KGMM, Zimmet PZ for the WHO consultations. Definition, diagnosis and classification of diabetes mellitus and its complications. Part 1. Diagnosis and classification of diabetes mellitus. Provisional report of a WHO consultation. Diabetic Med 1998; 15: 539–553.

Carr A, Samaras K, Thorisdottir A et al. Diagnosis, prediction, and natural course of HIV-1 protease-inhibitor-associated lipodystrophy, hyperlipidaemia, and diabetes mellitus: a cohort study. Lancet 1999; 353: 2093–2099.

Hales CN, Barker DJ. Type 2 (non-insulin-dependent) diabetes mellitus: the thrifty phenotype hypothesis. Diabetologia 1992; 35: 595–601.

James O, Day C. Non-alcoholic steatohepatitis: another disease of affluence. Lancet 1999; 353: 1634–1636.

King H, Rewers M, WHO ad hoc diabetes reporting group. Global estimates for prevalence of diabetes mellitus and impaired glucose tolerance in adults. Diabetes Care 1993; 16: 157–177.

Krentz AJ. Insulin resistance. Br Med J 1996; 313: 1385–1389.

National Diabetes Data Group. Classification and diagnosis of diabetes mellitus and other categories of glucose intolerance. Diabetes 1979; 28: 1039–1057.

Neel JV. Diabetes mellitus: a 'thrifty' genotype rendered detrimental by 'progress'. Am J Hum Genet 1962; 14: 353–362.

The Expert Committee on the diagnosis and classification of diabetes mellitus. Report of the Expert Committee on the diagnosis and classification of diabetes mellitus. Diabetes Care 1997; 20: 1183–1197.

World Health Organization Expert Committee on diabetes mellitus. Technical report series 646. Geneva: World Health Organization; 1980.

World Health Organization. Diabetes mellitus. Report of a study group. Technical report series. Geneva: World Health Organization; 1985.

FURTHER READING

Arner P. Not all fat is alike. Lancet 1998; 351: 1301–1302.

Barker DJ, Hales CN, Fall CHD et al. Type 2 (non-insulin-dependent) diabetes mellitus, hypertension, and hyperlipidaemia (syndrome X): relation to reduced fetal growth. Diabetologia 1993; 36: 62–67.

Bingley PJ, Bonifacio E, Gale EAM. Can we really predict IDDM? Diabetes 1993; 42: 213–220.

Caro JF, Sinha MK, Kolaczynski JW, Zhang PL, Considine RV. Leptin: the tale of an obesity gene. Diabetes 1996; 45: 1355–1462.

Gerbitz K-D, Gempel K, Brdiczka D. Mitochondria and diabetes. Diabetes 1996; 45: 113–126.

Hattersley AT. Maturity-onset diabetes of the young: clinical heterogeneity explained by genetic heterogeneity. Diabetic Med 1998; 15: 15–24.

Iourno MJ, Nestler JE. The polycystic ovary syndrome: treatment with insulin sensitizing agents. Diabetes, Obesity Metab 1999; 1: 127–136.

Kahn SE, Andrikopoulos S, Verchere CB. Islet amyloid. A long-recognized but underappreciated pathological feature of type 2 diabetes. Diabetes 1999; 48: 241–253.

Krentz AJ. Insulin resistance—a handbook for clinicians. Oxford, Blackwell Science (in press).

Nelson RG, Bennett PH, Tuomilehto J, Schersten B, Pettit DJ. Preventing non-insulin dependent diabetes. Diabetes 1995; 44: 483–488.

Reaven GM. Role of insulin resistance in human disease. Diabetes 1988; 37: 1595–1607.

Reaven GM, Laws A. Insulin resistance: the metabolic syndrome X. Totowa, Humana Press; 1999.

Rosenbloom AL, Joe JR, Young RS, Winter WE. Emerging epidemic of type 2 diabetes in youth. Diabetes Care 1999; 22: 345–354.

Shepherd PR, Kahn BB. Glucose transporters and insulin action. N Engl J Med 1999; 341: 248–257.

SECTION 2

REFERENCES AND BIBLIOGRAPHY

Evans JMM, Newton RW, Ruta DA et al. Frequency of blood glucose monitoring in relation to glycaemic control; observational study with diabetes database. Br Med J 1999; 319: 83–86.

Pickup J. Sensitive glucose sensing in diabetes. Lancet 2000; 355: 426–427.

St Vincent Declaration. Diabetes care and research in Europe. Diabetic Med 1990; 7: 370.

The Diabetes Control and Complications Trial Research Group. The effect of intensive treatment of diabetes on the development and progression of long-term complications in insulin-dependent diabetes mellitus. N Engl J Med 1993; 329: 977–986.

The Lisbon Statement. Diabetic Med 1997; 14: 517–518.

UK Prospective Diabetes Study Group. Intensive blood-glucose control with sulphonylureas or insulin compared with conventional treatment and risk of complications in patients with type 2 diabetes (UKPDS 33). Lancet 1998; 352: 837–853.

UK Prospective Diabetes Study Group. Effect of intensive blood-glucose control with metformin on complications in overweight patients with type 2 diabetes (UKPDS 34). Lancet 1998; 352: 854–865.

World Health Organization. Definition, diagnosis and classification of diabetes mellitus and its complications. Part 1. Diagnosis and classification of diabetes mellitus. Geneva: World Health Organization; 1999

FURTHER READING

Coutinho M, Wang Y, Gerstein HC, Yusuf S. The relationship between glucose and incident cardiovascular events. Diabetes Care 1999; 22: 233–240.

Davies M. New diagnostic criteria for diabetes – are they doing what they should? Lancet 1999; 354: 610–611.

Goldstein DE, Little RR, Lorenz RA et al. Tests of glycemia in diabetes (technical review). Diabetes Care 1995; 18: 896–909.

Klein R. Hyperglycemia and microvascular and macrovascular disease in diabetes. Diabetes Care 1995; 18: 258–268.

Krentz AJ. UKPDS and beyond: into the next millennium. Diabetes, Obesity Metab 1999; 1: 13–22.

Wareham NJ, O'Rahilly S. The changing classification and diagnosis of diabetes. Br Med J 1998; 317: 359–360.

SECTION 3

REFERENCES AND BIBLIOGRAPHY

Day C. Thiazolidinediones: a new class of oral antidiabetic drugs. Diabetic Med 1999; 16: 179–192.

Eriksson J, Lindström J, Valle T et al. Prevention of type II diabetes in subjects with impaired glucose tolerance: the Diabetes Prevention Study (DPS) in Finland. Diabetologia 1999; 42: 793–801.

Krentz AJ. Oral antidiabetic drugs: actions, adverse effects and pharmacokinetics. Prescriber 1998; 9: 67–78.

Lean MEJ, Han TS, Seidell JC. Impairment of health and quality of life in people with large waist circumference. Lancet 1998; 351: 853–856.

Manson JE, Colditz GA, Meir J et al. A prospective study of obesity and risk of coronary heart disease in women. N Engl J Med 1990; 322: 882–889.

Nutrition Subcommittee of the British Diabetic Association's Professional Advisory Committee. Dietary recommendations for people with diabetes: an update for the 1990s. Diabetic Med 1992; 9: 189–202.

Perry IJ, Wannamethee SG, Walker MK, Thomson AG, Whincup PH, Shaper AG. Prospective study of risk factors for development of non-insulin-dependent diabetes in middle-aged British men. Br Med J 1995; 310: 560–564.

Rimm EB, Chan J, Stampfer MJ, Colditz GA, Willett WC. Prospective study of cigarette smoking, alcohol use, and the risk of diabetes in men. Br Med J 1995; 310: 555–559.

United Kingdom Prospective Diabetes Study Group. United Kingdom Prospective Diabetes Study (UKPDS) 13: relative efficacy of randomly allocated diet, sulphonylurea, insulin, or metformin in patients with newly diagnosed non-insulin-dependent diabetes followed for three years. Br Med J 1995; 310: 83–88.

United Kingdom Prospective Diabetes Study Group. UK Prospective Diabetes Study 7: response of fasting glucose to diet therapy in newly presenting type II diabetic patients. Metabolism 1990; 39: 905–912.

WHO Expert Committee. Physical status: the use and interpretation of anthropometry. WHO Technical Report Series no. 854. Geneva: WHO; 1995.

Valmadrid CT, Klein R, Moss SE, Klein BEK, Cruickshanks KJ. Alcohol intake and the risk of coronary heart disease mortality in persons with older-onset diabetes mellitus. JAMA 1999; 282: 239–246.

FURTHER READING

Barman Balfour JA, Plosker GL. Rosiglitazone. Drugs 1999; 57: 921–930.

Deveraux RB. Appetite suppressants and valvular heart disease. N Engl J Med 1998; 339: 765–766.

Evans A, Krentz AJ. Benefits and risks of transfer from oral agents to insulin in type 2 diabetes. Drug Safety 1999; 21: 7–22.

Franz MJ, Horton ES, Bantle JP et al. Nutrition principles for the management of diabetes and related complications (technical review). Diabetes Care 1994; 17: 490–518.

Krentz AJ, Ferner RE, Bailey CJ. Comparative tolerability profiles of oral antidiabetic agents. Drug Safety 1994; 11: 223–241.

Kumar A, Newstead CG, Lodge JPA, Davison AM. Combined kidney and pancreatic transplantation. Br Med J 1999; 318: 886–887.

Riddle MC. Learning to use troglitazone. Diabetes Care 1998; 21: 1389–1390.

Selam JL. Implantable insulin pumps. Lancet 1999; 354: 178–179.

White SA, Nicholson ML, London NJM. Vacularized pancreas allotransplantation – clinical indications and outcome. Diabetic Med 1999; 16: 533–543.

SECTION 4

REFERENCES AND BIBLIOGRAPHY

Austin EJ, Deary IJ. Effects of repeated hypoglycaemia on cognitive function. Diabetes Care 1999; 22: 1273–1277.

Cryer PE, Fisher JN, Shamoon H. Hypoglycemia (technical review). Diabetes Care 1994; 17: 734–755.

EURODIAB Study Group. Microvascular and acute complications in IDDM patients. The EURODIAB IDDM Complications Study. Diabetologia 1994; 37: 278–285.

Jones TW, Porter P, Sherwin RS et al. Decreased epinephrine responses to hypoglycaemia during sleep. N Engl J. Med 1998; 338: 1657–1662.

Krentz AJ, Boyle PJ, Justice KM, Wright AD, Schade DS. Successful treatment of severe refractory sulfonylurea-induced hypoglycaemia with octreotide. Diabetes Care 1993; 16: 184–186.

Laing SP, Swerdlow AJ, Slater SD et al. The British Diabetic Association cohort study, II: cause-specific mortality in patients with insulin-treated diabetes mellitus. Diabetic Med 1999; 16: 466–471.

Morris AD, Boyle DIR, McMahon AD et al. Adherence to insulin treatment, glycaemic control, and ketoacidosis in insulin-dependent diabetes mellitus. Lancet 1997; 350: 1505–1510.

FURTHER READING

Amiel SA. Hypoglycaemia avoidance – technology and knowledge. Lancet 1998; 352: 502–503.

Burge MR, Sood V, Sohby TA, Rassam AG, Schade DS. Sulphonylurea-induced hypoglycaemia in type 2 diabetes mellitus: a review. Diabetes, Obesity Metab 1999; 1: 199–206.

Krentz AJ. Diabetic ketoacidosis, hyperosmolar coma and lactic acidosis. In: Föex P, Garrard C, Westaby S (eds). Principles and practice of critical care. Oxford: Blackwell Science; 1997: 637–648.

McNally PG, Lawrence IG, Panerai RB, Weston PJ, Thurston H. Sudden death in type 1 diabetes. Diabetes, Obesity Metab 1999; 1: 151–158.

SECTION 5

REFERENCES AND BIBLIOGRAPHY

American Diabetes Association. Management of dyslipidaemia in adult with diabetes. Diabetes Care 2000; 23 (suppl 1): S57–S60.

Curb JD, Pressel SL, Cutler JA et al for the systolic hypertension in the elderly program cooperative research group. Effect of diuretic-based antihypertensive treatment on cardiovascular disease risk in older patients with systolic hypertension. JAMA 1996; 276: 1886–1892.

Ferris FL III, Davis MD, Aiello LM. Treatment of diabetic retinopathy. N Engl J Med 1999; 341: 667–678.

Frick MH, Elo O, Haapa K et al. Helsinki heart study: primary prevention trial with gemfibrozil in middle-aged men with dyslipidemia. N Engl J Med 1987; 317: 1237–1245.

Gaede P, Vedel P, Parving H-H, Pederson O. Intensified multifactorial intervention in patients with type 2 diabetes mellitus and microalbuminuria; the Steno type 2 randomized study. Lancet 1999; 353: 617–622.

Goldberg RB, Mellies MJ, Sacks FM et al. Cardiovascular events and their reduction with pravastatin in diabetic and glucose intolerant myocardial infarction survivors with average cholesterol levels: subgroup analyses in the cholesterol and recurrent events (CARE) trial. Circulation 1998; 98: 2513–2519.

Guidelines subcommittee. World Health Organization–International Society for Hypertension guidelines for the management of hypertension. J Hypertens 1999; 17: 151–183.

Haffner SM, Lehto S, Ronnemaa T, Pyörälä K, Laasko M. Mortality from coronary heart disease in subjects with type 2 diabetes and in non-diabetic subjects with and without prior myocardial infarction. N Engl J Med 1998; 339: 229–234.

Hansson L, Zanchetti A, Carruthers SG et al for the HOT study group. Effects of intensive blood-pressure lowering and low-dose aspirin in patients with hypertension: principal results of the hypertension optimal treatment (HOT) randomised trial. Lancet 1998; 351: 1755–1762.

Joint British recommendations on prevention of coronary heart disease in clinical practice. Heart 1998; 80 (suppl 2): S1–S29.

Kannel WB, McGee DL. Diabetes and glucose tolerance as risk factors for cardiovascular disease: the Framingham study. Diabetes Care 1979; 2: 120–126.

Kohner E, Allwinkle J, Andrews J et al. Saint Vincent and improving diabetes care. Report of the visual handicap group. Diabetic Med 1996; 13: S13–S26.

Koskinen P, Manttari M, Manninen V et al. Coronary heart disease incidence in NIDDM patients in the Helsinki heart study. Diabetes Care 1992; 15: 820–825.

Malmberg K for the DIGAMI (Diabetes Melllitus, Insulin Glucose Infusion in Acute Myocardial Infarction) Study Group. Prospecive randomised study of intensive insulin treatment on long-term survival in patients with diabetes mellitus. Br Med J 1997; 314: 1512–1515.

Ramsay LE, Williams B, Johnston DG et al. Guidelines for management of hypertension: report of the third working party of the British Hypertension Society. J Hum Hypertens 1999; 13: 569–592.

Rubins HB, Robins SJ, Collins D et al. Gemfibrozil for the secondary prevention of coronary heart disease in men with low levels of high-density lipoprotein cholesterol. N Engl J Med 1999; 341: 410–418.

Skarfors ET, Lithell HO, Selenius I, Åbery H. Do antihypertensive drugs precipitate diabetes in predisposed men? Br Med J 1989; 298: 1147–1152.

Staessen JA, Fagard R, Lutgarde T et al for the systolic hypertension in Europe (Sys-Eur) trial investigators. Randomised double-blind comparison of placebo and active treatment for older patients wtith isolated systolic hypertension. Lancet 1997; 350: 757–764.

The Heart Outcome Prevention Evaluation (HOPE) Study Investigators. Effects of ramipril on cardiovascular and microvascular outcomes in people with diabetes mellitus: results of the HOPE and MICRO-HOPE study. Lancet 2000; 355: 253–259.

The Heart Outcome Prevention Evaluation Study Investigators. Effects of an angiotensin-converting-enzyme inhibitor, rampiril, on cardiovascular events in high-risk patients. N Engl J Med 2000; 342: 145–153.

Tuomilheto J, Rastenyte D, Birkenhäger WH et al for the systolic hypertension in Europe trial investigators. Effects of calcium-channel blockade in older patients with diabetes and systolic hypertension. N Engl J Med 1999; 340: 677–684.

UK Prospective Diabetes Study Group. Tight blood pressure control and risk of macrovascular and microvascular complications in type 2 diabetes (UKPDS 38). Br Med J 1998; 317: 703–713.

UK Prospective Diabetes Study Group. Efficacy of atenolol and captopril in reducing risk of macrovascular and microvascular complications in type 2 diabetes (UKPDS 39). Br Med J 1998; 317: 713–720.

Viberti G-C, Marshall S, Beech R et al. Saint Vincent and improving diabetes care. Report on renal disease in diabetes. Diabetic Med 1996; 13: S6–S12.

Wieman TJ, Smiell JM, Su Y. Efficacy and safety of a topical gel formulation of recombinant human platelet-derived growth factor-BB (becaplermin) in patients with chronic neuropathic diabetic ulcers. Diabetes Care 1998; 21: 822–827.

Yudkin JS. Which diabetic patients should be taking aspirin? Br Med J 1995; 311: 641–642.

FURTHER READING

Aiello LP, Gardner TW, King GL et al. Diabetic retinopathy (technical review). Diabetes Care 1998; 21: 143–156.

Armitage J. Lipid-lowering trials in diabetes. Eur Heart J 1999; 1 (suppl M): M13–M17.

Clark CM Jr, Lee DA. Prevention and treatment of the complications of diabetes melllitus. N Engl J Med 1995; 332: 1210–1217.

Conn J, Betteridge DJ. Insulin resistance in cardiovascular disease. Br J Cardiol 1998; 5: 329–337.

Cooper ME. Pathogenesis, prevention, and treatment of diabetic nephropathy. Lancet 1998; 352: 213–219.

Cullen P, Von Eckardstein A, Souris S, Schulte H, Assmann G. Dyslipidaemia and cardiovascular risk in diabetes. Diabetes, Obesity Metab 1999; 1: 189–198.

Edmonds ME. Progress in the care of the diabetic foot. Lancet 1999; 354: 270–272.

Fisher BM. Interventional cardiology in people with diabetes. Diabetic Med 1999; 16: 531–532.

Groeneveld Y, Petri H, Hermans J, Springer MP. Relationship between between blood glucose level and mortality in type 2 diabetes mellitus: a systematic review. Diabetic Med 1999; 16: 2–13.

Houston MC. Treatment of hypertension in diabetes mellitus. Am Heart J 1989; 118: 819–829.

Kendall MJ. Conventional versus newer hypertensive therapies—a draw. Lancet 1999; 354: 1744–1745.

Kennon B, Petrie JR, Small M, Connell JMC. Angiotensin-converting enzyme gene and diabetes mellitus. Diabetic Med 1999; 16: 448–458.

Lithell HO. Effect of antihypertensive drugs on insulin, glucose, and lipid metabolism. Diabetes Care 1991; 14: 203–209.

Mayfield JA, Reiber GE, Sanders LJ, Janisse D, Pogach LM. Preventive foot care in people with diabetes (technical review). Diabetes Care 1998; 21: 2161–2177.

Mason RP, Mason PE. Calcium antagonists and cardiovascular risk in diabetes. Diabetes Care 1999; 22: 1206–1208.

Viberti G-C. A glycemic threshold for diabetic complications? N Engl J Med 1995; 332: 1293–1294.

Yudkin JS. Managing the diabetic patient with acute myocardial infarction. Diabetic Med 1998; 15: 276–281.

SECTION 6

REFERENCES AND BIBLIOGRAPHY

Carson CA, Kelnar CJH. The adolescent with diabetes. J R Coll Physicians Lond 2000; 34: 24–17.

Casson IF, Clarke CA, Howard CV et al. Outcomes of pregnancy in insulin dependent diabetic women: results of a five year population cohort study. Br Med J 1997; 315: 275–278.

Edge JA, Ford-Adams ME, Dunger DB. Causes of death in children with insulin-dependent diabetes 1990–96. Arch Dis Child 1999; 81: 318–323.

Fruhbeck G. Childhood obesity: time for action, not complacency. Br Med J 2000; 320: 328–329.

Jardine Brown C, Dawson A, Dodds R et al. Saint Vincent and improving diabetes care. Report of the pregnancy and neonatal care group. Diabetic Med 1996; 13 (suppl 4): S43–S53.

Jovanovic L, Ilic S, Pettit DJ et al. Metabolic and immunologic effects of insulin lispro in gestational diabetes. Diabetes Care 1999; 22: 1422–1427.

MacLeod KM. Diabetes and driving: towards equitable, evidence-based decision-making. Diabetic Med 1999; 16: 282–290.

Metzger BE, Coustan DR (eds). Proceedings of the fourth international workshop-conference on gestational diabetes. Diabetes Care 1998; 21 (suppl 2): B1–B167.

O'Sullivan JB, Mahon CM, Charles D, Dandrow RV. Screening criteria for high-risk gestational diabetes patients. Am J Obstet Gynecol 1973; 116: 894–895.

Ryan CM. Memory and metabolic control in children. Diabetes Care 1999; 22: 1239–1241.

FURTHER READING

Alberti KGMM. Diabetes and surgery. Anesthesiology 1991; 74: 209–211.

Bargiota A, Corrall RJM. Monitoring blood glucose control in gestational diabetes. Br Med J 1997; 314: 3–4.

Deary IJ, Frier BM. Severe hypoglycaemia and cognitive impairment in diabetes. Br Med J 1996; 313: 767–768.

Finucane P, Sinclair AJ. Diabetes in old age. Chichester: Wiley; 1995.

Hirsch IB, Paauw DS, Brunzell J. Inpatient management of adults with diabetes. Diabetes Care 1995; 18: 870–879.

Jarrett RJ. Should we screen for gestational diabetes? Br Med J 1997; 315: 736–737.

MacGowan B. Churchill's pocket book of obstetrics and gynaecology. Edinburgh: Churchill Livingstone; 1997.

McNally PG, Raymond NT, Swift PGF, Hearnshaw JR, Burden AC. Does the prepubertal duration of diabetes influence the onset of microvascular complications? Diabetic Med 1993; 10: 906–908.

Stewart R, Liolitsa D. Type 2 diabetes mellitus, cognitive impairment and dementia. Diabetic Med 1999; 16: 93–112.

Index